ADVANCES IN SURGICAL PATHOLOGY: BREAST CANCER

ADVANCES IN SURGICAL PATHOLOGY: BREAST CANCER

Omar Hameed, MD

Associate Professor of Pathology, Microbiology, and Immunology
Associate Professor of Urologic Surgery
Vanderbilt University School of Medicine
Executive Medical Director, Anatomic and Surgical Pathology
Program Director, Surgical Pathology Fellowship
Vanderbilt University Medical Center
Nashville, Tennessee

Shi Wei, MD, PhD

Associate Professor of Pathology
The University of Alabama at Birmingham
Medical Director, Immunohistochemistry Laboratory
University of Alabama at Birmingham Hospital
Birmingham, Alabama

Mohamed Mokhtar Desouki, MD, PhD

Assistant Professor of Pathology, Microbiology, and Immunology
Vanderbilt University School of Medicine
Nashville, Tennessee

Heidi R. Umphrey, MD

Associate Professor of Radiology
Chief, Breast Imaging
Program Director, Breast Imaging Fellowship
The University of Alabama at Birmingham
Birmingham, Alabama

SERIES EDITORS

Philip T. Cagle, MD

Professor of Pathology and Laboratory Medicine
Weill Medical College of Cornell University
New York, New York
Director, Pulmonary Pathology
Houston Methodist Hospital
Houston, Texas

Timothy Craig Allen, MD, JD

Professor, Department of Pathology
Director of Anatomic Pathology
The University of Texas Medical Branch
Galveston, Texas

Wolters Kluwer

Philadelphia • Baltimore • New York • London
Buenos Aires • Hong Kong • Sydney • Tokyo

Acquisitions Editor: Ryan Shaw
Product Development Editor: Kate Marshall
Production Project Manager: Bridgett Dougherty
Design Coordinator: Stephen Druding
Senior Manufacturing Coordinator: Beth Welsh
Strategic Marketing Manager: Daniel Dressler
Prepress Vendor: SPi Global

9 8 7 6 5 4 3 2 1

Printed in China

Library of Congress Cataloging-in-Publication Data
Hameed, Omar, author.
Advances in surgical pathology. Breast cancer / Omar Hameed, Shi Wei, Mohamed Mokhtar Desouki, Heidi Umphrey.
p. ; cm. — (Advances in surgical pathology)
Breast cancer
Includes bibliographical references and index.
ISBN 978-1-4511-9171-4 (hardback)
I. Wei, Shi, 1964- , author. II. Desouki, Mohamed Mokhtar, author. III. Umphrey, Heidi, author. IV. Title. V. Title: Breast cancer. VI. Series: Advances in surgical pathology series.
[DNLM: 1. Breast Neoplasms—pathology. 2. Breast Neoplasms—surgery. WP 870]
RC280.B8
616.99'449—dc23

2014046116

LWW.com

RRS1503

Series Overview

Expectations for the pathologist practicing today exceed those for pathologists in practice only a few years ago. In addition to the rapid growth of knowledge and new technologies in the field of pathology, recent years have seen the emergence of many trends that significantly impact the traditional practice of pathology including the subspecialized multidisciplinary approach to patient care, personalized therapeutics including targeted molecular therapies, and imaging techniques such as endoscopic microscopy, molecular radiology, and imaging multimodality theranostics that compete with conventional light microscopy. In order to remain a viable member of the patient care team, the pathologist must keep up with growing knowledge in traditional subjects as well as in new areas of expertise such as molecular testing. Additionally, the pathologist is subject to an increasing number of credentialing requirements and, for those now completing training, Self-Assessment Modules for Maintenance of Certification, which require the pathologist to be examined on the recent advances in pathology in order to sustain their qualifications to practice.

Each volume in the series *Advances in Surgical Pathology* focuses on a specific subject in pathology that has undergone recent advancement in terms of knowledge, technical procedures, application, and/or integration as part of current trends in pathology and medicine. This series of books not only updates the pathologist on recently acquired knowledge but emphasizes the new uses of that knowledge within the context of the changing landscape of pathology practice in the 21st century. Rather than information in a vacuum, the pathologist is educated on how to apply the new knowledge as part of a subspecialized multidisciplinary team and for purposes of personalized patient therapy.

Each volume in the series will be divided into the following sections: (1) Overview—updates the pathologist on the general topic, including epidemiology, bringing the pathologist generally up to date on a topic as a basis for the more specialized sections that follow. (2) Histopathology—reviews histopathology and specific recent changes that warrant more description and more illustration, for example, recently described entities and recent revisions in classifications. This will also emphasize histopathology figures to illustrate recently described entities and to demonstrate the basis for classification changes so that the pathologist is able to understand and recognize these changes. (3) Imaging—reviews the impact of imaging techniques on histopathologic diagnosis and on the practice of pathology. An example of the former is the use of increasingly sensitive high-resolution CT scan in the diagnosis of interstitial lung diseases. An example of the latter is the use of multimodality theranostics rather than traditional histopathology for the diagnosis and treatment of lung cancer. Figures linking the radiologic images to the histopathology will be emphasized. (4) Molecular Pathology—a review and update on specific molecular pathology as it applies to specific diseases for the practicing pathologist in regard to molecular diagnostics and molecular therapeutics. An example of the former is the identification of a specific fusion gene to diagnose synovial sarcoma. An example of the latter is the identification of specific EGFR mutations in pulmonary adenocarcinoma and its relationship to treatment with EGFR antagonists. (5) For those volumes dealing with cancers (Lung Cancer, Breast Cancer, Prostate Cancer, Colon Cancer, etc.), additional sections will include Preneoplastic and Preinvasive Lesions, which will emphasize histopathologic figures and staging, particularly emphasizing the new staging systems and to illustrate specific problems in staging.

These books will assist the pathologist in daily practice in the modern setting and provide a basis for interacting with other physicians in patient care. They will also provide the timely updates in knowledge that are necessary for daily practice, for current credentialing and for Maintenance of Certification. As such, this series is invaluable to pathologists in practice at all levels of experience who need to keep up with advances for their daily performance and their periodic credentialing and to pathologists-in-training who will apply this knowledge to their boards and their future practice. In the latter case, this series will serve as a useful library for pathology training programs.

DEDICATION

To my beloved Chura for her unwavering love and support, and to our wonderful Shilan and Sara—OH

To my dear wife, Mei, and our wonderful children, Johnny and Erica—SW

To my wife and our lovely kids Aya, Mayar, Mokhtar, and Sarah—MMD

To my sunshine, Noah, Annalise, and Maxmartin—HRU

Preface

The management of breast cancer has significantly evolved from the Halstedian concepts of the last century in which breast cancer was thought to be potentially cured by more and more expansive surgery or that adjuvant systemic therapy should be withheld until metastasis develops. Instead, more limited surgery including lumpectomy (+/– radiation) has become the standard practice, as has neoadjuvant and adjuvant treatment protocols that are tailored to patients at higher risk for development of recurrent/metastatic disease. All this is a reflection of our better knowledge and understanding of the pathology, pathobiology, and natural history of breast cancer.

Similar to other monographs in this series, this book is devoted to presenting the key epidemiologic, histopathologic, radiologic, and molecular pathologic features of breast cancer, specifically addressing recent advances in these fields. Also included is a section that discusses issues in staging as well as one devoted to preneoplastic and preinvasive lesions. In no way does this book attempt to provide a comprehensive review of all the clinical, pathologic, radiologic, and investigational information related to breast cancer, not does it go into the entire range of breast disorders that one may encounter.

The goal of this book is to provide readers with a succinct and comprehensive overview on the pathology of breast cancer and related disciplines to be used for routine practice and for examination review such as boards and maintenance of certification. A significant emphasis has been placed on providing the most updated information, and the text is supplanted by numerous high-resolution color images to further highlight the various pathologic and radiologic features discussed.

This work would not have been possible without the significant contributions from different teams that deal with breast cancer including radiologists, pathologists, surgeons, medical oncologists, radiation oncologists, as well as basic and translational researchers in the field. We would also like to thank colleagues who provided microscopic images, especially Amberly Nunez who provided almost all of the cytology images, as well as Kate Marshall and other members of the publication team for their guidance and patience throughout the different phases of this book.

Omar Hameed
Shi Wei
Mohamed Mokhtar Desouki
Heidi R. Umphrey

Contents

SECTION IV. Molecular Pathology, Predictive and Prognostic Markers

SECTION V. Staging

SECTION VI. Precursor/Associated Lesions

ADVANCES IN SURGICAL PATHOLOGY: BREAST CANCER

SECTION

I

Overview

Overview of Breast Cancer

1

Constituting 16% of all female cancers, breast cancer (BC) is the commonest cancer in women worldwide. The incidence is higher in developed countries supposedly related to increase in life expectancy, urbanization, and western lifestyles. In the majority of cases, however, it is difficult to identify specific risk factors.[1] Accordingly, improving BC outcomes has focused on early detection strategies including increasing public awareness of early signs and symptoms, self- and clinical examination, and mammography screening.[2]

EPIDEMIOLOGY AND RISK FACTORS

Incidence of Breast Cancer

The incidence of BC varies greatly worldwide, with high rates in North America (~100 per 100,000) and Western Europe, low rates in African countries, and intermediate rates in Eastern Europe, South America, and Western Asia. In 2013, it was estimated that there would be 232,340 new cases of invasive BC, 64,640 new cases of *in situ* BC, and 39,620 BC deaths among US women.[3] The incidence of BC is much lower in men with corresponding US estimates being 2,240 new cases of invasive carcinoma and 410 deaths,[3] so women are 100 times more likely to develop BC than are men.[4] With the advent of mammography screening, more cases of BC have been identified at earlier stages, whereas the incidence of advanced-stage BC has remained stable.[4]

There are also significant racial and geographical differences in the incidence rates of BC, with higher incidence in Caucasian women compared to other races, and in Northern America and Western Europe compared to Asia and Africa.[3] Invasive carcinoma of no special type (NST) is the most common invasive mammary tumor, constituting about 80% of BCs, whereas invasive lobular carcinoma (ILC) represents about 5% to 15%. ILC has continued to rise in incidence, especially in women aged greater than 50 years. Of note, the mean age of patients with ILC is slightly higher than that of invasive carcinoma of NST.[5]

Survival of Breast Cancer

In terms of patient survival, the rates vary greatly worldwide. Because of lack of early detection programs and relative scarcity of diagnosis and treatment facilities,[6] survival rates in developing countries are about half of those in developed countries such as those in North America and Scandinavia. The latter survival rates are about 82% and 72% 5 and 10 years after initial diagnosis, respectively.[7,8] The most important determinant of survival is stage at diagnosis with 5-year survival rates in the US dropping from 84% in localized disease to 23% in cases with distant metastasis.[9] Other prognostic factors associated with better survival include younger age, lower histologic grade, estrogen and progesterone expression, and lack of HER2 overexpression/amplification.[10] Although the mortality rates of BC in the United States have been declining since the mid-1990s, this decline has been slower in Black compared to White women.[4]

Risk Factors

Age and Race

The incidence of BC is very closely related to age; the older a woman is, the more likely she will develop BC. The incidence begins to increase after the age of 40 years and is highest in women over the age of 70. The incidence of BC rates in the United States also varies by race and ethnicity: Between 2004 and 2008, this has been reported in the United States to be 125.4, 116.1, 89.2, and 84.9 per 100,000 non-Hispanic Whites, African American, Hispanic, and Asian American women, respectively. These racial differences in BC incidence rates may be related to such factors thought to be associated with BC such as age at menarche, age at menopause, age at first birth, body mass index, number of children, postmenopausal hormone use, and others.[11]

Although the overall incidence of BC in African American women is lower than that in Whites, the incidence of *premenopausal* BC is *higher* in this group, which may be related to particular risk factors such as earlier age at menarche and higher blood estrogen levels, a higher incidence of particular forms of BC,[12] or both.

Family History of Cancer

A family history of breast, ovarian, or prostate cancer is associated with a risk of developing BC that is two to three times that of the general population. This increased risk may be related to genetic factors, environmental factors, or both. Nevertheless, most patients with BC (87%) do not have a family history of the disease in an immediate female relative (mother, sister, or daughter).[13]

Inherited Genetic Mutations

Families with a strong family history of BC often carry inherited genetic mutation(s). Such mutations account for about 5% to 10% of BC cases.[3] In particular, patients with mutations in *BRCA1* and *BRCA2, p53, PTEN/MMAC1, CHEK2,* and *ATM* genes are at a high risk of developing BC, with *BRCA1* and *BRCA2* as the most well-known genes linked to cancer risk. In the United States, between 1 in 400 and 1 in 800 people in the general population carry a *BRCA1 or BRCA2* mutation; however, the prevalence varies by ethnic group.[14] Women who carry *BRCA1* or *BRCA2* gene mutations have 50% to 70% or 40% to 60% risk of developing BC by the age of 70, respectively,[13] compared to about 7% in the general population.[3]

Breast Density

Women with "high breast density" are reportedly up to four to five times more likely to develop BC than are women with low breast density.[15] "High" breast density, however, is not well defined, and there are no consistent ways of measurement.

Personal History of Breast Cancer

Survivors of BC have an increased risk of a second primary BC compared to those who have never had BC. Five percent of women develop a second carcinoma within 8 years of their initial diagnosis and about 8% to 12% within 20 to 25 years. Twenty to 30% of patients with low-grade ductal carcinoma *in situ* (DCIS) and the great majority of high-grade DCIS will progress to invasive BC if left untreated.[16]

Breast Lesions

Certain pathologic findings in biopsied or excised breast tissue are associated with an elevated risk of BC. The risk of usual ductal hyperplasia is 1.5 to 2 times that in the general population, atypical hyperplasia of ductal (ADH) and lobular (ALH) types is 4 to 5 times that, and lobular carcinoma *in situ* (LCIS) is associated with an even greater relative risk (7 to 12 times).[17,18]

Reproductive History

Prolonged exposure to endogenous estrogens in cases of early menarche, late menopause, and late age at first childbirth is among the most important reproductive risk factors for BC.

Exogenous steroids in oral contraceptive and hormone replacement therapy also put the user at a higher risk, while breast-feeding has a protective effect.[1]

Lifestyle

Alcohol use, smoking, poor diet habit, overweight and obesity, and physical inactivity are among modifiable lifestyles that are linked to increased risk of BC especially in developed countries. In developing countries, the risk factors of BC attribute mainly to physical inactivity.[19] The differences in BC incidence between developed and developing countries may be related to dietary factors, late first childbirth, low parity, and shorter breast-feeding in developed countries.[20]

PREVENTION, EARLY DETECTION, AND SCREENING

Comprehensive BC control involves prevention, early detection, diagnosis, and treatment. Raising public awareness and available screening programs as well as advocating for appropriate policies are key elements of successful BC control.[2]

Prevention

Control of modifiable lifestyle risk factors, including healthy diet, physical activity, and control of alcohol intake, smoking, overweight, and obesity, could have a positive impact in reducing the incidence of BC.[21]

Breast Self-Examination and Mammography Screening

Early detection and treatment are crucial to improve BC outcome and survival rates. Awareness of early signs and symptoms and periodic screening are the cornerstones for early detection. Identifying the right cohort and high-risk patients will lead to cost-effective and successful programs for early detection.[22]

The sensitivity and specificity of breast self-examination are limited in detecting early BC lesions. However, self-examination has been seen to empower women, especially those at risk, to take the responsibility and awareness for more effective screening methods.[2]

Mammography screening is one of the most effective screening methods for early detection of BC. Mammography screening reduced BC mortality by 25% to 30% in women over 40 years in developed countries between 1986 and 2008.[23–25] Most mammography screening programs focus on low-risk women aged 50 to 69 years with screening every other year. The participation rate is over 66.5% in the United States.[26]

References

1. Lacey JV Jr, Kreimer AR, Buys SS, et al. Breast cancer epidemiology according to recognized breast cancer risk factors in the Prostate, Lung, Colorectal and Ovarian (PLCO) Cancer Screening Trial Cohort. *BMC Cancer* 2009;9:84.
2. The Susan G. Komen Breast Cancer Foundation I; Susan G. Komen for the cure official page. http://ww5.komen.org/Default.aspx. Retrieved September 2, 2013. Dallas, TX.
3. American Cancer Society. *Cancer Facts & Figures 2013*. Atlanta, GA: American Cancer Society; 2013.
4. Howlader N, Noone AM, Krapcho M, et al. SEER Cancer Statistics Review, 1975–2009. In: Howlader N, Noone A, Krapcho M, et al., eds. Bethesda, MD: National Cancer Institute; 2012.
5. Arpino G, Bardou VJ, Clark GM, et al. Infiltrating lobular carcinoma of the breast: tumor characteristics and clinical outcome. *Breast Cancer Res* 2004;6:R149–R156.
6. Coleman MP, Quaresma M, Berrino F, et al. Cancer survival in five continents: a worldwide population-based study (CONCORD). *Lancet Oncol* 2008;9:730–756.
7. Baade PD, Youlden DR, Chambers SK. When do I know I am cured? Using conditional estimates to provide better information about cancer survival prospects. *Med J Aust* 2011;194:73–77.

8. Youlden DR, Cramb SM, Dunn NA, et al. The descriptive epidemiology of female breast cancer: an international comparison of screening, incidence, survival and mortality. *Cancer Epidemiol* 2012;36:237–248.
9. Brenner H, Francisci S, de Angelis R, et al. Long-term survival expectations of cancer patients in Europe in 2000–2002. *Eur J Cancer* 2009;45:1028–1041.
10. Cianfrocca M, Goldstein LJ. Prognostic and predictive factors in early-stage breast cancer. *Oncologist* 2004;9:606–616.
11. American Cancer Society. *Cancer Facts & Figures 2011–2012.* Atlanta, GA: American Cancer Society; 2011.
12. Stark A, Kleer CG, Martin I, et al. African ancestry and higher prevalence of triple-negative breast cancer: findings from an international study. *Cancer* 2010;116:4926–4932.
13. Antoniou AC, Cunningham AP, Peto J, et al. The BOADICEA model of genetic susceptibility to breast and ovarian cancers: updates and extensions. *Br J Cancer* 2008;98:1457–1466.
14. National Cancer Institute. Genetics of Breast and Gynecologic Cancers (PDQ®). High-penetrance breast and/or gynecologic cancer susceptibility genes. http://www.cancer.gov/cancertopics/pdq/genetics/breast-and-ovarian/HealthProfessional/page2. Retrieved January 15, 2015.
15. Pollan M, Ascunce N, Ederra M, et al. Mammographic density and risk of breast cancer according to tumor characteristics and mode of detection: a Spanish population-based case–control study. *Breast Cancer Res* 2013;15:R9.
16. Nsouli-Maktabi HH, Henson DE, Younes N, et al. Second primary breast, endometrial, and ovarian cancers in Black and White breast cancer survivors over a 35-year time span: effect of age. *Breast Cancer Res Treat* 2011;129:963–969.
17. Cote ML, Ruterbusch JJ, Alosh B, et al. Benign breast disease and the risk of subsequent breast cancer in African American women. *Cancer Prev Res (Phila)* 2012;5:1375–1380.
18. Bagaria SP, Shamonki J, Kinnaird M, et al. The florid subtype of lobular carcinoma in situ: marker or precursor for invasive lobular carcinoma? *Ann Surg Oncol* 2011;18:1845–1851.
19. Danaei G, Vander Hoorn S, Lopez AD, et al. Causes of cancer in the world: comparative risk assessment of nine behavioural and environmental risk factors. *Lancet* 2005;366:1784–1793.
20. Peto J. Cancer epidemiology in the last century and the next decade. *Nature* 2001;411:390–395.
21. Wiseman M. The second World Cancer Research Fund/American Institute for Cancer Research expert report. Food, nutrition, physical activity, and the prevention of cancer: a global perspective. *Proc Nutr Soc.* 2008;67:253–256.
22. Anderson BO, Yip CH, Smith RA, et al. Guideline implementation for breast healthcare in low-income and middle-income countries: overview of the Breast Health Global Initiative Global Summit 2007. *Cancer* 2008;113:2221–2243.
23. Hellquist BN, Duffy SW, Abdsaleh S, et al. Effectiveness of population-based service screening with mammography for women ages 40 to 49 years: evaluation of the Swedish Mammography Screening in Young Women (SCRY) cohort. *Cancer* 2011;117:714–722.
24. Bleyer A, Welch HG. Effect of three decades of screening mammography on breast-cancer incidence. *N Engl J Med* 2012;367:1998–2005.
25. Schopper D, de Wolf C. How effective are breast cancer screening programmes by mammography? Review of the current evidence. *Eur J Cancer* 2009;45:1916–1923.
26. International Cancer Screening Network. Participation rates and target populations for breast cancer screening programs in 27 ICNS countries, 2012. http://appliedresearch.cancer.gov/icsn/breast/screening.html. Accessed January 15, 2015.

SECTION

II

Histopathology

Carcinoma *In Situ*

2

DUCTAL CARCINOMA *IN SITU*

Ductal carcinoma *in situ* (DCIS) is a noninvasive form of breast cancer, where the neoplastic epithelial cells remain confined to the ductal–lobular system with intact basement membrane and myoepithelial cells.[1] The diagnosis of DCIS has tremendously increased after the widespread introduction of screening programs and now accounts for 20% to 25% of screen-detected cancers in western countries[2] and 15% to 20% of all breast cancers detected. DCIS is most common in Caucasians[3,4] and in women over the age of 50 years. Risk factors for developing DCIS are the same as those of invasive carcinoma of no special type, including a family history of breast cancer, nulliparity, older age at birth of first child, and *BRCA1* or *BRCA2* mutations (Chapter 1).[5]

Three-dimensional studies have shown that, in the vast majority of cases, DCIS is a unicentric disease process.[1] In the premammography era, most patients presented with large palpable masses, whereas the majority of patients now present with abnormal findings (most frequently calcifications) on mammographic screening and about 10% present with Paget disease of the nipple, nipple discharge, or a palpable mass.[1] These latter presentations are more likely to be seen with extensive DCIS or in association with a component of invasive cancer.[1]

DUCTAL CARCINOMA *IN SITU*, CYTOLOGY

The cytologic features of DCIS are similar to those described for invasive carcinoma and include moderate-to-abundant cellularity, noncohesive cells including isolated cells with intact cytoplasm (as opposed to myoepithelial cells that appear as naked nuclei). Nuclear pleomorphism, conspicuous nucleoli, nuclear membrane irregularity, and mitotic figures are variable criteria of malignancy. The background may also include cellular debris, necrosis, and inflammatory cells.[6]

DUCTAL CARCINOMA *IN SITU*, IMAGING AND GROSS FEATURES

Microcalcifications are the most common abnormality identified by mammography. The calcium has a characteristic branched, linear, casting pattern highly suspicious for malignancy (Figure 2-1). Additionally, few cases of DCIS present with architectural distortion, ill-defined masses (Figure 2-2), nodules, or breast asymmetry. Most cases of DCIS are not visible grossly; however, high-grade DCIS can form a large mass with oozing of necrotic debris (comedo-like) from the ducts.[7]

DUCTAL CARCINOMA *IN SITU*, HISTOLOGY

DCIS has been traditionally classified based on architectural growth pattern into solid, comedo, cribriform, micropapillary, and other subtypes. However, more than one pattern in the same lesion is the norm rather than the exception. Other classification systems incorporate cell morphology,

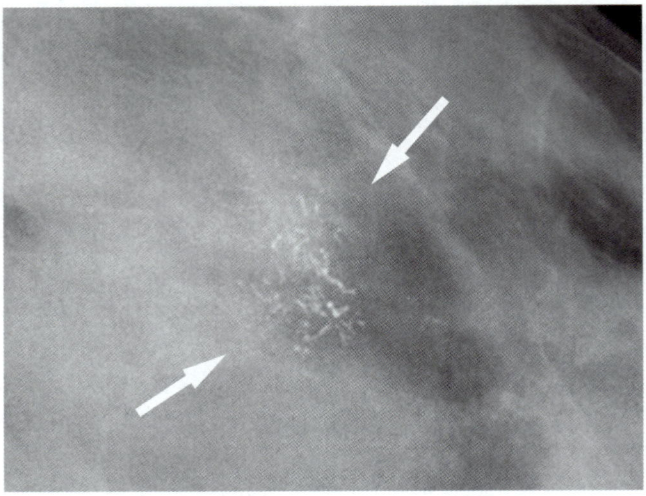

FIGURE 2-1: Craniocaudal mammogram image reveals fine pleomorphic and linear branching calcifications (*arrows*) in a grouped distribution characteristic of ductal carcinoma *in situ*.

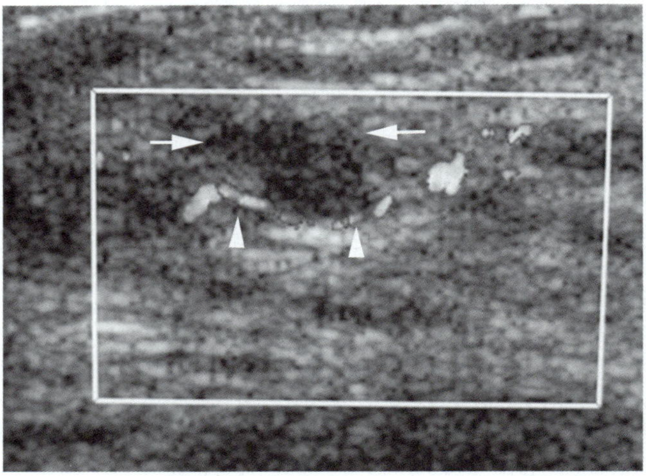

FIGURE 2-2: Ultrasound image reveals an irregular hypoechoic mass (*arrows*) with indistinct margins and peripheral vascularity (*arrowheads*). Excision showed high-grade ductal carcinoma *in situ*.

necrosis, and volume.[1] The current internationally accepted and reproducible classification system with clinical relevance regarding the probability of progression to invasive carcinoma is based on nuclear grade.[3] Other recommended elements for reporting DCIS include the clinical history, surgical procedure, specimen laterality, lymph node sampling and status, site and size (extent), architectural pattern, presence of necrosis and microcalcifications, margin status, treatment effect, pathologic staging, and results of ancillary studies (e.g., hormone receptor status) if available.[8]

Architectural Patterns of DCIS

Common Patterns

Comedo-type DCIS is characterized by the presence of intermediate- to high-grade nuclei (see below) with associated intraluminal zonal comedo-like necrosis. This is frequently associated with calcifications, periductal fibrosis, and chronic inflammation (Figure 2-3).

Solid DCIS appears as a compact proliferation of (usually) low- to intermediate-grade nuclei that fills the entire duct space. The cytoplasm can be clear, granular, amphophilic, or eosinophilic in nature. Necrosis and calcifications are infrequent (Figure 2-4).

Cribriform DCIS shows the neoplastic cells growing in a sieve-like or fenestrated pattern in which the lumens are rounded and rigid. So-called Roman arches, "bridges" and rosette-like structures may also be formed.[9] The nuclei are usually low grade, evenly spaced, nonoverlapping, and with evenly distributed chromatin; however, higher-grade nuclei may also be seen (Figure 2-5).

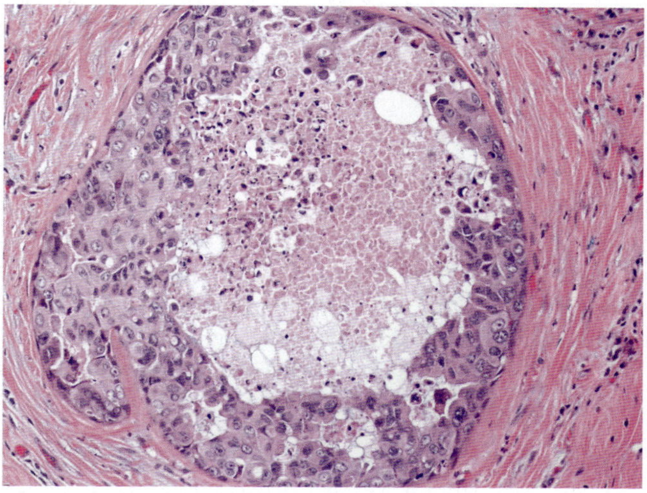

FIGURE 2-3: High-grade ductal carcinoma *in situ*, comedo type with characteristic central necrosis.

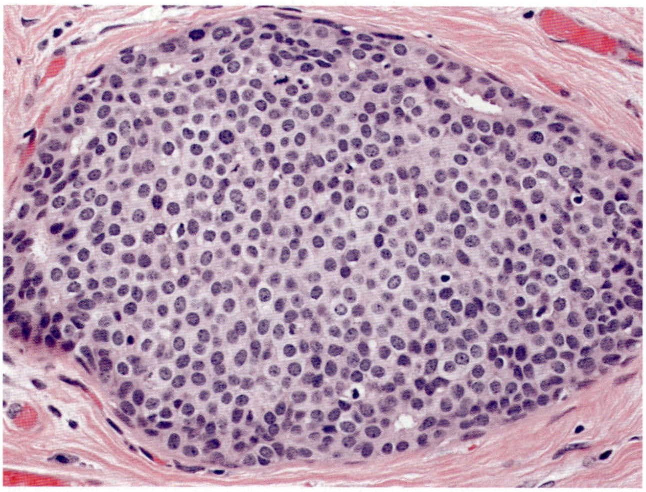

FIGURE 2-4: Low-grade ductal carcinoma *in situ*, solid type.

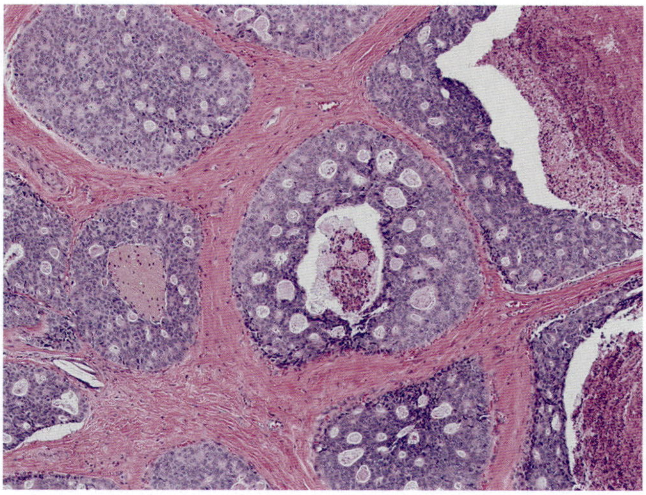

FIGURE 2-5: Intermediate-grade ductal carcinoma *in situ*, cribriform type.

Micropapillary DCIS is characterized by minute papillary fronds lacking fibrovascular cores (Figure 2-6). Areas similar to cribriform DCIS may also be present. Micropapillary DCIS can be extensive.[3]

Less Common Patterns

There are other less common types of DCIS that, although usually displaying one or more of the patterns above, have distinguishing cytologic features. Apocrine DCIS is characterized by the presence of cells with abundant, granular, and eosinophilic (or sometimes vacuolated/clear) cytoplasm with enlarged nuclei and eosinophilic macronucleoli (Figure 2-7). Although usually composed of intermediate- to high-grade nuclei (often with necrosis), lower-grade apocrine DCIS is often intermixed, which, when seen in isolation, can be difficult to distinguish from apocrine metaplasia. Other variants include clear cell DCIS (Figure 2-8), so-called "flat" or "clinging" DCIS (Figure 2-9), neuroendocrine/endocrine DCIS,[10] and signet-ring DCIS.

Grading of DCIS

DCIS is graded as low, intermediate, or high grade primarily based on nuclear features, similar to how nuclear features are used for grading invasive carcinoma. Low-grade lesions exhibit monomorphic cells with rounded nuclei displaying regular chromatin and inconspicuous nucleoli; cell polarization is well maintained (Figures 2-4, 2-8 and 2-10). On the other hand, high-grade DCIS is characterized by large, pleomorphic, poorly polarized nuclei with irregular nuclear contours,

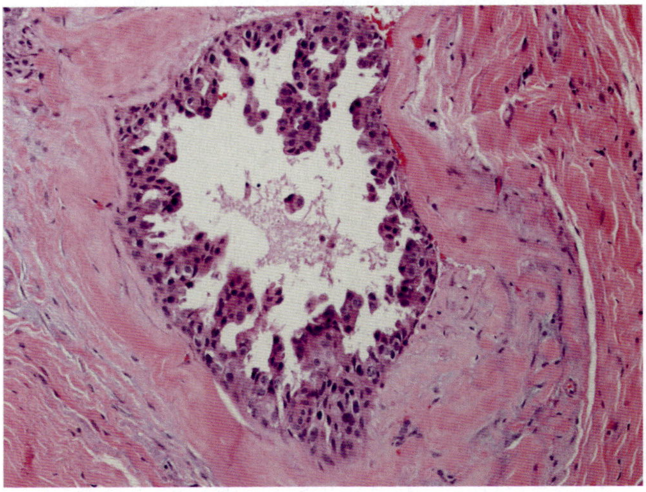

FIGURE 2-6: Intermediate-grade ductal carcinoma *in situ*, micropapillary type.

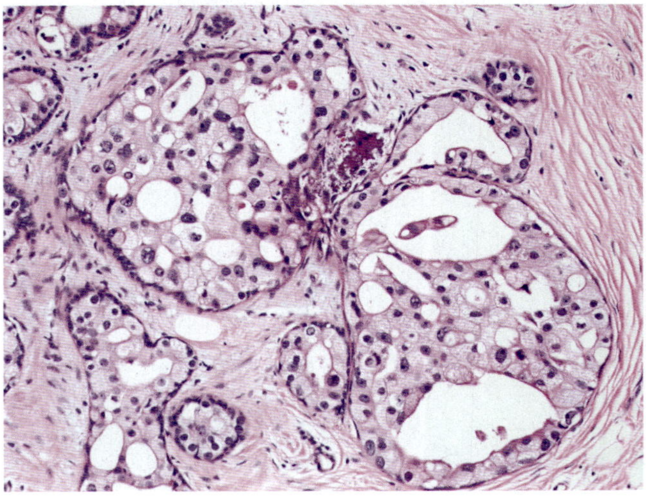

FIGURE 2-7: Intermediate- to high-grade ductal carcinoma *in situ* with apocrine features displaying cells with abundant, granular, eosinophilic, and vacuolated cytoplasm with enlarged nuclei and eosinophilic prominent nucleoli.

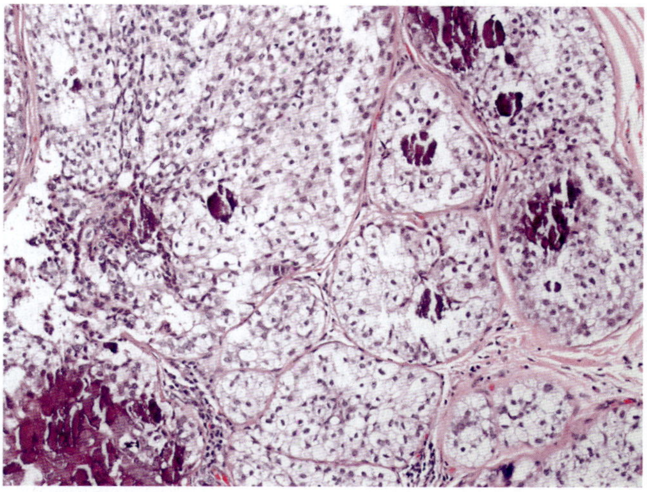

FIGURE 2-8: Low-grade ductal carcinoma *in situ* with clear cell changes and associated laminated microcalcifications.

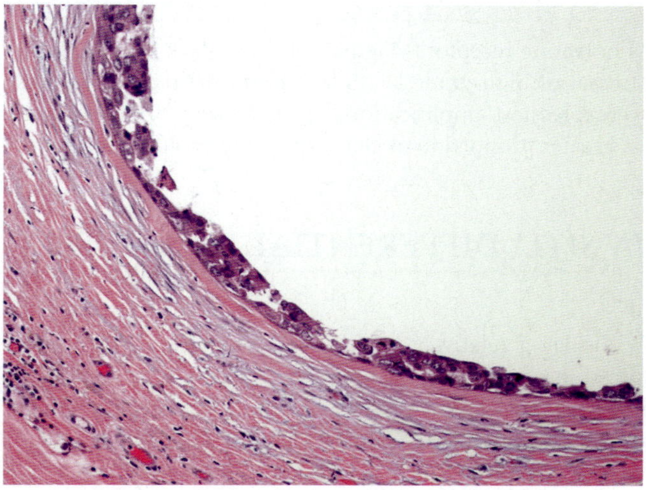

FIGURE 2-9: High-grade ductal carcinoma *in situ* with flattened growth pattern.

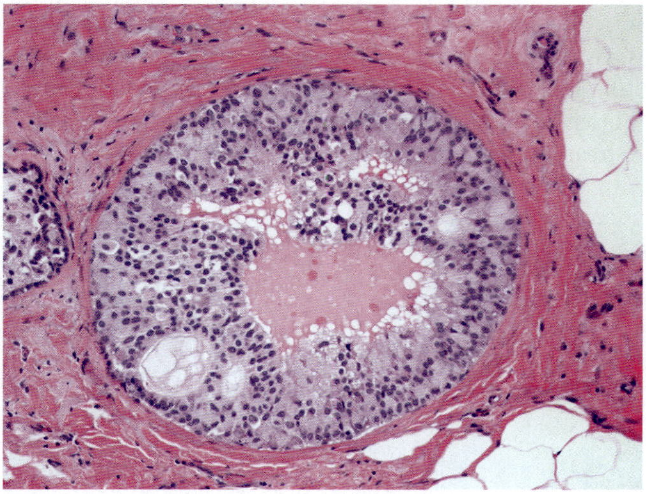

FIGURE 2-10: Low-grade cribriform ductal carcinoma *in situ*.

coarse/clumped chromatin, and prominent nucleoli with high mitotic and apoptotic bodies (Figure 2-3). Intermediate-grade DCIS lies in between where there is mild-to-moderate variability in size, shape, and placement of cells and nuclei, with variably coarse chromatin and visible nucleoli (Figures 2-5 and 2-6).

Size/extent and Margin Status of DCIS

Determination of the size/extent of DCIS is an important factor for patient management and prognosis.[11] Residual disease, positive margin status, local recurrence, and the possibility of missed invasion are directly proportional to the extent of DCIS.[12] Methods for estimating the extent of DCIS include[13] (a) measurement of the linear extent of DCIS in the glass slide if the lesion is present in one block; (b) in serial sequential sampling with DCIS, the extent can be calculated by using a diagram of the specimen and the thickness of the slices; (c) if DCIS involves or is close to two margins, the distance between the margins can be used as the extent of the DCIS; and (d) finally, in few cases of DCIS, there may be a gross lesion that can be measured and reported. Extent of DCIS and adequacy of excision (margin status) are reflected in the Van Nuys Prognostic Index, which incorporates these factors into a numerical system to predict which patients are more likely to recur after conservative therapy.[14] Negative margins should be obtained after breast-conserving surgery for DCIS. A margin of 2 mm has been found to be as good as a larger margin when breast-conserving surgery is combined with radiation therapy.[15]

DUCTAL CARCINOMA *IN SITU*, IMMUNOHISTOCHEMISTRY

Most low-grade DCIS lesions express hormone receptors (Figure 2-11) and lack HER2 overexpression/amplification, whereas most cases of high-grade DCIS lack hormone receptor expression and frequently display HER2 overexpression/amplification.[16] p53 is also more likely to be expressed in high-grade lesions, with a greater proportion of cells expressing proliferation markers such as Ki-67.[17]

DUCTAL CARCINOMA *IN SITU*, DIFFERENTIAL DIAGNOSIS

Invasive Mammary Carcinoma

Invasive carcinoma may occasionally display a relatively large nested pattern of growth with round aggregates of tumor cells. Expression of myoepithelial markers, such as p63, basal cytokeratins, and smooth muscle myosin heavy chain around DCIS (Figure 2-12) can always be used to substantiate the diagnosis whenever invasive carcinoma is in the differential diagnosis.

Usual and Atypical Duct Hyperplasia

Usual duct hyperplasia (UDH) and atypical duct hyperplasia (ADH) are in the differential diagnosis of DCIS. Usual ductal hyperplasia is characterized by increased cellularity of ductal epithelium supported by peripheral myoepithelial layer. The cells often form syncytial growth pattern with indistinct cell borders and basally oriented nuclei at the perimeter of the ducts. The nuclei are often overlapping and distributed in a streaming pattern (cells oriented parallel to the long axis of

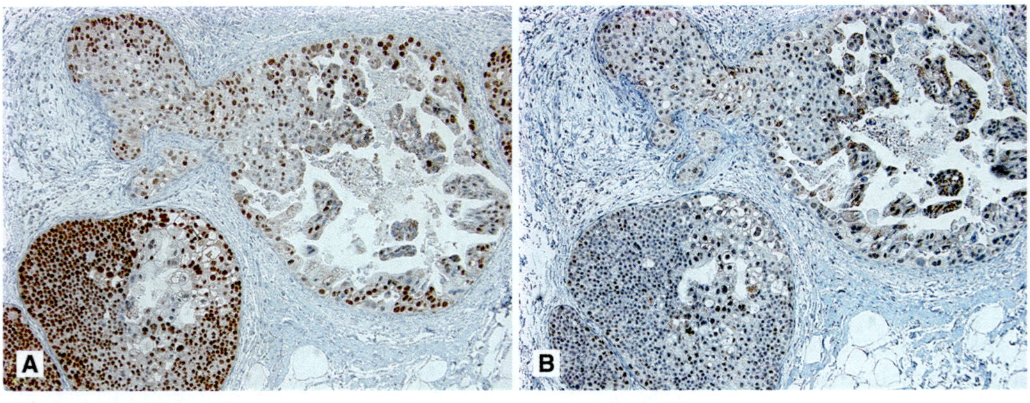

FIGURE 2-11: Estrogen (**A**) and progesterone (**B**) receptor–positive ductal carcinoma *in situ*.

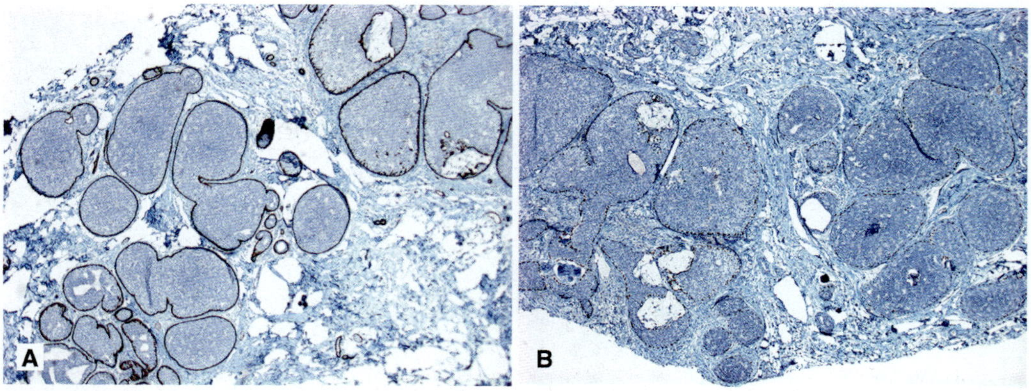

FIGURE 2-12: Myoepithelial markers such as smooth muscle myosin heavy chain in (**A**) and p63 (**B**) can be helpful to delineate myoepithelial cells in ductal carcinoma *in situ*.

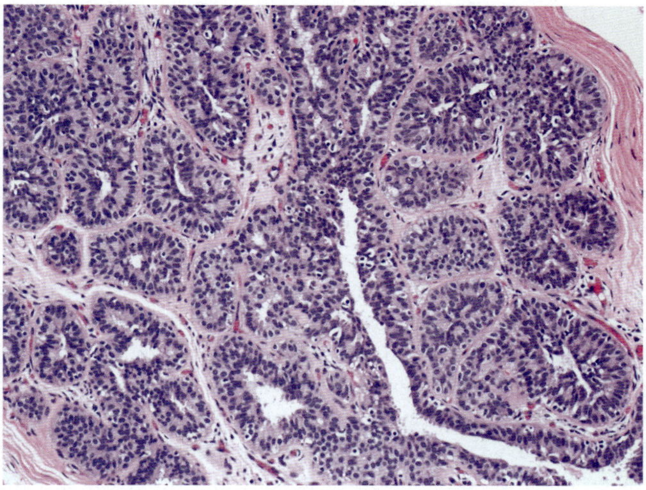

FIGURE 2-13: Usual ductal hyperplasia. Notice slit-like fenestrations, streaming of nuclei, and cellular heterogeneity. Compare to the monotonous population of cells and rigid spaces of ductal carcinoma *in situ* as shown in Figure 2-5.

the duct). If fenestrations are present, they tend to be slit-like and irregular (Figure 2-13) and very different from the crisp, punched out, well-defined spaces seen in cribriform DCIS (Figure 2-5). Cytokeratin 5/cytokeratin 6 may prove helpful to distinguish UDH from DCIS lesions. Most of the epithelial cells of the former express cytokeratin 5/cytokeratin 6 compared to negative/patchy staining in DCIS lesions.[18] A gray zone exists between low-grade DCIS and ADH. The latter is described as a lesion showing some but not all of the histologic features of low-grade DCIS. These changes may fall short of DCIS qualitatively or quantitatively (Chapter 27).[19,20]

Classic Lobular Carcinoma *In Situ* and Low-Grade DCIS, Solid Growth Pattern

Most cases of lobular carcinoma *in situ* (LCIS) are readily distinguished from low-grade DCIS with hematoxylin–eosin stain. Dyshesive growth pattern and the presence of prominent intracytoplasmic vacuoles favor the former (Figure 2-14). On the other hand, the presence of microacinar formations supports a diagnosis of DCIS. In ambiguous cases, immunohistochemistry (IHC) can be of utility (see differential diagnosis of LCIS below).

Pleomorphic LCIS and High-Grade DCIS

Pleomorphic LCIS (PLCIS) is very easily confused with high-grade DCIS, particularly when there is associated central necrosis and calcifications. Again, the dyshesive appearance of the cells (Figure 2-14) and IHC can be utilized to aid in the distinction. Since PLCIS and high-grade DCIS are currently managed similarly, there is minimal added value in distinguishing between them.[21]

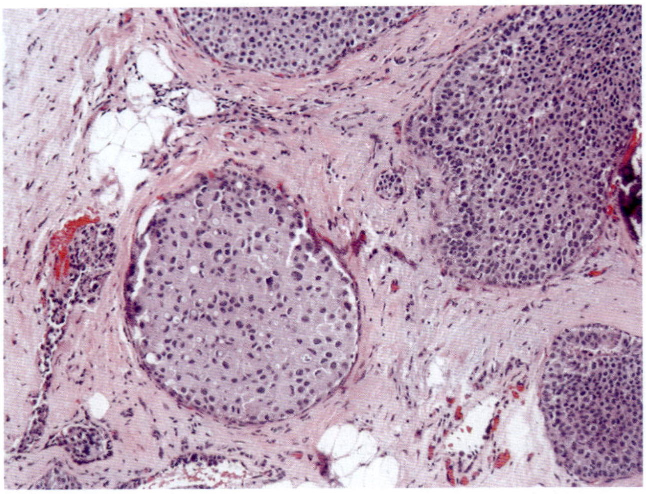

FIGURE 2-14: Lobular carcinoma *in situ*, classic and pleomorphic patterns. Notice the dyscohesive monotonous cells in both classic (*ducts to the right*) and pleomorphic (*duct to the left*) patterns. PLCIS shows greater degree of pleomorphism with abundant eosinophilic cytoplasm, which could more easily be mistaken for ductal carcinoma *in situ*.

DUCTAL CARCINOMA *IN SITU*, MOLECULAR GENETICS

The developmental pathway of non-high–grade lesions (including low- and intermediate-grade DCIS) is thought to differ biologically and cytogenetically from that of high-grade disease. There is convincing genetic evidence to suggest that low-grade and high-grade DCIS evolve through distinct evolutionary pathways.[22] Low-grade DCIS lesions are usually diploid and harbor recurrent loss of chromosome 16q and gains of chromosome 1q. In contrast, high-grade breast cancers are usually aneuploid with complex genetic profiles and infrequent deletion of 16q and more often shows 17q gain.[23] In high-grade DCIS, even when loss of 16q is present, the underlying genetic mechanism is distinct from that seen in low-grade ones. ADH is thought to be a precursor lesion of low-grade DCIS. On the other hand, high-grade DCIS has no obvious precursor lesion. Low-grade DCIS stays dormant in most cases and, if it progresses, tends to develop into low-grade invasive cancer, whereas high-grade DCIS progresses to high-grade invasive disease in a significant proportion of cases.[24] Taken together, these findings suggest that progression from low-grade breast carcinoma to high-grade breast cancers is an unlikely biologic phenomenon and that low-grade cancers are a distinct class of breast cancer.[9]

LOBULAR CARCINOMA *IN SITU* AND ATYPICAL LOBULAR HYPERPLASIA

Lobular lesions of the breast include atypical lobular hyperplasia (ALH), lobular carcinoma *in situ* (LCIS), and invasive lobular carcinoma (ILC). The term lobular neoplasia (LN) was introduced to clearly separate ALH and LCIS from ductal neoplasia and emphasize the importance of utilizing a conservative rather than surgical approach in dealing with these lesions.[25]

Lobular neoplasia has been regarded as a risk factor and a non-obligate precursor for subsequent development of invasive carcinoma. Compared to the general population, the risk of developing breast cancer is elevated up to 5-fold and 10-fold after a diagnosis of ALH and LCIS, respectively.[26] Breast cancer may manifest more than 15 years after the initial diagnosis of LN. The risk of developing breast cancer is significantly higher in both breasts. However, the risk is higher in ipsilateral breast with previous diagnosis of LN.[27]

Lobular neoplasia predominantly arises in women between 40 and 50 years of age[27] and is typically asymptomatic and often multicentric and bilateral.[28] Data from the Surveillance, Epidemiology and End Results Program[29] have shown that the age-adjusted rates of LCIS among women in the United States have increased fourfold between the late 1970s (0.9 per 100,000 person years) and late 1990s (3.2 per 100,000 person years), which may be a reflection of increased pathologic sampling of mammographically detected abnormalities.[30]

LOBULAR CARCINOMA *IN SITU*, CYTOLOGY

Due to low cellularity, LCIS can easily be missed in cytology preparations. Nevertheless, the appearance is that of a monomorphic population of single cells or loosely cohesive clusters of cells with scant cytoplasm and well-defined cytoplasmic borders. Intracytoplasmic lumens may be prominent and signet-ring cells may also be identified. The nucleus is small and often eccentric with fine and evenly distributed chromatin, mildly irregular nuclear membranes, and inconspicuous nucleoli. The pleomorphic variant of LCIS exhibits a greater degree of cytologic atypia.[31]

LOBULAR CARCINOMA *IN SITU*, IMAGING AND GROSS FEATURES

The diagnosis of LN is exclusively pathologic since it does not have any specific radiologic characteristics, making its detection almost completely incidental in the workup of other mammographic lesions as calcifications, in association with a mass lesion or architectural distortion.[30] There are also no gross pathologic findings that might point toward LN.[27]

LOBULAR NEOPLASIA, HISTOLOGY

The characteristic feature is the presence a uniform population of neoplastic cells replacing the normal epithelium of acini and intralobular ductules, causing expansion and enlargement of the lobules.[27] The distinction between ALH and LCIS is quantitative. More than half of the acini of a lobular unit needs to be distended (not just filled) and distorted by the neoplastic cells for a diagnosis of LCIS; anything less than that is ALH.[32] Of note, LN (and DCIS) can arise in or involve preexisting breast lesions such as fibroadenomas, papillomas, radial scars, and sclerosing adenosis.

Classic LCIS

As described in cytology section above, classic LCIS is composed of small, rounded, monomorphic, dyshesive cells with an increased nuclear to cytoplasmic ratio (Figures 2-15 to 2-17). Intracytoplasmic vacuoles are common finding and can be a prominent feature. Associated histiocytes (Figure 2-18) and clear cell changes may be seen in LN.[28] Pagetoid spread along ducts can produce a cloverleaf-like pattern of growth (Figure 2-19).

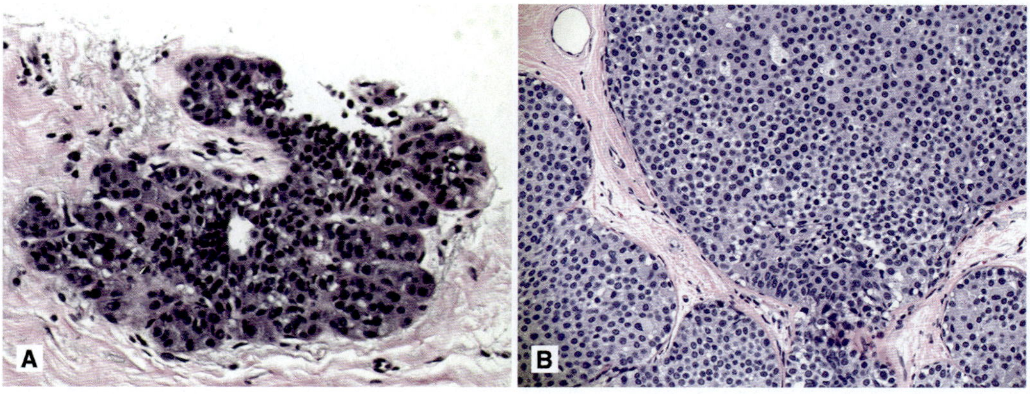

FIGURE 2-15: Lobular neoplasia. Note the extent of lobular expansion by the characteristic loosely cohesive cells. Atypical lobular hyperplasia is less well-developed lesion without distension (**A**) compared to distension of more than 50% of the acini in LCIS (**B**).

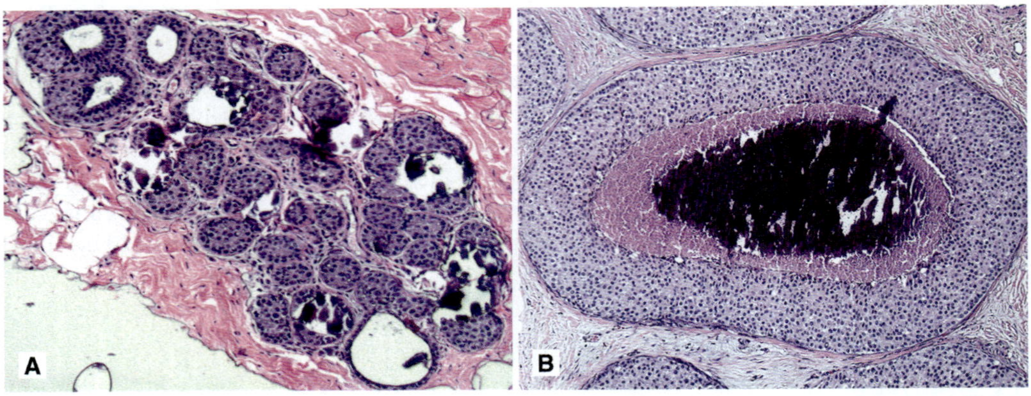

FIGURE 2-16: Atypical lobular hyperplasia (**A**) and classic lobular carcinoma *in situ* with necrosis (**B**), both with associated microcalcifications.

FIGURE 2-17: Lobular carcinoma *in situ* with necrosis.

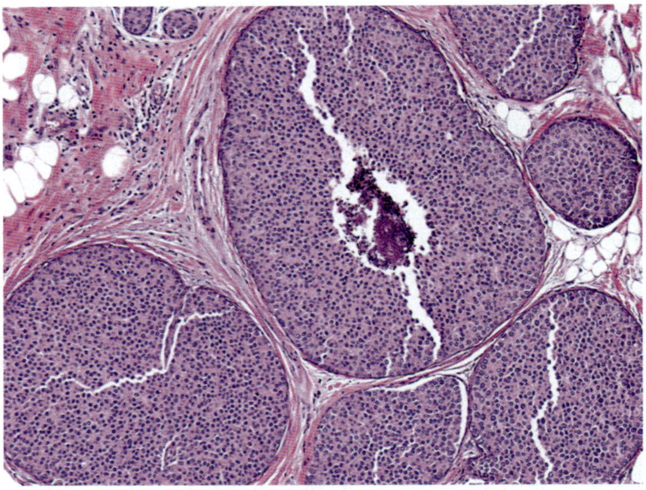

FIGURE 2-18: Lobular carcinoma *in situ* with associated histiocytes.

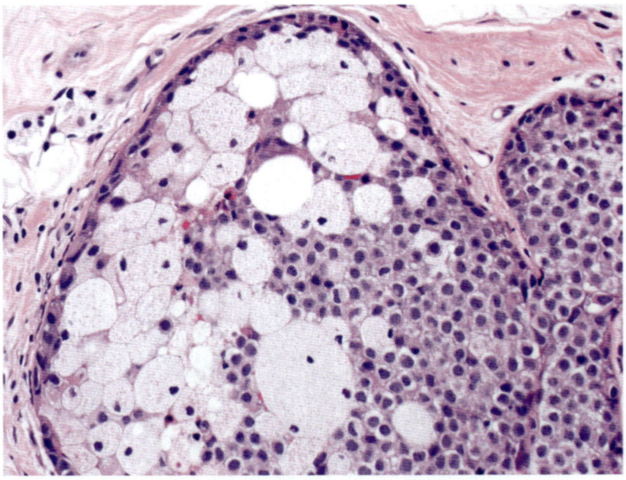

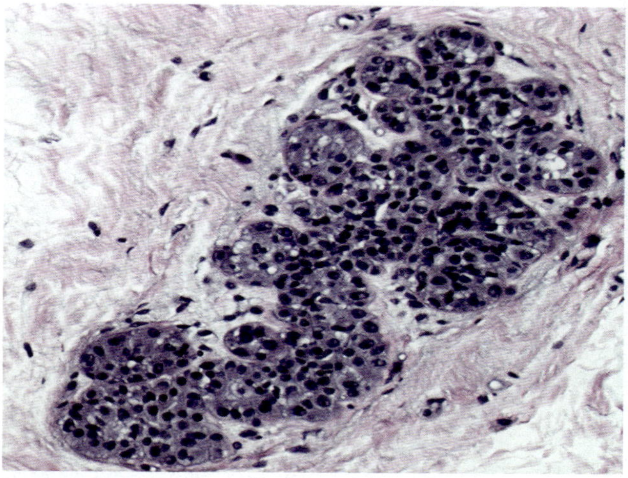

FIGURE 2-19: Lobular neoplasia with a cloverleaf-like pattern of growth in terminal duct lobular units.

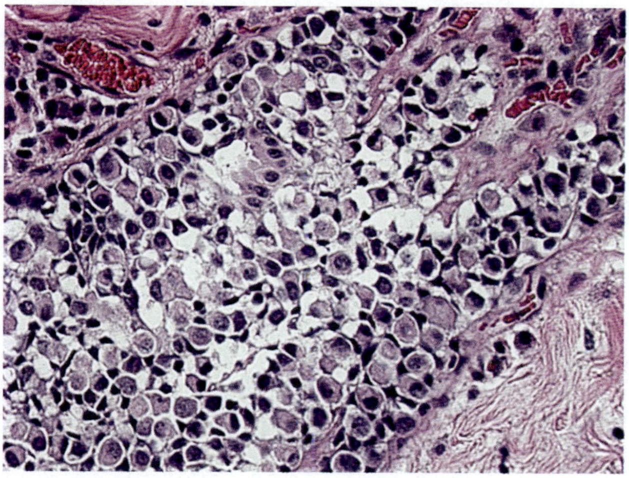

FIGURE 2-20: Pleomorphic lobular carcinoma *in situ*.

Pleomorphic LCIS

PLCIS, introduced as a distinct entity by Eusebi et al.,[33] is usually associated with ILC and cytologically different from classic LCIS. The cells appear dyshesive as in classic LCIS; however, they exhibit a greater degree of nuclear pleomorphism and usually contain abundant cytoplasm (Figure 2-20). Occasionally, the cytoplasm appears eosinophilic and finely granular, giving the cells an apocrine appearance (pleomorphic apocrine LCIS). Central (zonal) comedo necrosis and calcifications are quite commonly associated with these lesions and can be confused with comedo DCIS (Figure 2-21).

LCIS with Comedo Necrosis

These lesions are composed of identical cells to those of classic LCIS, namely, small, uniform cells with intracytoplasmic lumina and a dyshesive growth pattern, but in addition, contain central areas of comedo necrosis with or without associated calcifications[34] (Figures 2-16, 2-17, and 2-22).

LOBULAR CARCINOMA *IN SITU*, IHC

Almost all cases of LN express estrogen (ER) and progesterone (PR) receptors and lack for membranous E-cadherin and p120 expression by IHC.[35] Classic LCIS is usually negative for HER2 protein overexpression/gene amplification, lacks p53 mutations, and has a low Ki-67 labeling index. In contrast, PLCIS may show HER2 protein overexpression/gene amplification, p53 expression,

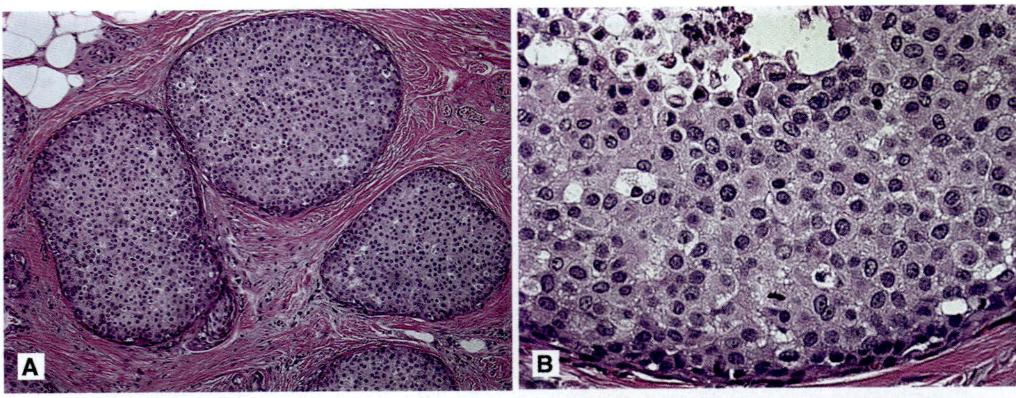

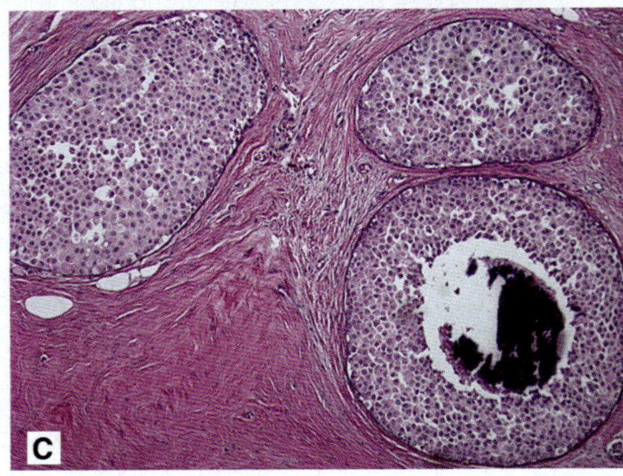

FIGURE 2-21: Pleomorphic lobular carcinoma *in situ*. The cells appear dyshesive as in classic lobular carcinoma *in situ*; however, they exhibit a greater degree of nuclear pleomorphism with eosinophilic cytoplasm giving the cells an apocrine appearance (**A, B**). Note the calcifications (**C**) commonly associated with these lesions.

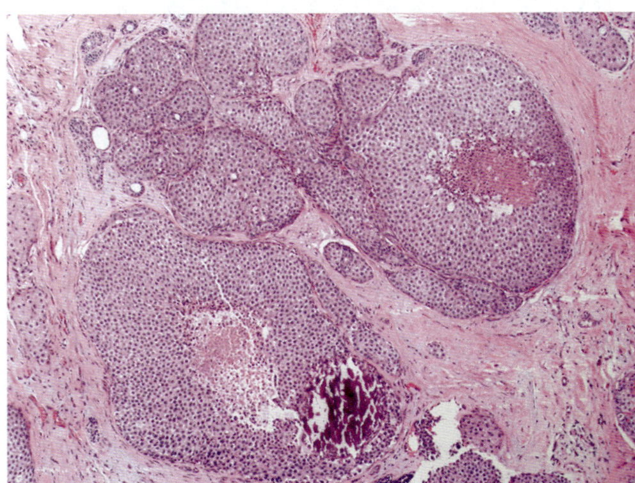

FIGURE 2-22: Lobular carcinoma *in situ* with necrosis resembling ductal carcinoma *in situ* with necrosis.

and a moderate to high Ki-67 labeling index.[36] E-cadherin is very useful as an adjunct in differentiating ductal from lobular lesions, with morphologically unequivocal cases of LN only rarely shown to demonstrate focal E-cadherin positivity.[37] p120 catenin IHC can also be very useful to confirm the diagnosis of both classic and pleomorphic variants of LCIS. Characteristically, there is diffuse cytoplasmic expression in LN, which contrasts with the preserved membranous expression in normal breast and ductal proliferations[35] (Figure 2-23). Expression of high molecular weight keratins may also be useful in characterizing LN. High molecular weight cytokeratins, highlighted by the 34betaE12 antibody (targeting cytokeratins 1, 5, 10, and 14), are commonly expressed by LN and are usually absent or minimally expressed by ductal carcinoma.[38]

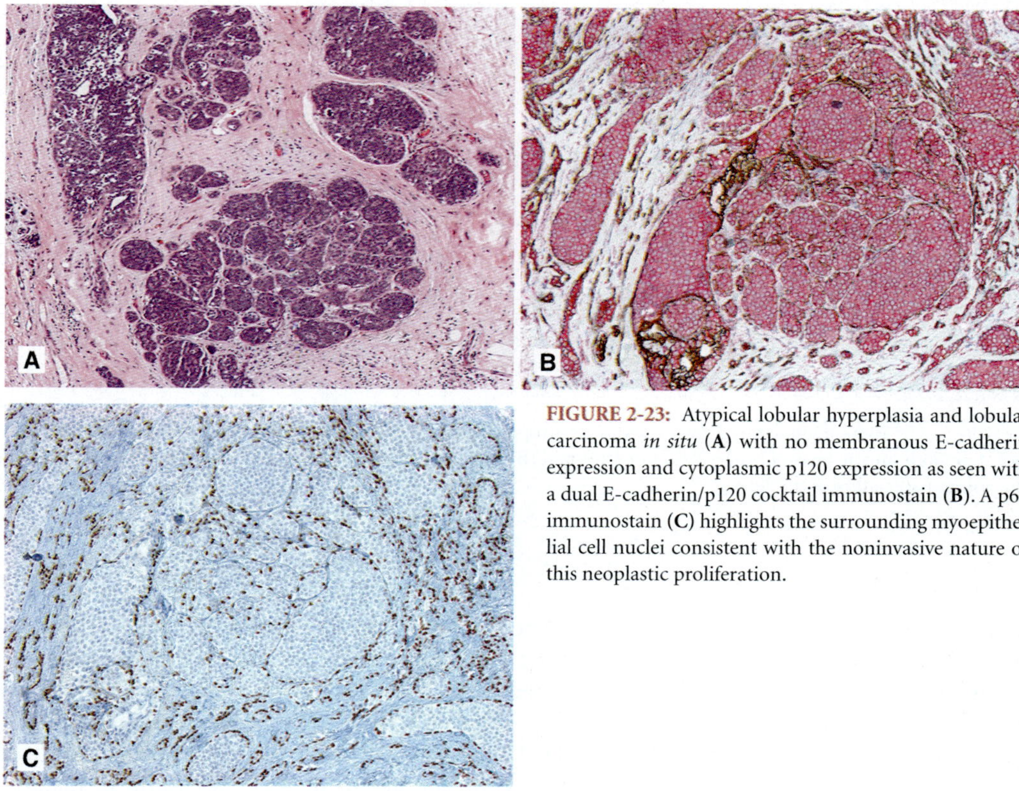

FIGURE 2-23: Atypical lobular hyperplasia and lobular carcinoma *in situ* (**A**) with no membranous E-cadherin expression and cytoplasmic p120 expression as seen with a dual E-cadherin/p120 cocktail immunostain (**B**). A p63 immunostain (**C**) highlights the surrounding myoepithelial cell nuclei consistent with the noninvasive nature of this neoplastic proliferation.

LOBULAR CARCINOMA *IN SITU*, DIFFERENTIAL DIAGNOSIS

Lobular carcinoma *in situ* has been described in association with collagenous spherulosis,[39] and this unusual pattern arises through the confluence of LN and spherulosis (Figure 2-24). This association might be confused with cribriform DCIS. Pathologists must remain alert to this form of mimicry because classification of *in situ* carcinoma of the breast carries important clinical implications. The identification of LN in this setting should be interpreted based on morphology with or without the utilization of E-cadherin IHC stain (see above). Association of LN with atrophic lobules and sclerosing adenosis may mimic ILC. Myoepithelial markers can help to delineate the presence of myoepithelial cells in the vicinity of LCIS[40] (Figure 2-25).

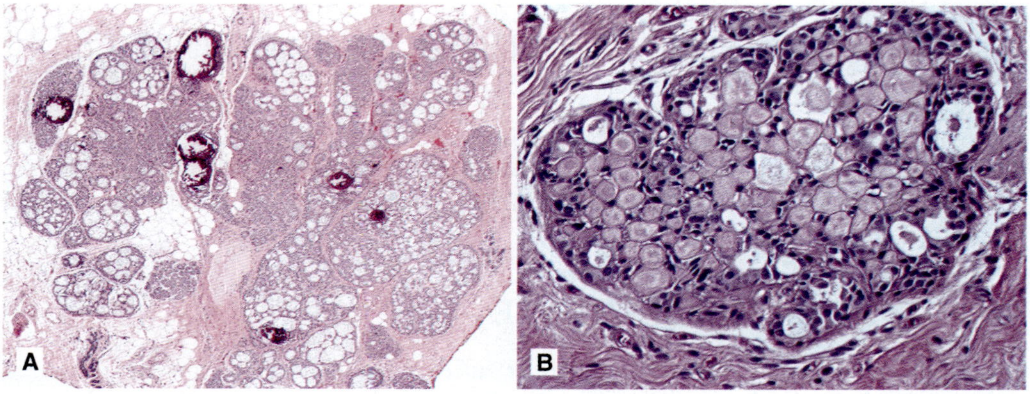

FIGURE 2-24: Lobular carcinoma *in situ* with collagenous spherulosis (**A,B**).

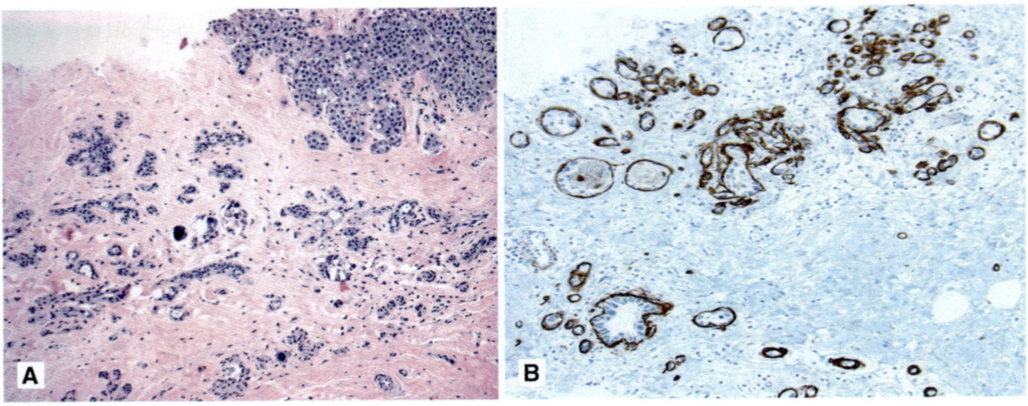

FIGURE 2-25: Atypical lobular hyperplasia involving atrophic lobules, which may be confused with an invasive process (**A**). A smooth muscle myosin heavy chain immunostain (**B**) highlights the myoepithelial cells present, thus supporting the noninvasive nature of this lesion.

DCIS

Differentiating LCIS from DCIS is important because of markedly different management[41] and, in most cases, is straightforward. A dyshesive growth pattern and prominent intracytoplasmic vacuoles favor LN, while well-defined cell borders and microacinar formation favor DCIS. In ambiguous cases, use of IHC may be helpful (see above) in the context of morphologic features. PLCIS is easily confused with high-grade DCIS, particularly when there is associated central necrosis and calcifications. Again, the dyshesive appearance of the cells is helpful in making this diagnosis, as is the lack of E-cadherin staining. As noted earlier, PLCIS and high-grade DCIS are currently managed similarly, and hence, distinguishing between them has minimal clinical impact. Again, PLCIS is most readily identified by the presence of classic LCIS in the nearby vicinity. Like classic LCIS, PLCIS exhibits loss of E-cadherin staining and cytoplasmic redistribution of p120 catenin, and hence, these two stains are useful to confirm a suspected diagnosis.[42]

Invasive Carcinoma

Lobular carcinoma *in situ* sometimes is confused with ILC especially the alveolar and solid patterns (Chapter 6). Myoepithelial markers such as p63 and smooth muscle myosin heavy chain along with others are helpful to delineate myoepithelial cells around LCIS compared to absent staining in invasive carcinoma.

LOBULAR CARCINOMA *IN SITU*, MOLECULAR GENETICS

Loss of heterozygosity and mutations in CDH1, the gene encoding E-cadherin, has been identified in both LN and ILC.[43] Alterations at chromosomes 1, 6, 16, 17, and 22 in LN have been identified by array comparative genomic hybridization (CGH).[44] On the other hand, few molecular genetic studies of PLCIS exist. PLCIS shows HER2 and MYC amplification, deletion of 13q, and gain of 20q.[45,46]

PAGET DISEASE OF THE NIPPLE

Paget disease, observed in 1% to 4% of all breast cancers, is an *in situ* adenocarcinoma localized within the epidermis of the nipple/areola region. The mean age of patients with Paget disease is 57 years,[47] and males can be afflicted as well.[48]

In most cases, Paget disease is associated with an underlying invasive and/or *in situ* carcinoma. Fifteen to 25% of patients report symptoms such as itching, tingling, burning sensation, or pain. Hard breast nodules, reflecting the existence of an underlying tumor, are found on palpation in up to 50% of cases. In the other 50%, the underlying carcinoma is detected by imaging techniques or by histopathologic examination of surgical specimens. Paget disease can also be an incidental histopathologic finding in patients initially presenting with a mammary tumor and no clinically obvious skin lesions.[49]

PAGET DISEASE, GROSS FEATURES

Clinically, early lesions of Paget disease consist of scaly, fissured, or oozing erythema of the nipple and areola with surface ulceration and crust formation. Advanced lesions present as a well-demarcated, round/ovoid eczema-like plaques. The lesions are usually unilateral and only rarely bilateral.[49]

PAGET DISEASE, HISTOLOGY

The characteristic feature of Paget disease is the presence within the epidermis of malignant epithelial cells with abundant, clear cytoplasm, and enlarged hyperchromatic nuclei with prominent nucleoli. The malignant cells are more abundant within the lower epidermal layers, where they may form gland-like structures and surround adnexal structures. Such cells become more dispersed within the upper epidermis including the keratinized layer (Figure 2-26). Intracytoplasmic mucin may also be evident within the tumor cells. Acanthosis with orthokeratosis or parakeratosis, with or without ulceration, may be present. The dermis may be edematous and/or telangiectatic with or without infiltration with polymorphous inflammatory cells. The in situ or invasive mammary carcinomas associated with Paget disease are often multifocal[50] and usually close to the areola.

PAGET DISEASE, IHC AND DIFFERENTIAL DIAGNOSIS

Aside from other clinical mimics of Paget disease, the histopathologic differential diagnosis includes other intraepidermal lesions with clear cells, specifically Bowen disease, pagetoid melanoma, and Toker cells. Aside from Toker cells, IHC is very helpful in this regard as the neoplastic

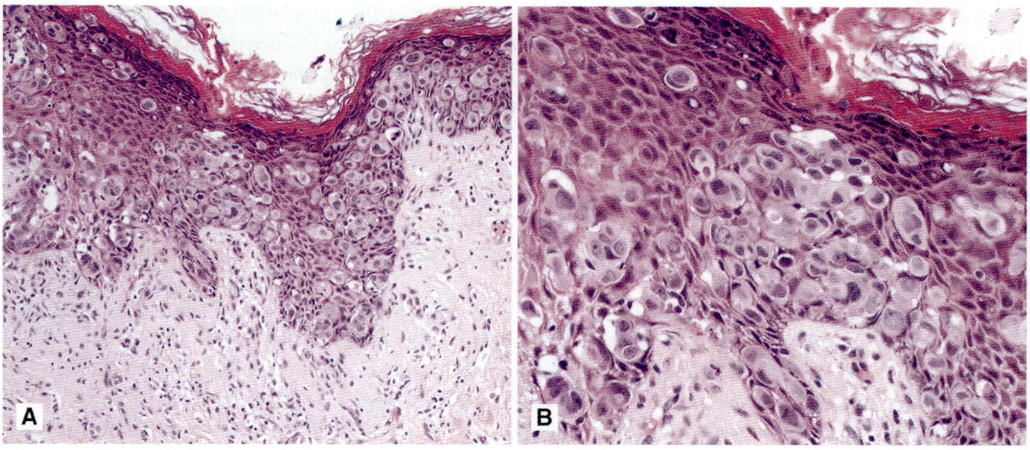

FIGURE 2-26: Paget disease of the nipple. Low-power caption (**A**) shows the lower epidermis infiltrated with malignant epithelial cells with abundant clear cytoplasm and enlarged hyperchromatic atypical nuclei. In the upper epidermis, the malignant cells are more scattered. High-power caption (**B**) shows the full-thickness epidermis is infiltrated with malignant epithelial cells. This particular case was associated with an underlying high-grade ductal carcinoma *in situ* depicted in Figure 2-3.

cells in Paget disease express low molecular weight cytokeratins, EMA, CEA, GCDFP-15, and frequently HER2,[51] but lack expression of high molecular weight cytokeratins and melanocytic markers, expected to be expressed in Bowen disease and melanoma, respectively. Toker cells and Toker cell hyperplasia are more difficult to distinguish from Paget disease because of overlapping morphology and IHC. In such situations, significant cytologic atypia and HER2 overexpression are the two findings that can help substantiate a diagnosis of Paget disease.

References

1. Allred DC. Ductal carcinoma in situ: terminology, classification, and natural history. *J Natl Cancer Inst Monogr* 2010;2010:134–138.
2. Ernster VL, Barclay J. Increases in ductal carcinoma in situ (DCIS) of the breast in relation to mammography: a dilemma. *J Natl Cancer Inst Monogr* 1997:151–156.
3. Schnitt S, Allred C, Britton P, et al. Intraductal proliferative lesions: ductal carcinoma in situ. In: Lakhani S, Ellis IO, Schnitt SJ, et al., eds. *WHO Classification of Tumours of the Breast.* 4th ed. Lyon, France: International Agency for Research and Cancer (IARC); 2012:90–94.
4. Allegra CJ, Aberle DR, Ganschow P, et al. National Institutes of Health State-of-the-Science Conference statement: diagnosis and management of ductal carcinoma in situ, September 22–24, 2009. *J Natl Cancer Inst* 2010;102:161–169.
5. Claus EB, Petruzella S, Matloff E, et al. Prevalence of BRCA1 and BRCA2 mutations in women diagnosed with ductal carcinoma in situ. *JAMA* 2005;293:964–969.
6. Sauer T, Lomo J, Garred O, et al. Cytologic features of ductal carcinoma in situ in fine-needle aspiration of the breast mirror the histopathologic growth pattern heterogeneity and grading. *Cancer* 2005;105:21–27.
7. Hermann G, Keller RJ, Drossman S, et al. Mammographic pattern of microcalcifications in the preoperative diagnosis of comedo ductal carcinoma in situ: histopathologic correlation. *Can Assoc Radiol J* 1999;50:235–240.
8. Edge B, Byrd RD, Compton CC, et al. *AJCC Cancer Staging Manual (Edge, AJCC Cancer Staging Manual).* 7th ed. New York: Springer; 2011.
9. Ellis IO. Intraductal proliferative lesions of the breast: morphology, associated risk and molecular biology. *Mod Pathol* 2010;23(suppl 2):S1–S7.
10. Cross AS, Azzopardi JG, Krausz T, et al. A morphological and immunocytochemical study of a distinctive variant of ductal carcinoma in-situ of the breast. *Histopathology* 1985;9:21–37.
11. Silverstein MJ, Recht A, Lagios MD, et al. Special report: consensus conference III. Image-detected breast cancer: state-of-the-art diagnosis and treatment. *J Am Coll Surg* 2009;209:504–520.
12. Wei S, Kragel CP, Zhang K, et al. Factors associated with residual disease after initial breast-conserving surgery for ductal carcinoma in situ. *Hum Pathol* 2012;43:986–993.
13. College of American Pathologists. Protocol for the examination of specimens from patients with ductal carcinoma in situ (DCIS) of the Breast. 2013. http://www.cap.org/ShowProperty?nodePath=/UCMCon/Contribution Folders/WebContent/pdf/cp-breast-dcis-13protocol-3200.pdf. Accessed January 15, 2015.
14. Silverstein MJ, Poller DN, Waisman JR, et al. Prognostic classification of breast ductal carcinoma-in-situ. *Lancet* 1995;345:1154–1157.
15. Dunne C, Burke JP, Morrow M, et al. Effect of margin status on local recurrence after breast conservation and radiation therapy for ductal carcinoma in situ. *J Clin Oncol* 2009;27:1615–1620.
16. Kapucuoglu N, Losi L, Eusebi V. Immunohistochemical localization of Bcl-2 and Bax proteins in in situ and invasive duct breast carcinomas. *Virchows Arch* 1997;430:17–22.
17. Allred DC, Clark GM, Molina R, et al. Overexpression of HER-2/neu and its relationship with other prognostic factors change during the progression of in situ to invasive breast cancer. *Hum Pathol* 1992;23:974–979.
18. Rabban JT, Koerner FC, Lerwill MF. Solid papillary ductal carcinoma in situ versus usual ductal hyperplasia in the breast: a potentially difficult distinction resolved by cytokeratin 5/6. *Hum Pathol* 2006;37:787–793.
19. Page DL, Rogers LW. Combined histologic and cytologic criteria for the diagnosis of mammary atypical ductal hyperplasia. *Hum Pathol* 1992;23:1095–1097.

20. Tavassoli FA, Norris HJ. A comparison of the results of long-term follow-up for atypical intraductal hyperplasia and intraductal hyperplasia of the breast. *Cancer* 1990;65:518–529.
21. Khoury T, Karabakhtsian RG, Mattson D, et al. Pleomorphic lobular carcinoma in situ of the breast: clinicopathological review of 47 cases. *Histopathology* 2013;64:981–993.
22. Simpson PT, Reis-Filho JS, Gale T, et al. Molecular evolution of breast cancer. *J Pathol* 2005;205:248–254.
23. Hwang ES, DeVries S, Chew KL, et al. Patterns of chromosomal alterations in breast ductal carcinoma in situ. *Clin Cancer Res* 2004;10:5160–5167.
24. American College of Radiology. Practice guideline for the management of ductal carcinoma in-situ of the breast (DCIS). *J Am Coll Surg* 2007;205:145–161.
25. Haagensen CD, Lane N, Lattes R, et al. Lobular neoplasia (so-called lobular carcinoma in situ) of the breast. *Cancer* 1978;42:737–769.
26. Page DL, Dupont WD, Rogers LW, et al. Atypical hyperplastic lesions of the female breast. A long-term follow-up study. *Cancer* 1985;55:2698–2708.
27. Rosen PP, Kosloff C, Lieberman PH, et al. Lobular carcinoma in situ of the breast. Detailed analysis of 99 patients with average follow-up of 24 years. *Am J Surg Pathol* 1978;2:225–251.
28. Beute BJ, Kalisher L, Hutter RV. Lobular carcinoma in situ of the breast: clinical, pathologic, and mammographic features. *AJR Am J Roentgenol* 1991;157:257–265.
29. Li CI, Anderson BO, Daling JR, et al. Changing incidence of lobular carcinoma in situ of the breast. *Breast Cancer Res Treat* 2002;75:259–268.
30. Cocquyt V, Van Belle S. Lobular carcinoma in situ and invasive lobular cancer of the breast. *Curr Opin Obstet Gynecol* 2005;17:55–60.
31. Rajesh L, Dey P, Joshi K. Fine needle aspiration cytology of lobular breast carcinoma. Comparison with other breast lesions. *Acta Cytol* 2003;47:177–182.
32. Page DL, Kidd TE Jr, Dupont WD, et al. Lobular neoplasia of the breast: higher risk for subsequent invasive cancer predicted by more extensive disease. *Hum Pathol* 1991;22:1232–1239.
33. Eusebi V, Magalhaes F, Azzopardi JG. Pleomorphic lobular carcinoma of the breast: an aggressive tumor showing apocrine differentiation. *Hum Pathol* 1992;23:655–662.
34. Fadare O, Dadmanesh F, Alvarado-Cabrero I, et al. Lobular intraepithelial neoplasia [lobular carcinoma in situ] with comedo-type necrosis: a clinicopathologic study of 18 cases. *Am J Surg Pathol* 2006;30:1445–1453.
35. Dabbs DJ, Kaplai M, Chivukula M, et al. The spectrum of morphomolecular abnormalities of the E-cadherin/catenin complex in pleomorphic lobular carcinoma of the breast. *Appl Immunohistochem Mol Morphol* 2007;15:260–266.
36. Sneige N, Wang J, Baker BA, et al. Clinical, histopathologic, and biologic features of pleomorphic lobular (ductal-lobular) carcinoma in situ of the breast: a report of 24 cases. *Mod Pathol* 2002;15:1044–1050.
37. Goldstein NS, Bassi D, Watts JC, et al. E-cadherin reactivity of 95 noninvasive ductal and lobular lesions of the breast. Implications for the interpretation of problematic lesions. *Am J Clin Pathol* 2001;115:534–542.
38. Bratthauer GL, Miettinen M, Tavassoli FA. Cytokeratin immunoreactivity in lobular intraepithelial neoplasia. *J Histochem Cytochem* 2003;51:1527–1531.
39. Sgroi D, Koerner FC. Involvement of collagenous spherulosis by lobular carcinoma in situ. Potential confusion with cribriform ductal carcinoma in situ. *Am J Surg Pathol* 1995;19:1366–1370.
40. Jung WH, Noh TW, Kim HJ, et al. Lobular carcinoma in situ in sclerosing adenosis. *Yonsei Med J* 2000;41:293–297.
41. Apple SK, Matin M, Olsen EP, et al. Significance of lobular intraepithelial neoplasia at margins of breast conservation specimens: a report of 38 cases and literature review. *Diagn Pathol* 2010;5:54.
42. Dabbs DJ, Bhargava R, Chivukula M. Lobular versus ductal breast neoplasms: the diagnostic utility of p120 catenin. *Am J Surg Pathol* 2007;31:427–437.
43. Mastracci TL, Tjan S, Bane AL, et al. E-cadherin alterations in atypical lobular hyperplasia and lobular carcinoma in situ of the breast. *Mod Pathol* 2005;18:741–751.
44. Mastracci TL, Shadeo A, Colby SM, et al. Genomic alterations in lobular neoplasia: a microarray comparative genomic hybridization signature for early neoplastic proliferation in the breast. *Genes Chromosomes Cancer* 2006;45:1007–1017.
45. Raju U, Mei L, Seema S, et al. Molecular classification of breast carcinoma in situ. *Curr Genomics* 2006;7:523–532.
46. Reis-Filho JS, Simpson PT, Jones C, et al. Pleomorphic lobular carcinoma of the breast: role of comprehensive molecular pathology in characterization of an entity. *J Pathol* 2005;207:1–13.

47. Kawase K, Dimaio DJ, Tucker SL, et al. Paget's disease of the breast: there is a role for breast-conserving therapy. *Ann Surg Oncol* 2005;12:391–397.
48. Goodman MT, Tung KH, Wilkens LR. Comparative epidemiology of breast cancer among men and women in the US, 1996 to 2000. *Cancer Causes Control* 2006;17:127–136.
49. Ascenso AC, Marques MS, Capitao-Mor M. Paget's disease of the nipple. Clinical and pathological review of 109 female patients. *Dermatologica* 1985;170:170–179.
50. Kothari AS, Beechey-Newman N, Hamed H, et al. Paget disease of the nipple: a multifocal manifestation of higher-risk disease. *Cancer* 2002;95:1–7.
51. Fu W, Lobocki CA, Silberberg BK, et al. Molecular markers in Paget disease of the breast. *J Surg Oncol* 2001;77:171–178.

Microinvasive Carcinoma 3

Microinvasive carcinoma is defined by the presence of one or more microscopic foci of invasive carcinoma, none more than 1 mm in size.[1,2] In most cases, microinvasive carcinoma is associated with an *in situ* carcinoma, usually high-grade ductal carcinoma *in situ* (DCIS) and less frequently non-high–grade DCIS or lobular carcinoma *in situ*.[3] The prognosis of microinvasive carcinoma is similar to that of DCIS of equivalent grade, and the clinical management is not different from that of high-grade DCIS.[1]

MICROINVASIVE CARCINOMA, GROSS FEATURES

Although microinvasive carcinoma by itself is not associated with particular gross findings, associated high-grade DCIS, especially when extensive, may produce a firm mass-like lesion.

MICROINVASIVE CARCINOMA, HISTOLOGY

Microinvasive carcinoma is most commonly seen in the background of extensive, high-grade DCIS (Figure 3-1). Periductal stromal reactions, such as desmoplasia and lymphocytic response, are frequent. Microinvasion can be unifocal or multifocal (with no focus >1 mm) and manifests as isolated tumor cells, solid clusters or glandular structures. Tumor cells typically exhibit similar cytologic features to those in coexisting DCIS. It is important to point out that foci of microinvasion could potentially be obscured by the amount of associated inflammatory reaction (Figures 3-2 and 3-3). Accordingly, areas of inflammation in close proximity to high-grade DCIS should always be carefully scrutinized to exclude this possibility. Evaluation of additional histologic levels may also be useful in this regard.

MICROINVASIVE CARCINOMA, DIFFERENTIAL DIAGNOSIS

The main differential diagnosis of microinvasive carcinoma essentially is pure DCIS without invasive carcinoma. In DCIS with lobular cancerization, areas of acinar branching can be cut tangentially and mimic microinvasion. In such cases, however, the lobulocentric configuration is typically maintained on low-power view, and the nests of tumor cells usually demonstrate rounded contours as they are confined within lobular acini. DCIS arising in a background of sclerosing adenosis or other sclerosing lesions is sometimes troublesome as the involved ducts or acini can be markedly compressed and distorted by densely fibrotic stroma, thus imparting an erroneous impression of microinvasive or frankly invasive carcinoma. Crush and cautery artifacts may also result in similar appearance. Once again, the preserved lobular architecture on low magnification, along with the presence of myoepithelial cells associated with tumor cell nests by histomorphology or immunohistochemistry, can help resolve any uncertainty.

Not uncommonly, benign epithelial cells of proliferative lesions (particularly from papillomas) or tumor cells of DCIS (particularly papillary and micropapillary types) can be mechanically

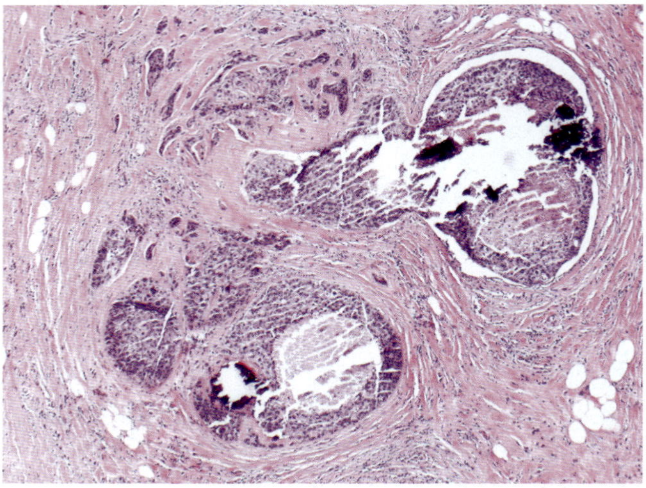

FIGURE 3-1: A small focus of invasive carcinoma arises in the background of high-grade DCIS with comedo necrosis. A desmoplastic stroma is evident.

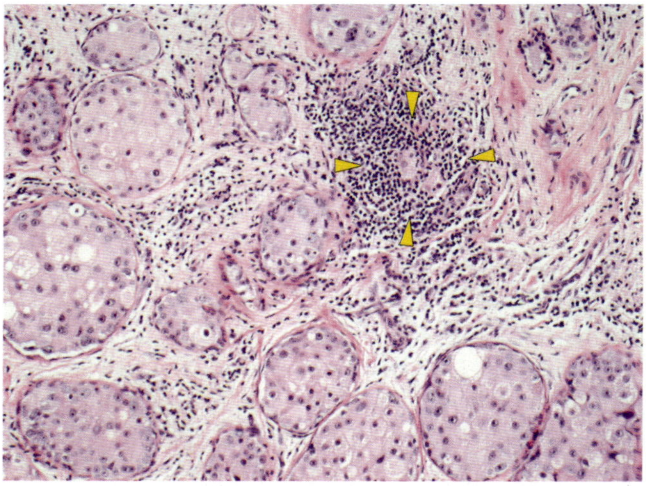

FIGURE 3-2: An intermediate power view showing extensive, high-grade DCIS with lobular cancerization. Note that even at this magnification, a few single cells with cytologic features identical to those in DCIS are seen within the inflammatory infiltrate (*arrowheads*).

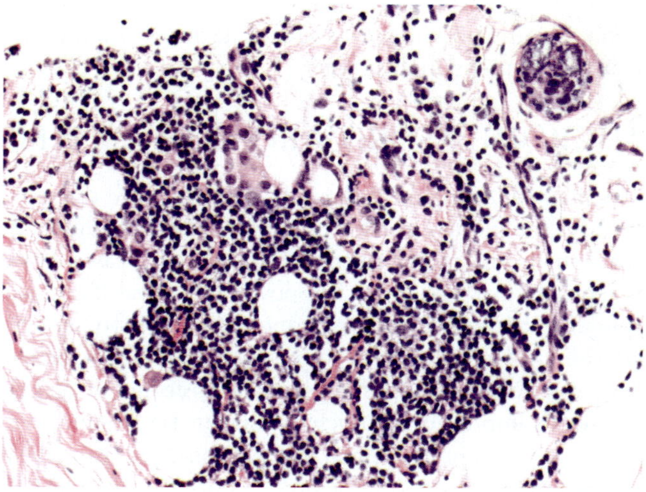

FIGURE 3-3: A higher magnification from the deeper levels shown in Figure 3-2 reveals larger invasive cell clusters surrounded by a dense lymphocytic infiltrate.

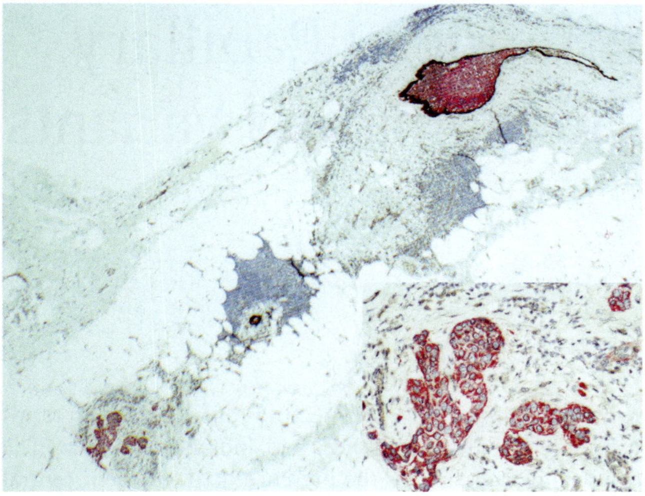

FIGURE 3-4: Immunohistochemistry may be of value in distinguishing true microinvasion from its mimics. An antibody cocktail comprising luminal markers (CK7 and CK18; red chromogen) and basal/myoepithelial markers (CK5, CK14, p63; brown chromogen) was utilized in this case. In contrast to the focus of DCIS (**right upper corner**), the focus of microinvasion (**left lower corner**; **inset**, higher magnification) shows only luminal cytokeratin expression with no surrounding basal/myoepithelial marker expression.

displaced into stroma by needling procedures such as needle core biopsy or fine needle aspiration. The tumor cell clusters in the absence of myoepithelial cells give rise to the appearance of microinvasion. The findings that the cells of interest are only present in the needle tract associated with biopsy site changes (e.g., fat necrosis, hemosiderin, and histiocytic or giant cell reaction) should point to the correct diagnosis. This phenomenon is discussed in greater detail in Chapter 18.

It should be noted that if the focus indefinite for microinvasion is no longer present in the subsequent levels or immunostains, the lesion should be regarded as *in situ* carcinoma, and a diagnosis of microinvasive carcinoma should not be rendered.

MICROINVASIVE CARCINOMA, IMMUNOHISTOCHEMISTRY

Immunohistochemical stains can be useful to confirm the diagnosis of invasive carcinoma in problematic cases. The tumor cells, be they single or in clusters/nests, can be highlighted by broad-spectrum or low molecular weight cytokeratin markers, while certain markers (e.g., p63) can be used to support the absence of myoepithelial cells in the potential foci of microinvasive carcinoma. In this context, antibody "cocktails" (Figure 3-4) can be very advantageous to minimize loss of lesional tissue, frequently seen when multiple immunostains are performed on small foci.

References

1. Pinder SE, Ellis IO, Schnitt SJ, et al. Microinvasive carcinoma. In: Lakhani SR, Ellis IO, Schnitt SJ, et al., eds. *WHO Classification of Tumours of the Breast.* Lyon, France: IARC Press; 2012:96–97.
2. Prasad ML, Osborne MP, Hoda SA. Observations on the histopathologic diagnosis of microinvasive carcinoma of the breast. *Anat Pathol* 1998;3:209–232.
3. Nemoto T, Castillo N, Tsukada Y, et al. Lobular carcinoma in situ with microinvasion. *J Surg Oncol* 1998;67:41–46.

4 Intraductal Papillary Carcinoma and Variants

Intraductal papillary lesions of the breast encompass a wide spectrum of neoplasms in terms of their clinical presentation, histomorphologic appearance, and biologic potential. The characteristic defining feature of the papillary lesions is the presence of arborescent central fibrovascular cores of variable length and thickness lined by proliferative epithelial cells. Benign papillary lesions are characterized by the presence of an intervening myoepithelial cell layer in the fibrovascular fronds, whereas their malignant counterparts generally lack an intact myoepithelial cell layer within the papillae. The spectrum of intraductal papillary lesions includes intraductal papilloma, papilloma with atypia ductal hyperplasia (ADH) (atypical papilloma), papilloma with ductal carcinoma *in situ* (DCIS), and intraductal papillary carcinoma (papillary DCIS; papillary carcinoma, noninvasive), including two variants: intracystic/encapsulated papillary carcinoma and solid papillary carcinoma.

While histologically classifying a breast lesion as "papillary" is usually not challenging, the distinction between different papillary lesions is not always an easy task. Although characteristic of benign papillary lesions, the presence of myoepithelial cells in the fibrovascular fronds does not always exclude malignancy. The difficulty in categorizing papillary lesions is further confounded by variable terminology and lack of standardized criteria for a given entity. The classification and terminology of intraductal papillary lesions in this chapter are based on the 2012 WHO Classification of Tumors of the Breast.[1]

INTRADUCTAL PAPILLARY CARCINOMA, IMAGING AND GROSS FEATURES

There are no specific imaging features for intraductal papillary carcinoma. The tumor may appear as an irregular mass with increased vascularity (Figure 4-1). As discussed later in this chapter, atypical ductal hyperplasia (ADH) or DCIS can arise in a preexisting intraductal papilloma, which may originate from a central duct (central papilloma; large duct papilloma) or a peripheral duct (peripheral papilloma; small duct papilloma). In fact, intraductal papilloma extensively involved by DCIS is often morphologically indistinguishable from de novo intraductal papillary carcinoma and is not managed any differently. The patient may present with nipple discharge and/or a palpable mass. Macroscopically, the tumor is typically solitary and forms a tan-pink, well-circumscribed nodule in a cystically dilated space. The papillary appearance can be appreciated on gross examination (Figure 4-2). Conversely, those originating from peripheral ducts generally show occult macroscopic features unless they are associated with other findings.

INTRADUCTAL PAPILLARY CARCINOMA, HISTOLOGY

Microscopically, intraductal papillary carcinomas typically show ducts and/or terminal duct lobular units (TDLUs) filled with slender or branching fibrovascular cores lined by stratified columnar neoplastic epithelial cells without an intervening myoepithelial cell layer (Figure 4-3).

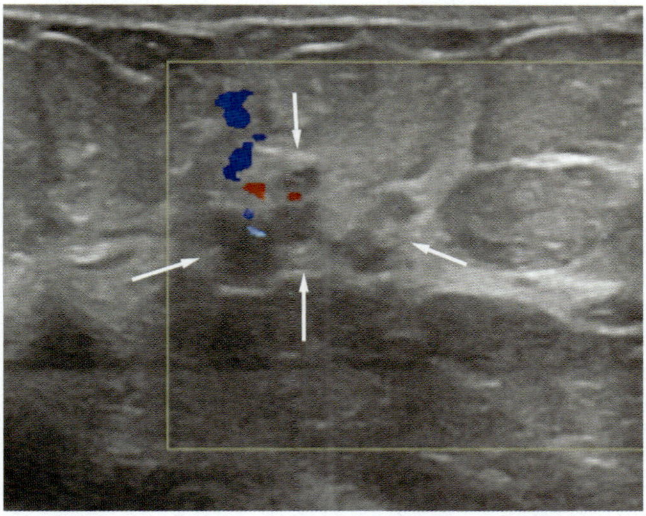

FIGURE 4-1: Intraductal papillary carcinoma. Ultrasound color Doppler image reveals an irregular solid mass (*arrows*) with increased vascularity.

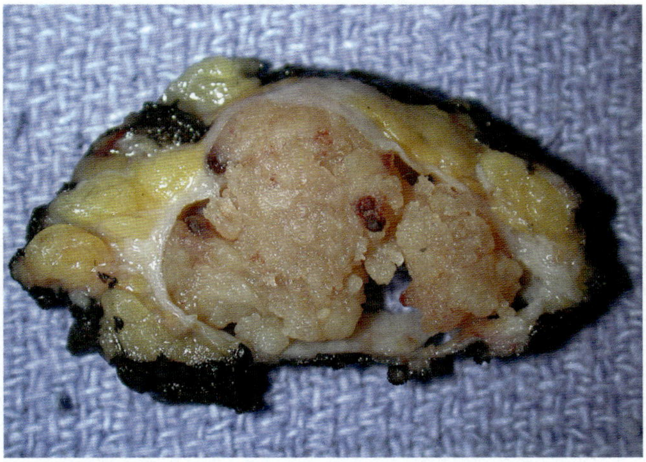

FIGURE 4-2: Gross pathologic features of an intraductal papillary neoplasm arising from a central duct. Note a tan-pink, circumscribed nodule protruding into a cystically dilated duct. The lesion has a frankly papillary configuration. The histologic examination revealed a papilloma with DCIS (Photograph courtesy of Erik Scott Young, Pennsylvania.)

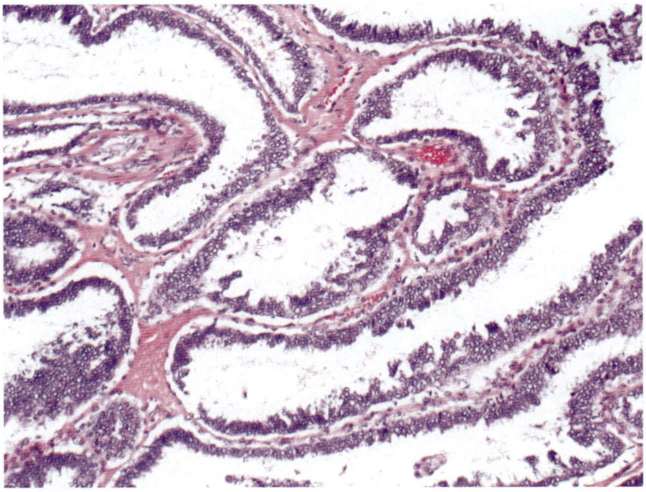

FIGURE 4-3: An example of intraductal papillary carcinoma showing arborizing and slender fibrovascular cores covered by a single population of stratified neoplastic epithelial cells.

The fibrovascular stalks are usually thin, delicate, and less fibrotic than are those of intraductal papillomas. Scant myoepithelial cells may rarely be present within the papillae beneath the epithelial proliferation (Figure 4-4).[2,3] Continuous growth of the epithelium may result in architectural complexity, such as solid, cribriform, and micropapillary patterns, and thus may obliterate the spaces between the papillae (Figure 4-5). At the periphery of the involved duct spaces, a myoepithelial cell layer is present, thus defining the *in situ* nature of the lesion (Figure 4-6). However, the myoepithelial layer may be attenuated or discontinuous, especially in larger lesions with markedly distended duct spaces.[4,5]

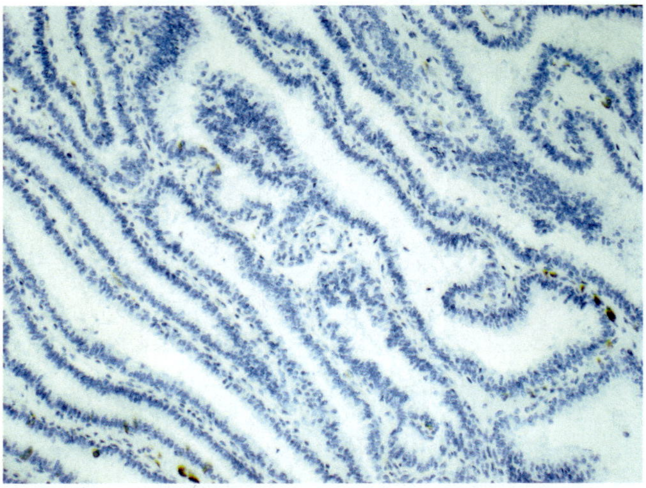

FIGURE 4-4: A p63 immunostain of the case shown in Figure 4-3 demonstrates the absence of myoepithelium in the papillary fronds. However, scant myoepithelial cells may rarely be present within the papillae beneath the epithelial proliferation, as illustrated.

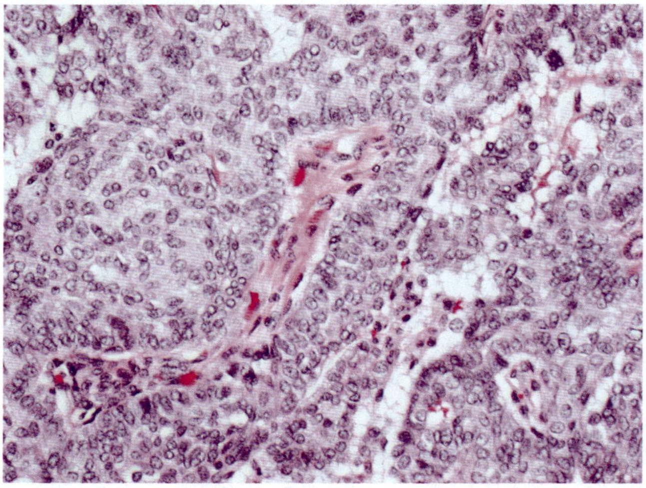

FIGURE 4-5: Intraductal papillary carcinoma showing neoplastic epithelial proliferation, which results in a solid pattern, thus obliterating the spaces between the papillae.

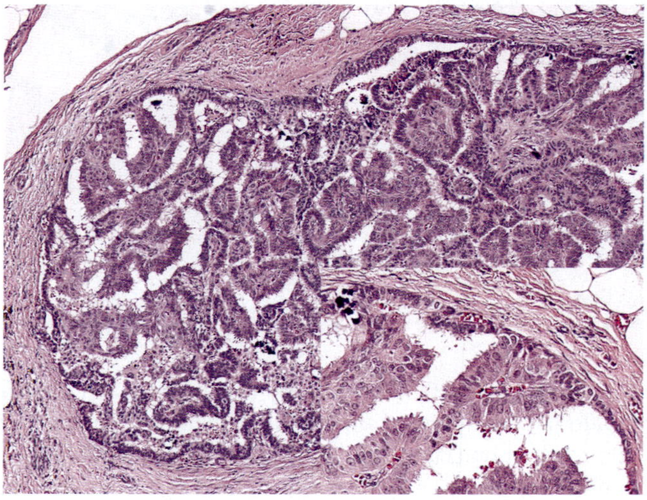

FIGURE 4-6: The presence of a myoepithelial cell layer at the periphery of the involved duct can be appreciated in this intraductal papillary carcinoma by routine hematoxylin–eosin (H&E) stain (**inset**, higher magnification).

The lesional cells are usually of low or intermediate nuclear grade and demonstrate a single, uniform cell population. However, a dimorphic cell population may be present in some examples, in which the second population consists of cells with clear cytoplasm, often in a basal location (Figure 4-7). These cells may be mistaken for myoepithelial cells and thus may potentially lead to an erroneous diagnosis of intraductal papilloma. When in doubt, immunohistochemical stains for ductal epithelial cells (i.e., low molecular weight cytokeratins) and myoepithelial cells (high molecular weight cytokeratins or p63) can be used to resolve the uncertainty.

INTRADUCTAL PAPILLARY CARCINOMA, DIFFERENTIAL DIAGNOSIS

The differential diagnosis of intraductal papillary carcinoma essentially includes all intraductal papillary lesions, namely, intraductal papilloma, papilloma with ADH, and papilloma with DCIS. The papillary fronds in benign papillomas are generally broad and may be variably sclerotic or, rarely, infracted (Figure 4-8). A prominent myoepithelial cell layer is invariably present in the papillae. Occasionally, myoepithelial cell hyperplasia may also be seen. Frequently, papillomas are associated with florid ductal epithelial proliferation and can be difficult to distinguish from their malignant counterpart. However, the epithelial proliferation in papillomas is typically a heterogeneous, nonneoplastic cell population with architectural and cytologic characteristics of usual

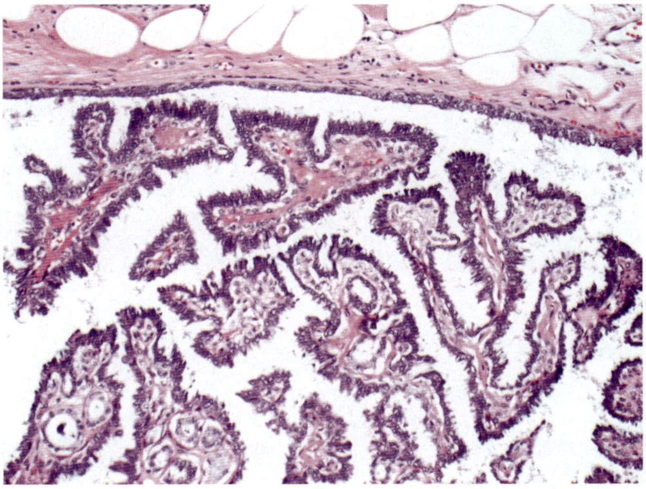

FIGURE 4-7: An intraductal papillary carcinoma with a dimorphic cell population. The second population of neoplastic cells with clear cytoplasm may lead to an erroneous impression of myoepithelial cells.

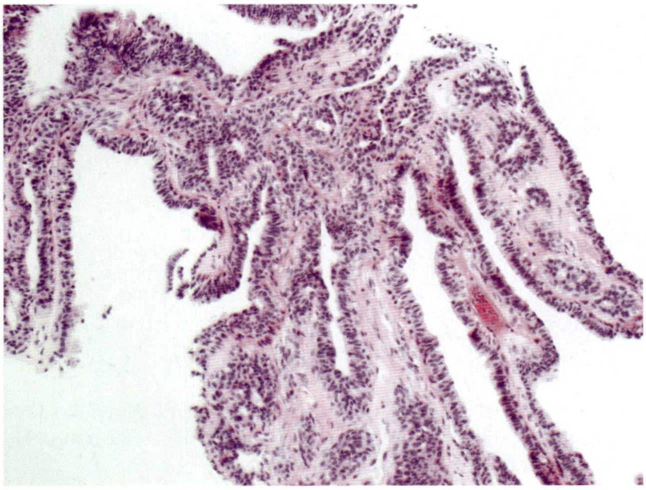

FIGURE 4-8: The papillary fronds in intraductal papillomas are generally thickened and variably sclerotic.

ductal hyperplasia (Figure 4-9). As in the latter, cytokeratin 5/6 staining often shows a patchy staining pattern, while p63 only highlights the myoepithelial cells and thus is most helpful in evaluating fibrovascular cores (Figure 4-10). Focal apocrine metaplasia and, less frequently, squamous metaplasia may be present within benign papillomas but are almost always absent in intraductal papillary carcinomas. It should be noted that collagenous spherulosis can involve papillomas, thus giving rise to a fenestrated appearance mimicking that of cribriform DCIS (Figure 4-11). Identification of the basement membrane material within the pseudoluminal spaces and recognizing the myoepithelial nature of the surrounding cells are essential to reach a correct diagnosis.

Foci within papillomas fulfilling the criteria for ADH or DCIS can be seen, more commonly associated with peripheral papillomas than those in the central location.[6,7] These lesions are referred to as papilloma with ADH and papilloma with DCIS, respectively.[1] The atypical features in these lesions include the presence of a monotonous population of epithelial cells characteristic of those in ADH and low-grade DCIS and a complex architecture pattern such as solid, cribriform,

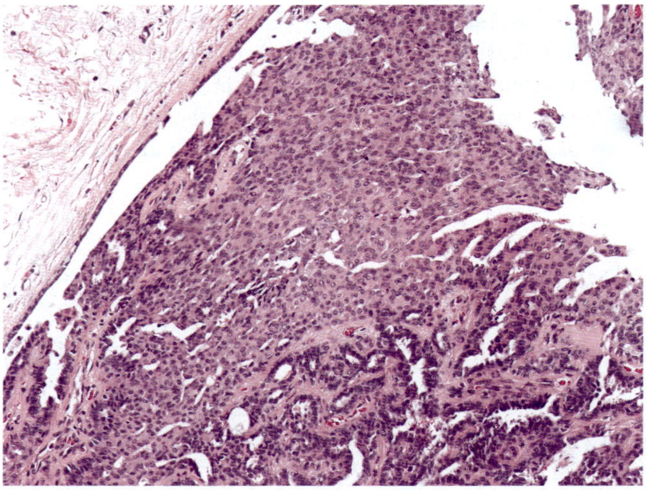

FIGURE 4-9: An intraductal papilloma with florid ductal epithelial proliferation showing a heterogeneous cell population intermixed with myoepithelial cells characteristics of usual ductal hyperplasia.

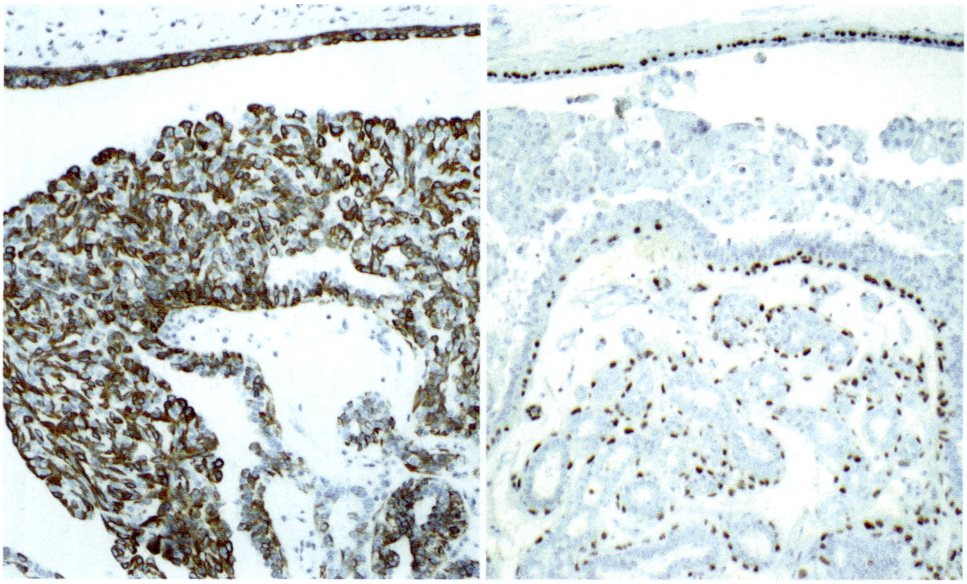

FIGURE 4-10: CK5/6 and p63 immunostains in an intraductal papilloma with usual ductal hyperplasia. While CK5/6 often shows a patchy staining pattern in the ductal epithelial proliferation (**left panel**), p63 only highlights the myoepithelial cells and thus is most helpful in evaluating fibrovascular cores (**right panel**).

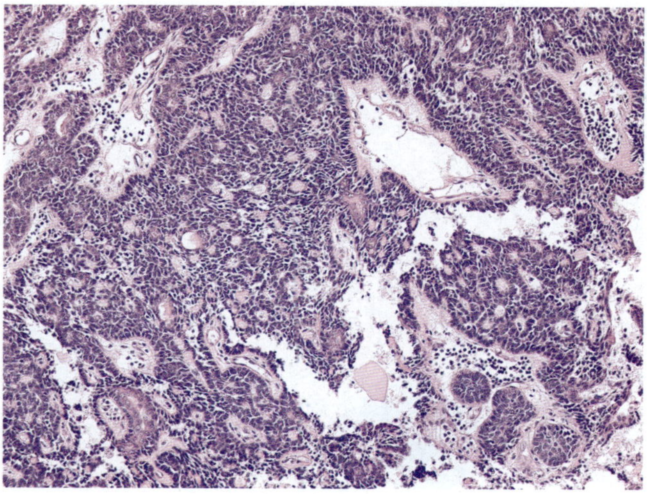

FIGURE 4-11: Collagenous spherulosis involving an intraductal papilloma. The fenestrated appearance results in close resemblance of a cribriform DCIS. Note the presence of the basement membrane material in the pseudoluminal spaces.

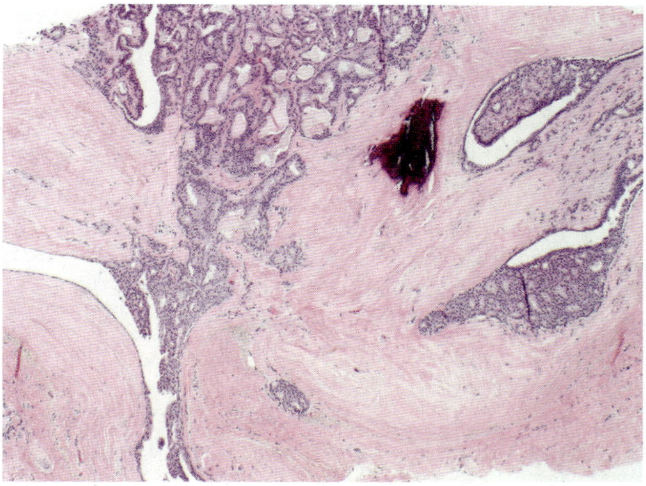

FIGURE 4-12: Papilloma with ADH. Note the presence of a monotonous population of epithelial cells in this sclerosing papilloma characteristic of those in ADH and low-grade DCIS.

or micropapillary (Figures 4-12 to 4-14). Myoepithelial cells are absent or scant in these atypical foci. The atypical epithelial proliferation usually shows lack of expression for high molecular weight cytokeratins (Figure 4-15) and strong staining for estrogen and progesterone receptors.[8] There are no universally accepted criteria for distinguishing papilloma with ADH and papilloma with DCIS, while extent and proportion criteria have been proposed. Some authorities have suggested using 3 mm as the extent cutoff; a papilloma with ADH is diagnosed when the atypical epithelial proliferation is <3 mm, while a papilloma with DCIS is diagnosed when the atypical focus is ≥3 mm.[9] The proportion cutoff proposed by some authors was 30%[10] and later revised to 90%.[11] The WHO Working Group was of the view that the extent-/size-based criteria should be utilized in routine practice.[1] It should be emphasized that when the atypical epithelial proliferation is that of intermediate or high nuclear grade, a diagnosis of papilloma with DCIS should be rendered regardless of its extent. In addition, the presence of DCIS in neighboring breast tissue is of help to support the diagnosis of DCIS within a papilloma. Papillomas with DCIS should be distinguished from intraductal papillary carcinoma, as the latter is considered, at least by some authorities, a *de novo in situ* malignant process that is more significant in predicting the patient's risk of subsequent breast cancer.[12] The prognosis of intraductal papillary carcinoma is similar to those for DCIS in general.[1] The clinical significance of papillomas with DCIS after complete excision remains unclear, but is thought to be at least equivalent to a diagnosis of ADH.[13] However, breast cancer risk is reportedly much higher in patients with multiple atypical papillomas.[14]

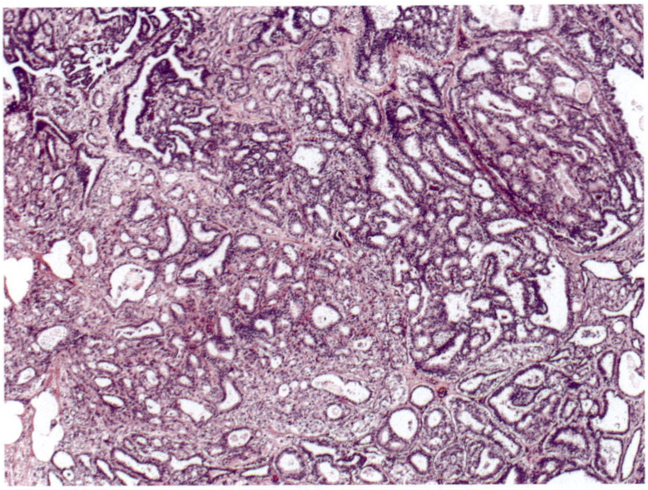

FIGURE 4-13: Papilloma with DCIS. A low-power view shows proliferation of small, uniform neoplastic cells in a significant proportion of tumor.

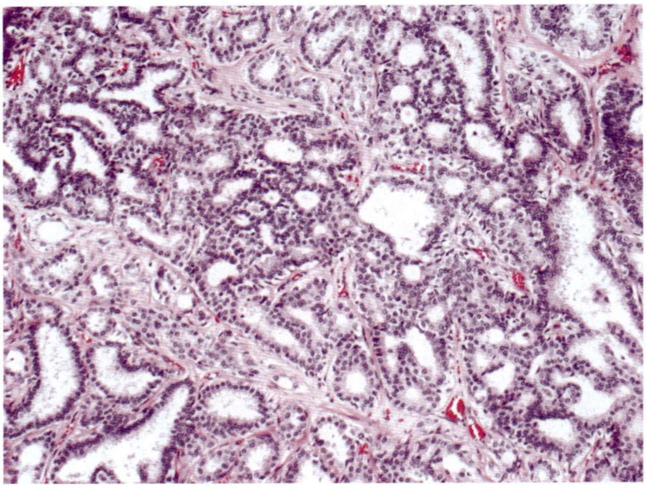

FIGURE 4-14: A higher magnification of the section seen in Figure 4-13 shows solid and cribriform architectural patterns.

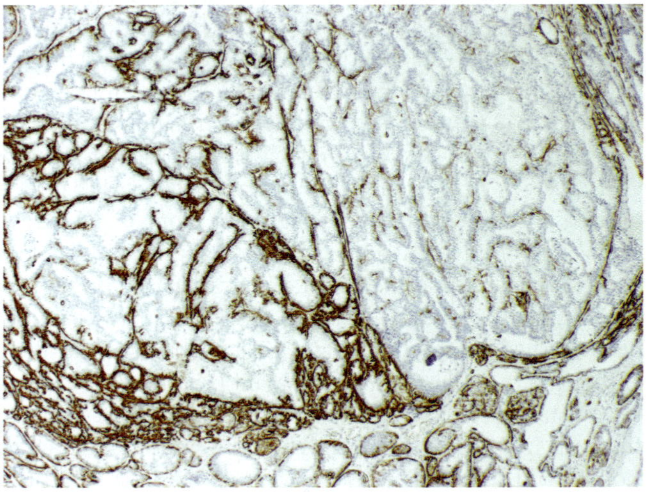

FIGURE 4-15: Papilloma with DCIS. A CK5/6 stain demonstrates reduced of expression in the areas with atypical epithelial proliferation.

INTRADUCTAL PAPILLARY CARCINOMA, IMMUNOHISTOCHEMISTRY

The absence of myoepithelial cells in the papillary fronds and the presence of a myoepithelial cell layer at the periphery of the involved ducts can be demonstrated by p63, high molecular weight cytokeratins (CK5/6, CK14, 34βE12/CK903), and smooth muscle markers (calponin, smooth muscle myosin heavy chain, etc.). A pitfall is that blood vessels juxtaposed to basal aspect of epithelial cells in the papillae can be misinterpreted as myoepithelial cells, as endothelial cells are immunoreactive with smooth muscle markers. Thus, p63 and high molecular weight cytokeratins are superior markers in this setting. The neoplastic epithelial cells are negative for high molecular weight cytokeratins[15] and typically show strong overexpression of ER and PR.

INTRADUCTAL PAPILLARY CARCINOMA, PATHOGENESIS

The pathogenesis of intraductal papillary carcinoma has long been a matter of debate. Some authorities believe that these lesions are fundamentally distinct from papillomas with DCIS in that the former is a *de novo* neoplastic proliferation.[12] Others advocate that they represent a neoplastic population resulting from a gradual malignant transformation and replacement of the epithelial component of a preexisting papilloma.[16]

ENCAPSULATED (INTRACYSTIC) PAPILLARY CARCINOMA, IMAGING AND GROSS FEATURES

Encapsulated papillary carcinoma is traditionally considered a variant of intraductal papillary carcinoma. It differs from the latter by lack of myoepithelial cells at the periphery of lesion, leading some to propose that the tumor may be invasive in nature. Given these lesions have an excellent prognosis with adequate local therapy alone, the consensus of the WHO Working Group was that such tumors should be staged and managed as *in situ* disease in the absence of conventional invasive carcinoma.[1]

Most frequently found in elderly patients, encapsulated papillary carcinoma is often seen as a retroareolar round or oval circumscribed mass on mammography (Figure 4-16) and a cystic

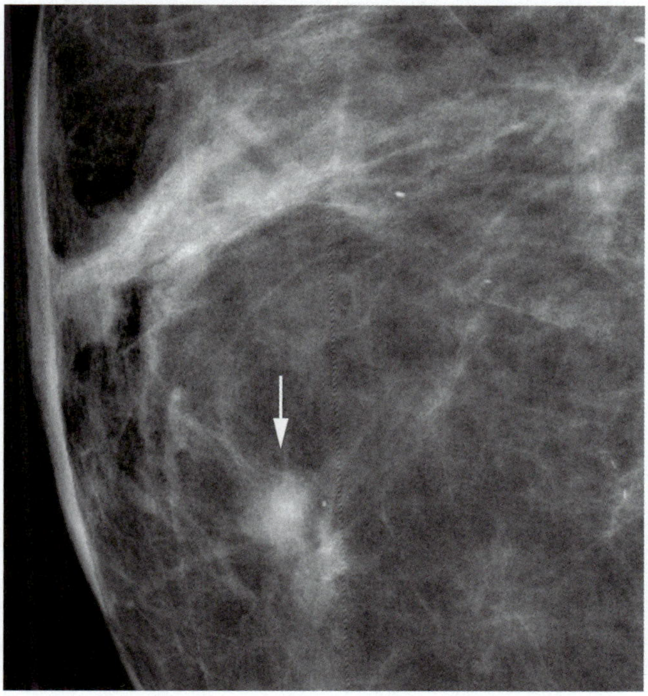

FIGURE 4-16: Encapsulated papillary carcinoma. A craniocaudal mammographic view shows an oval mass (*arrow*) in the retroareolar region with obscured margins.

lesion with solid components on US.[17,18] Grossly, the tumor often appears as a circumscribed friable mass within a cystic cavity and thus is also known as intracystic papillary carcinoma.

ENCAPSULATED PAPILLARY CARCINOMA, HISTOLOGY

At low magnification, the tumor is characterized by one or more nodules of papillary carcinoma within a cystically dilated duct surrounded by a fibrous capsule in which there may be variable degrees of inflammatory infiltrate (Figure 4-17). The neoplastic epithelial proliferation may be arranged in cribriform or solid patterns (Figure 4-18). The neoplastic cells more commonly have low- or intermediate-grade nuclei but may occasionally show high nuclear grade (Figure 4-19). The papillary fronds are lined by neoplastic columnar epithelial cells devoid of myoepithelial cells, as those in intraductal papillary carcinomas. In contrast to the latter, a layer of myoepithelial cells is absent at the periphery of the lesion (Figure 4-20).[4,19] The tumor may also be present in a cystically dilated space lined by stratified epithelial cells and thus closely resembles an intraductal papillary carcinoma (Figures 4-21 and 4-22). In contrast to myoepithelial cells that typically possess flat, cuboidal, or rounded nuclei, the lining cells may take on a more spindle cell appearance and show identical nuclear features with those covering the papillary fronds. Rarely, the lining cells contain subnuclear vacuoles and show reverse polarity, thus simulating piano keys. Again, the neoplastic (nonmyoepithelial) nature of these lining cells can be demonstrated by myoepithelial markers (Figure 4-23).

While encapsulated papillary carcinoma was originally classified as a variant of DCIS, the nature of this lesion remains a subject to debate. The absence of a myoepithelial cell layer at the

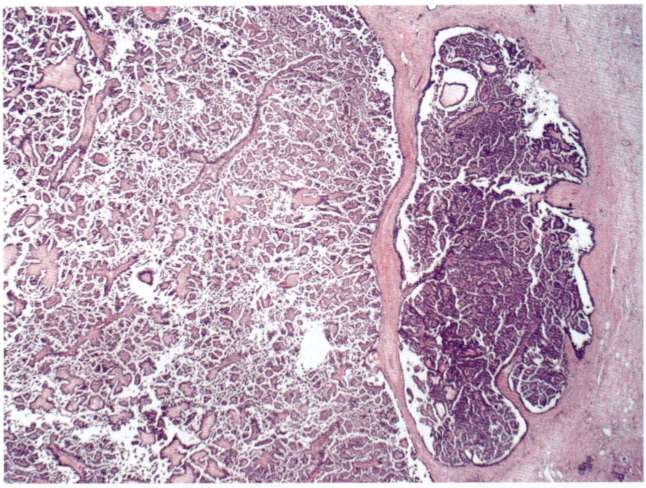

FIGURE 4-17: A low-power view of encapsulated papillary carcinoma showing tumoral nodules within cystically dilated duct spaces.

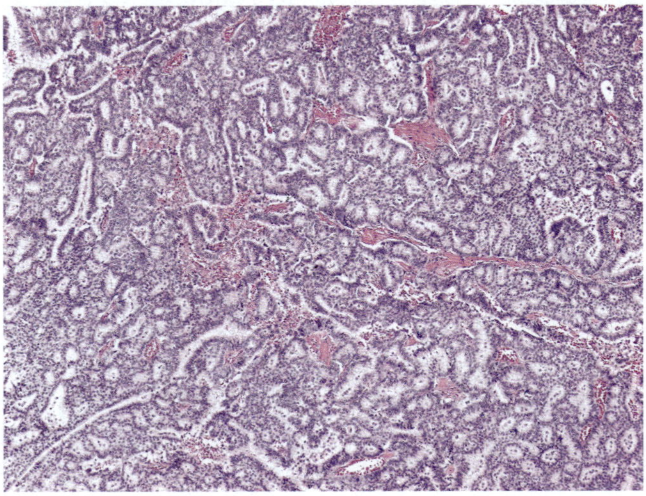

FIGURE 4-18: Encapsulated papillary carcinoma exhibiting a predominantly cribriform growth pattern. The tumor cells demonstrate low- to intermediate-grade nuclei.

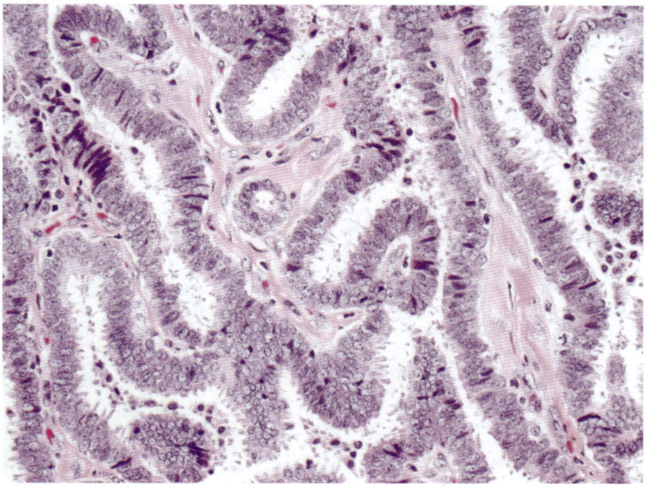

FIGURE 4-19: Encapsulated papillary carcinoma showing high nuclear grade.

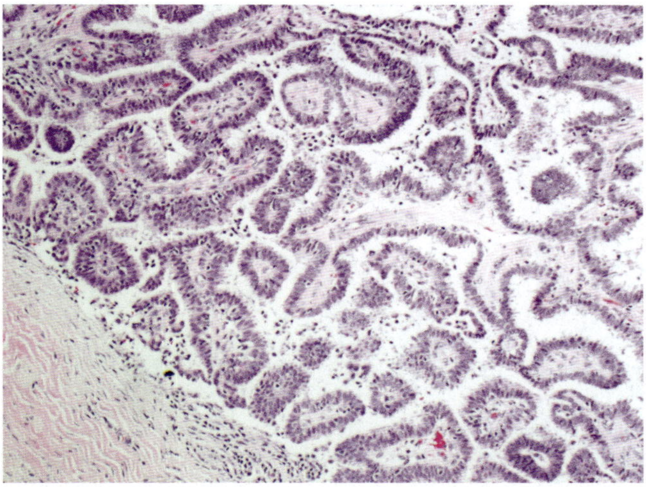

FIGURE 4-20: Encapsulated papillary carcinoma showing lack of a myoepithelial cell layer at the periphery of the lesion.

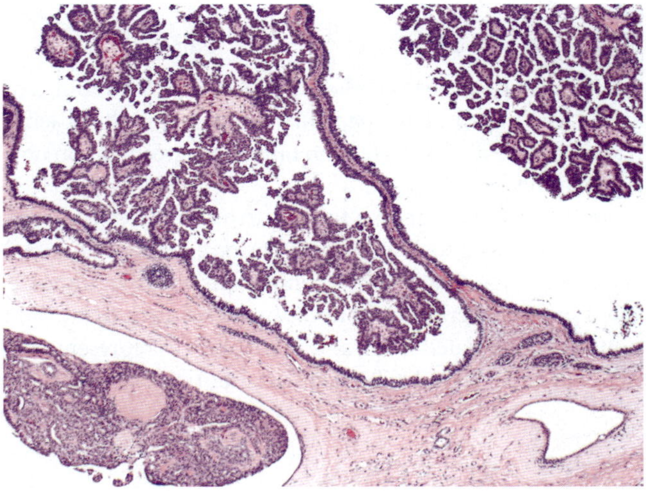

FIGURE 4-21: An encapsulated papillary carcinoma adjacent to a small intraductal papilloma. Note the presence of stratified epithelial cells lining the cystically dilated space closely simulating myoepithelium.

periphery of the tumor nodules on hematoxylin–eosin-stained sections as well as with a variety of myoepithelial markers argues against our current understanding of an *in situ* lesion. The findings raise the possibility by some authorities that these lesions may represent an indolent form of invasive carcinoma, while others have postulated that they may be in neoplastic progression

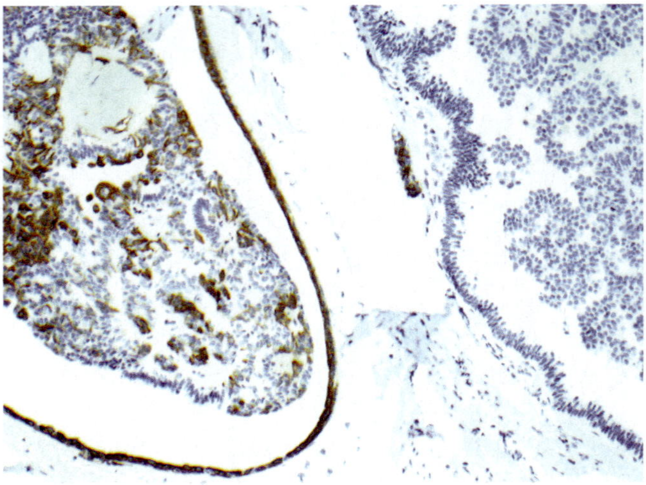

FIGURE 4-22: A CK5/6 stain of the section shown in Figure 4-21 demonstrates the absence of myoepithelial cells at the periphery of encapsulated papillary carcinoma, but highlights the myoepithelium at the periphery of the adjacent papilloma while showing a mosaic staining pattern in the ductal epithelial proliferation of the latter.

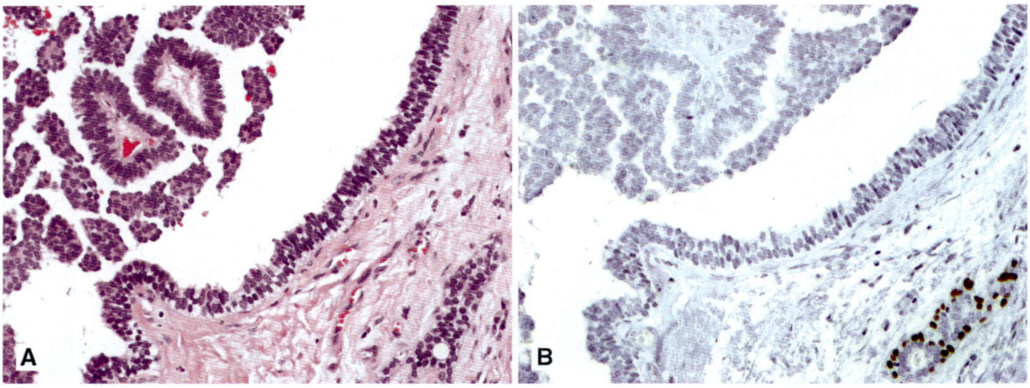

FIGURE 4-23: The nuclei of the "lining" cells at the periphery of encapsulated papillary carcinoma sometimes take on a more spindle cell appearance identical to those covering the papillary fronds. These cells may rarely contain subnuclear vacuoles and show reverse polarity simulating piano keys (**A**). A p63 stain on the section demonstrates the nonmyoepithelial nature of the lining cells (**B**). Note the presence of a myoepithelial cell layer in a group of benign glands in the right lower corner of this image serving as an internal control.

from *in situ* to invasive disease.[4,19,20] This concept has been further supported by the findings of axillary lymph node metastasis in patients with encapsulated papillary carcinoma in the absence of frankly invasive carcinoma.[21] Given these controversies, there is no universal agreement on how to stage encapsulated papillary carcinoma at this time.

In the absence of DCIS or unequivocal invasive carcinoma in the surrounding breast tissue, encapsulated papillary carcinoma has a favorable prognosis with adequate local therapy alone.[22–25] Thus, a diagnosis of invasive carcinoma should be made only when a frank invasive tumor is evident. However, the presence of isolated small clusters of tumor cells in the adjacent tissue (and axillary lymph nodes) should be cautiously differentiated from, and more likely to represent, displacement of the epithelium. The presence of concurrent DCIS in the neighboring breast tissue is reportedly associated with a higher risk of local recurrence.[26]

ENCAPSULATED PAPILLARY CARCINOMA, DIFFERENTIAL DIAGNOSIS

The differential diagnosis of encapsulated papillary carcinoma generally includes intraductal papillary carcinoma, solid papillary carcinoma, and intraductal papilloma. As previously discussed, myoepithelial cells are present around the periphery of involved ducts in intraductal papillary carcinoma. Solid papillary carcinomas also have a multinodular growth pattern and typically lack peripheral myoepithelial cell lining, but are more solid rather than cystic, often with inconspicuous and delicate fibrovascular cores. The neoplastic cells typically demonstrate neuroendocrine differentiation and are mostly immunoreactive for neuroendocrine markers such as chromogranin and synaptophysin. In intraductal papillomas, a well-developed myoepithelial cell layer is present within the papillae and surrounding the lesion.

ENCAPSULATED PAPILLARY CARCINOMA, IMMUNOHISTOCHEMISTRY

Myoepithelial cell markers can be used to confirm the absence of myoepithelial cells in papillary fronds and outer portion of the lesion. Moderate-to-intense collagen type IV expression in the capsule surrounding the tumor nodules was reportedly seen in all encapsulated papillary carcinomas.[20] The neoplastic cells are typically positive for ER and PR.

SOLID PAPILLARY CARCINOMA, IMAGING AND GROSS FEATURES

Solid papillary carcinoma usually appears as a well-defined mass on mammography and sonography (Figure 4-24).[17,18] The tumor is more likely to have one or more of the following sonographic features: nonparallel orientation, an echogenic halo, posterior acoustic enhancement, and associated microcalcifications.[27] On gross examination, solid papillary carcinoma may present as a fleshy firm or soft, well-circumscribed nodular mass with a tan-white or yellowish brown appearance (Figure 4-25). The sizes vary from a few millimeters to several centimeters. The tumor typically occurs in women of seventh and eighth decades.

SOLID PAPILLARY CARCINOMA, HISTOLOGY

As its name indicates, solid papillary carcinomas are seen as multiple solidified circumscribed nodules on low-power magnification (Figure 4-26). The tumor has long been considered a variant of DCIS as the tumoral nests appear noninvasive due to their circumscription and many lesions exhibit peripheral myoepithelial cell lining.[28] However, the tumor nodules frequently lack peripheral myoepithelium as demonstrated by immunohistochemistry (Figure 4-27) and thus raised the possibility that a subset of lesions may represent invasive carcinomas with "pushing-border" and expansile growth pattern rather than variants of DCIS.[29,30] This is further complicated by the fact that an intact myoepithelial cell layer may be present in some of the tumoral nests, especially in

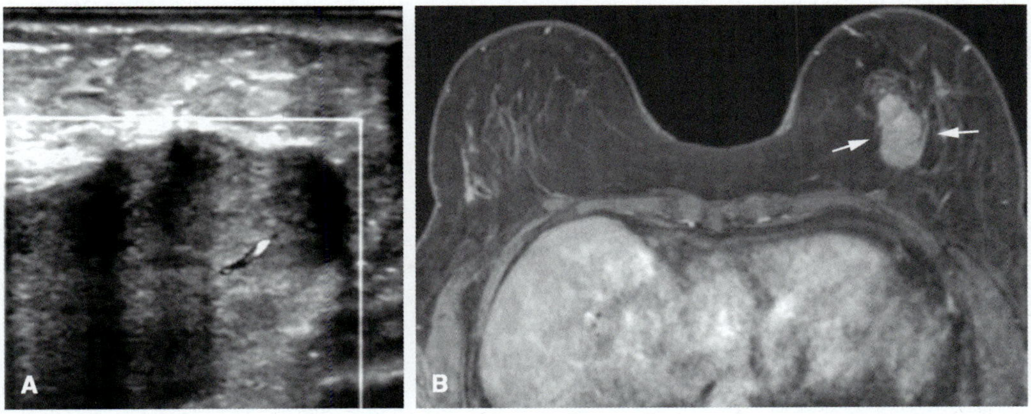

FIGURE 4-24: Imaging features of solid papillary carcinoma. An ultrasound image reveals a large hypoechoic mass with increased vascularity (**A**). An axial T1 delayed postcontrast fat-saturated image shows an enhancing oval mass with well-circumscribed margins (**B**).

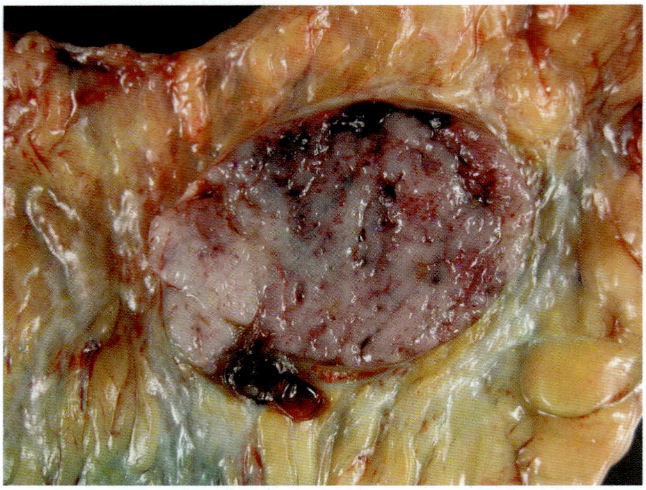

FIGURE 4-25: Gross pathologic appearance of solid papillary carcinoma. The tumor typically appears as single or multiple solid circumscribed masses (Photograph courtesy of Erik Scott Young, Pennsylvania.)

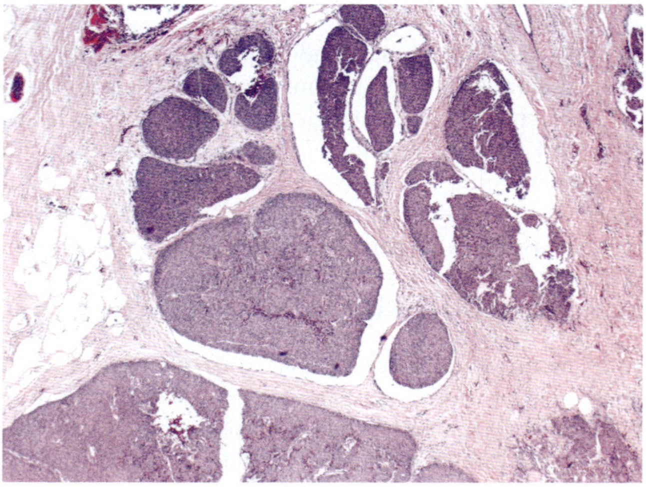

FIGURE 4-26: A low-power view of solid papillary carcinoma showing multiple solid nodules.

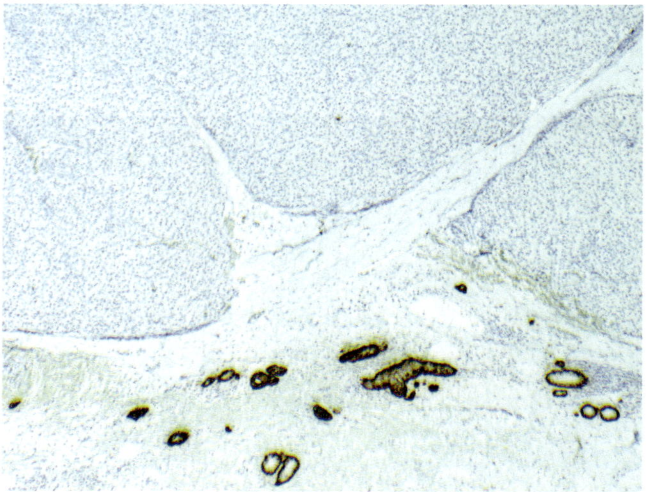

FIGURE 4-27: A peripheral myoepithelial cell layer is absent in this solid papillary carcinoma as demonstrated by a CK5/6 stain. Note the appropriate internal control in the neighboring normal glands.

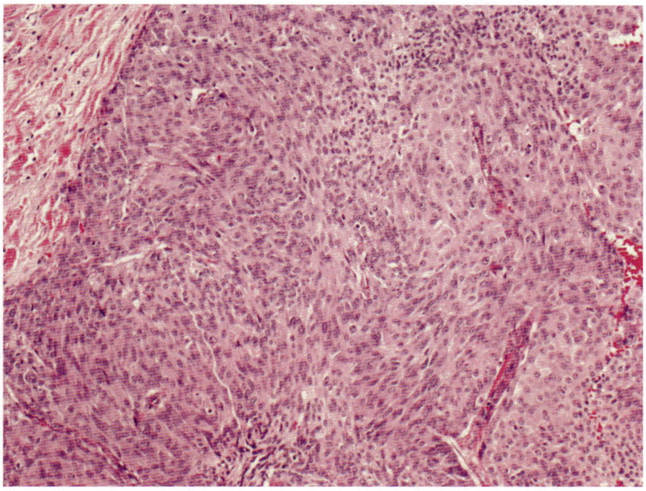

FIGURE 4-28: An intermediate power view of solid papillary carcinoma shows dense cellular proliferation. The neoplastic cells often take on the appearance of streaming bland spindle cells with eosinophilic cytoplasm and intermediate-grade nuclei. The fibrovascular cores are typically delicate or inconspicuous.

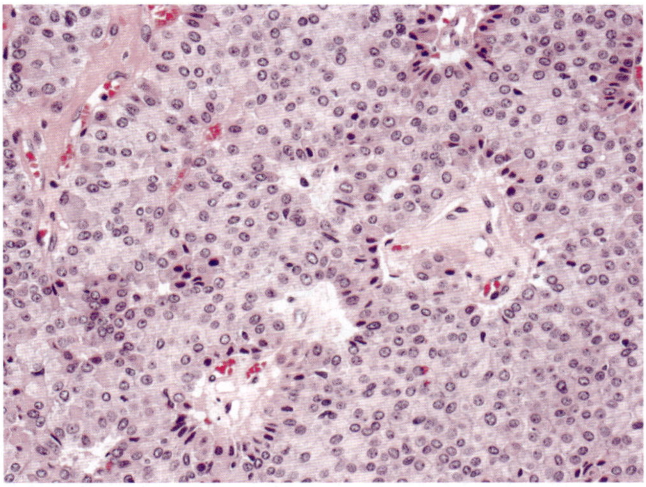

FIGURE 4-29: Solid papillary carcinoma showing variably collagenized fibrovascular cores with peripheral palisading of tumor cells forming perivascular pseudorosettes.

those of larger duct-like structures.[12,29] Thus, a precise distinction between *in situ* and invasive disease in these lesions is difficult and has been controversial. Nonetheless, given that solid papillary carcinomas without frankly invasive component have an indolent clinical course more similar to DCIS,[28,30] the general consensus is that these lesions should be regarded for staging purposes as *in situ* carcinoma.[1] Metastases from such tumors do occur but are rare.[29]

The proliferative tumor cells are densely cellular and monotonous. The fibrovascular cores are devoid of myoepithelial cells and are typically delicate or inconspicuous owing to the solid growth of tumor. The neoplastic epithelial cells often take on the appearance of streaming bland spindle cells with eosinophilic cytoplasm, similar to those seen in usual ductal hyperplasia (Figure 4-28). The fibrovascular cores can be variably collagenized, with peripheral palisading of tumor cells forming perivascular pseudorosettes (Figure 4-29). On higher magnification, the lesional cells often demonstrate neuroendocrine features, with finely granular eosinophilic cytoplasm and round-to-oval nuclei with "salt-and-pepper" chromatin pattern (Figure 4-30), and frequently show immunoreactivity for chromogranin and synaptophysin (Figure 4-31).[28] Mitotic figures are generally discernible but are not abundant. Intracellular and/or extracellular mucin production is a common feature (Figure 4-32).

The tumoral nests may have a geographic jigsaw growth pattern with irregular contours at the periphery, thus suggestive of invasive disease. Sometimes, such areas may merge into microinvasive and frankly invasive carcinoma (Figures 4-33 and 4-34). The coexisting invasive

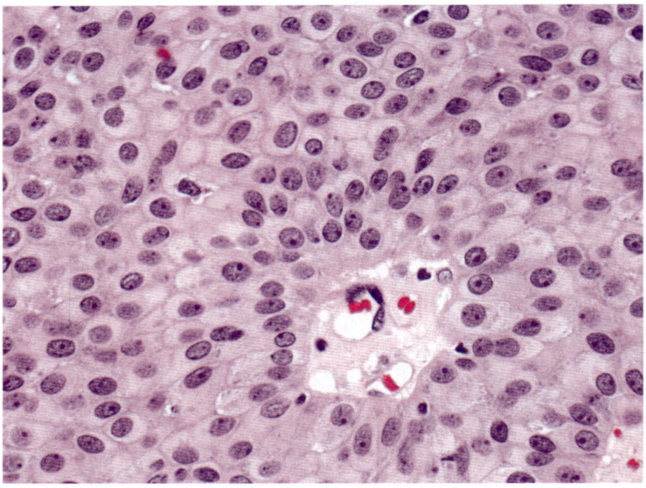

FIGURE 4-30: Solid papillary carcinoma exhibiting neuroendocrine features with finely granular eosinophilic cytoplasm and round-to-oval nuclei with "salt-and-pepper" chromatin.

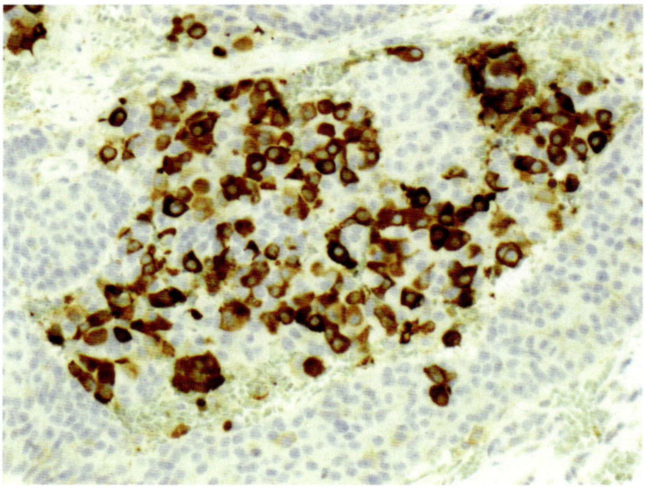

FIGURE 4-31: Focal or diffuse immunoreactivity for neuroendocrine markers such as synaptophysin (illustrated in this image), chromogranin, and neuron-specific enolase is frequently seen in solid papillary carcinoma.

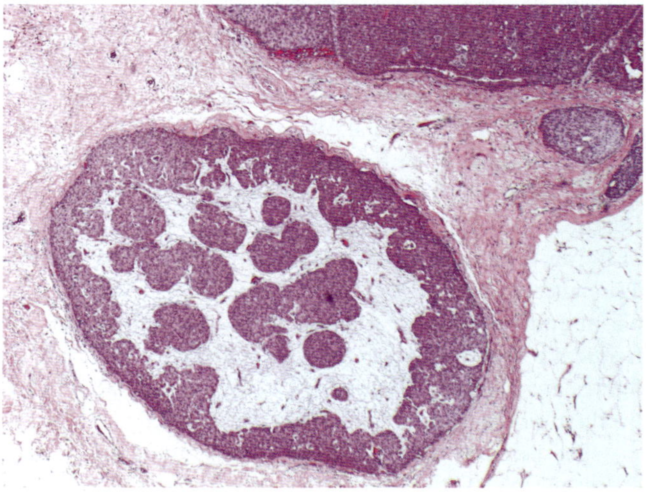

FIGURE 4-32: A solid papillary carcinoma showing extracellular mucin production.

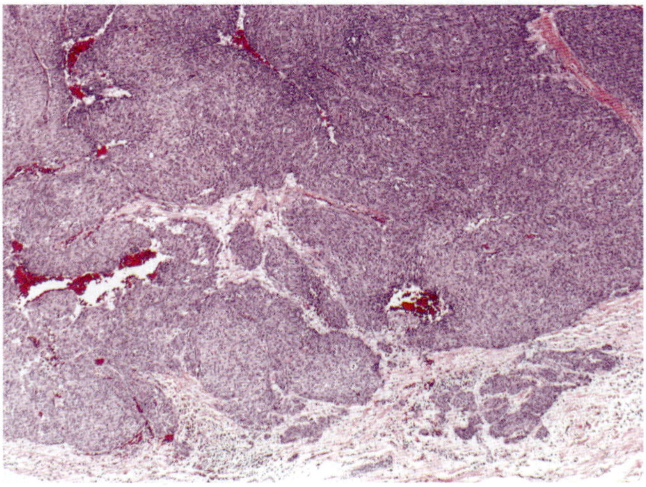

FIGURE 4-33: Solid papillary carcinoma with adjacent microinvasive carcinoma.

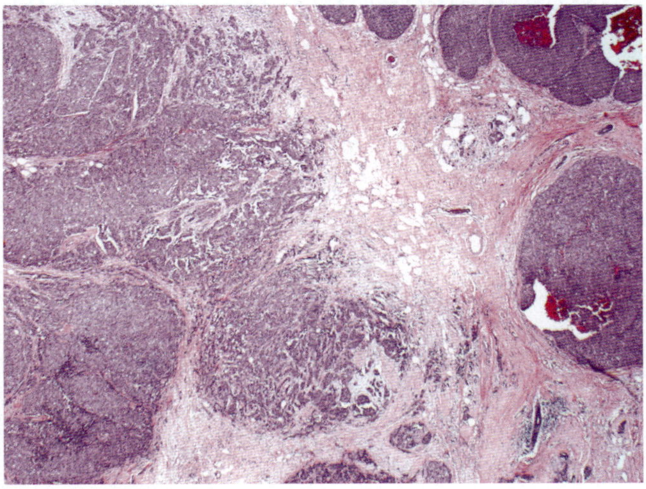

FIGURE 4-34: Solid papillary carcinoma merged into frankly invasive carcinoma.

carcinoma frequently has mucinous and/or endocrine features.[28] Other types of carcinoma may also be seen, such as ductal, lobular, and mixed histologic patterns.[30,31]

SOLID PAPILLARY CARCINOMA, DIFFERENTIAL DIAGNOSIS

The differential diagnostic considerations encountered chiefly include intraductal papilloma with florid usual ductal hyperplasia. The latter typically has broad fibrovascular cores in which the myoepithelial cells are frequently identifiable. The proliferative benign epithelia generally demonstrate significant heterogeneity but lack neuroendocrine features, increased mitotic activity, and mucin production. When in doubt, the absence of staining for high molecular weight keratins (i.e., CK5/6) in solid papillary carcinoma is typically of diagnostic value.[32] This is in contrast to the patchy and mosaic staining pattern in the benign ductal epithelial proliferation. In addition, the nature of "papillary carcinoma" can be demonstrated by a lack of myoepithelial cells in the papillary fronds by using p63 or high molecular weight keratins.

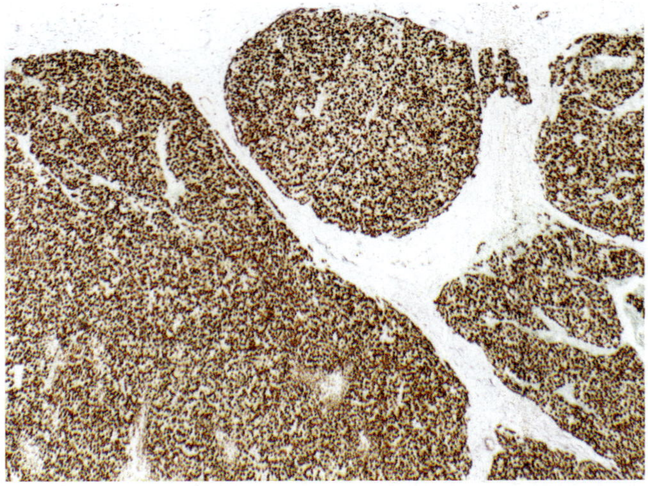

FIGURE 4-35: Solid papillary carcinoma showing diffuse and strong ER expression.

SOLID PAPILLARY CARCINOMA, IMMUNOHISTOCHEMISTRY

The immunohistochemical evidence of neuroendocrine differentiation has been reportedly observed in at least half of the cases.[31,33] Solid papillary carcinomas are positive for ER (Figure 4-35) and PR and lack HER2 overexpression/gene amplification. When an invasive carcinoma is coexistent, it usually shows a similar hormonal receptor expression pattern.[30]

References

1. Intraductal papillary lesions. In: Lakhani SR, Ellis IO, Schnitt SJ, et al., eds. *WHO Classification of Tumours of the Breast.* Lyon, France: IARC Press; 2012:99–110.
2. Raju UB, Lee MW, Zarbo RJ, et al. Papillary neoplasia of the breast: immunohistochemically defined myoepithelial cells in the diagnosis of benign and malignant papillary breast neoplasms. *Mod Pathol* 1989;2:569–576.
3. Papotti M, Eusebi V, Gugliotta P, et al. Immunohistochemical analysis of benign and malignant papillary lesions of the breast. *Am J Surg Pathol* 1983;7:451–461.
4. Hill CB, Yeh IT. Myoepithelial cell staining patterns of papillary breast lesions: from intraductal papillomas to invasive papillary carcinomas. *Am J Clin Pathol* 2005;123:36–44.
5. Tse GM, Tan PH, Lui PC, et al. The role of immunohistochemistry for smooth-muscle actin, p63, CD10 and cytokeratin 14 in the differential diagnosis of papillary lesions of the breast. *J Clin Pathol* 2007;60:315–320.
6. Ali-Fehmi R, Carolin K, Wallis T, et al. Clinicopathologic analysis of breast lesions associated with multiple papillomas. *Hum Pathol* 2003;34:234–239.
7. Ohuchi N, Abe R, Kasai M. Possible cancerous change of intraductal papillomas of the breast. A 3-D reconstruction study of 25 cases. *Cancer* 1984;54:605–611.
8. Ichihara S, Fujimoto T, Hashimoto K, et al. Double immunostaining with p63 and high-molecular-weight cytokeratins distinguishes borderline papillary lesions of the breast. *Pathol Int* 2007;57:126–132.
9. Page DL, Salhany KE, Jensen RA, et al. Subsequent breast carcinoma risk after biopsy with atypia in a breast papilloma. *Cancer* 1996;78:258–266.
10. Tavassoli FA. *Pathology of the Breast.* 2nd ed. Stamford, CT: Appleton & Lange; 1999.
11. Ueng SH, Mezzetti T, Tavassoli FA. Papillary neoplasms of the breast: a review. *Arch Pathol Lab Med* 2009;133:893–907.
12. Collins LC, Schnitt SJ. Papillary lesions of the breast: selected diagnostic and management issues. *Histopathology* 2008;52:20–29.

13. Raju U, Vertes D. Breast papillomas with atypical ductal hyperplasia: a clinicopathologic study. *Hum Pathol* 1996;27:1231–1238.
14. Lewis JT, Hartmann LC, Vierkant RA, et al. An analysis of breast cancer risk in women with single, multiple, and atypical papilloma. *Am J Surg Pathol* 2006;30:665–672.
15. Tan PH, Aw MY, Yip G, et al. Cytokeratins in papillary lesions of the breast: is there a role in distinguishing intraductal papilloma from papillary ductal carcinoma in situ? *Am J Surg Pathol* 2005;29:625–632.
16. MacGrogan G, Moinfar F, Raju U. Intraductal papillary neoplasms. In: Tavassoli FA, Devilee P, eds. *Tumors of the Breast and Female Genital Organs*. Lyon, France: IARC Press; 2003:76–80.
17. Knelson MH, el Yousef SJ, Goldberg RE, et al. Intracystic papillary carcinoma of the breast: mammographic, sonographic, and MR appearance with pathologic correlation. *J Comput Assist Tomogr* 1987;11:1074–1076.
18. Schneider JA. Invasive papillary breast carcinoma: mammographic and sonographic appearance. *Radiology* 1989;171:377–379.
19. Collins LC, Carlo VP, Hwang H, et al. Intracystic papillary carcinomas of the breast: a reevaluation using a panel of myoepithelial cell markers. *Am J Surg Pathol* 2006;30:1002–1007.
20. Esposito NN, Dabbs DJ, Bhargava R. Are encapsulated papillary carcinomas of the breast in situ or invasive? A basement membrane study of 27 cases. *Am J Clin Pathol* 2009;131:228–242.
21. Mulligan AM, O'Malley FP. Metastatic potential of encapsulated (intracystic) papillary carcinoma of the breast: a report of 2 cases with axillary lymph node micrometastases. *Int J Surg Pathol* 2007;15:143–147.
22. Calderaro J, Espie M, Duclos J, et al. Breast intracystic papillary carcinoma: an update. *Breast J* 2009;15:639–644.
23. Harris KP, Faliakou EC, Exon DJ, et al. Treatment and outcome of intracystic papillary carcinoma of the breast. *Br J Surg* 1999;86:1274.
24. Leal C, Costa I, Fonseca D, et al. Intracystic (encysted) papillary carcinoma of the breast: a clinical, pathological, and immunohistochemical study. *Hum Pathol* 1998;29:1097–1104.
25. Lefkowitz M, Lefkowitz W, Wargotz ES. Intraductal (intracystic) papillary carcinoma of the breast and its variants: a clinicopathological study of 77 cases. *Hum Pathol* 1994;25:802–809.
26. Carter D. Intraductal papillary tumors of the breast: a study of 78 cases. *Cancer* 1977;39:1689–1692.
27. Kim TH, Kang DK, Kim SY, et al. Sonographic differentiation of benign and malignant papillary lesions of the breast. *J Ultrasound Med* 2008;27:75–82.
28. Maluf HM, Koerner FC. Solid papillary carcinoma of the breast. A form of intraductal carcinoma with endocrine differentiation frequently associated with mucinous carcinoma. *Am J Surg Pathol* 1995;19:1237–1244.
29. Nicolas MM, Wu Y, Middleton LP, et al. Loss of myoepithelium is variable in solid papillary carcinoma of the breast. *Histopathology* 2007;51:657–665.
30. Nassar H, Qureshi H, Adsay NV, et al. Clinicopathologic analysis of solid papillary carcinoma of the breast and associated invasive carcinomas. *Am J Surg Pathol* 2006;30:501–507.
31. Otsuki Y, Yamada M, Shimizu S, et al. Solid-papillary carcinoma of the breast: clinicopathological study of 20 cases. *Pathol Int* 2007;57:421–429.
32. Rabban JT, Koerner FC, Lerwill MF. Solid papillary ductal carcinoma in situ versus usual ductal hyperplasia in the breast: a potentially difficult distinction resolved by cytokeratin 5/6. *Hum Pathol* 2006;37:787–793.
33. Tan PH, Lui GG, Chiang G, et al. Ductal carcinoma in situ with spindle cells: a potential diagnostic pitfall in the evaluation of breast lesions. *Histopathology* 2004;45:343–351.

5 Invasive Carcinoma of No Special Type

Invasive carcinoma of no special type (NST), traditionally known as invasive ductal carcinoma, has been known historically as scirrhous carcinoma, carcinoma simplex, and invasive carcinoma, not otherwise specified.[1,2]

Invasive carcinoma of NST is the most common invasive mammary tumor, comprising about 80% of breast carcinomas,[1] and is rare in patients younger than 40 years of age.[1] Studies have shown that the risk factors and genomic profile of invasive carcinoma of NST differ from those of invasive lobular carcinoma (ILC), the second most common type of invasive carcinoma.[3] Familial breast cancers associated with *BRCA1* or *BRCA2* mutations are mostly of NST type, often with basal-like features.[4] Invasive carcinoma of NST affects Black women at younger age (mean, 55 years) compared to White women (mean, 60 years). Black patients are also more likely to have larger tumors and tumors with associated necrosis.[5]

Due to widespread population-based screening, most cases in developed countries are asymptomatic. The most common presentation in symptomatic women is a breast lump that may or may not be associated with pain. Other presentations, for example, nipple abnormalities (discharge, retraction, or eczema), skin dimpling, or change in contour of the breast, are less common.[1]

INVASIVE CARCINOMA OF NO SPECIAL TYPE, CYTOLOGY

Differentiating invasive carcinoma of NST from ductal carcinoma in situ (DCIS) cannot be performed with certainty by cytologic examination of smears. The cytologic characteristics of such carcinomas include high cellularity and loosely cohesive groups arranged in syncytial pattern with loss of polarity and also as single cells. The malignant cells are usually larger than benign ductal cells with increased nuclear/cytoplasmic ratio, hyperchromatic nuclei with irregular and thickened nuclear membranes, and prominent nucleoli. The cytoplasm tends to be basophilic, finely to coarsely granular, or vacuolated with occasional intracellular lumina and signet-ring cells. Usually, there are no bipolar naked myoepithelial nuclei. The background can vary from bloody or necrotic to clean (Figure 5-1).[6]

INVASIVE CARCINOMA OF NO SPECIAL TYPE, IMAGING AND GROSS FEATURES

In approximately 50% of cases,[7] the mammographic appearance of invasive carcinoma of NST is that of a spiculated mass (Figure 5-2) architectural distortion and/or calcifications (Figures 5-3 to 5-5). Grossly, these invasive carcinomas usually have irregular, stellate or nodular configurations with infiltrating margins. Most tumors are firm in consistency and often gritty on sectioning. Forty to fifty percent of invasive carcinoma of NST occurs in the upper outer quadrant of the breast.[8]

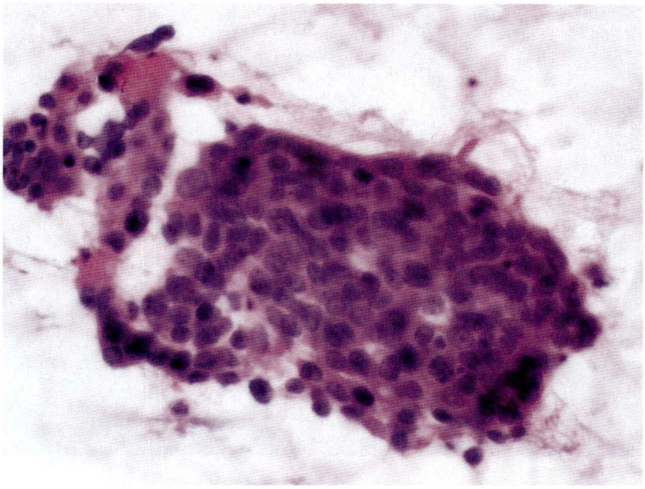

FIGURE 5-1: Fine needle aspiration showing highly atypical ductal cells with no naked nuclei (no myoepithelial cells) and background necrosis. This case proved to be invasive carcinoma of NST on breast excision.

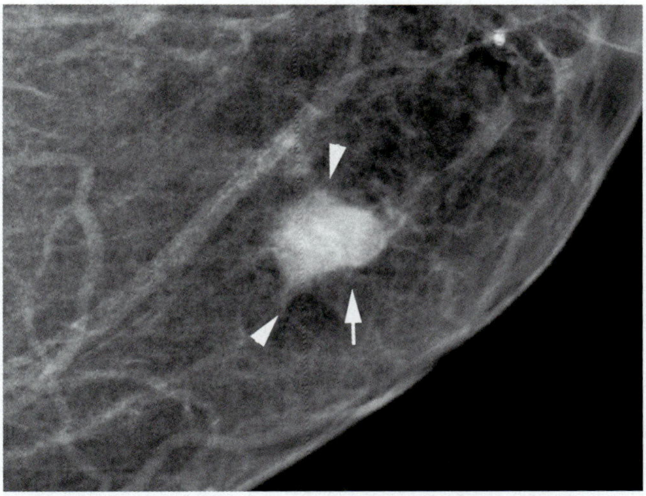

FIGURE 5-2: Left craniocaudal mammogram shows a hyperdense oval mass (*arrow*) with spiculated margins (*arrowheads*) in the medial left breast. This case proved to be invasive carcinoma of NST.

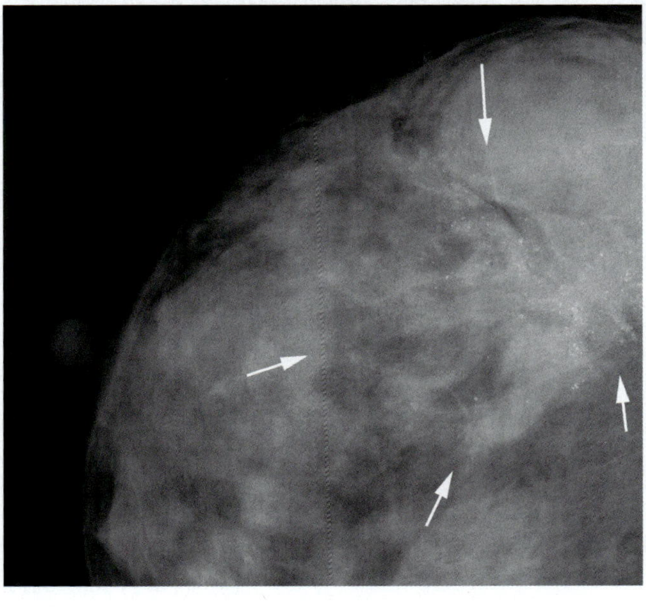

FIGURE 5-3: Right craniocaudal mammogram reveals architectural distortion (*arrows*) with associated pleomorphic calcifications in this extremely dense right lateral breast. Excision showed invasive carcinoma of NST.

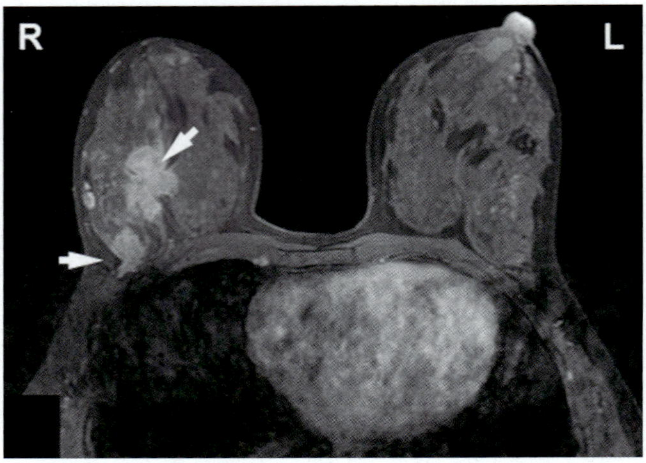

FIGURE 5-4: Axial T1-saturated post-contrast image reveals mammographic distortion and calcifications corresponding to multifocal irregular enhancing masses (*arrows*) of invasive carcinoma of NST in a patient with known brain metastases.

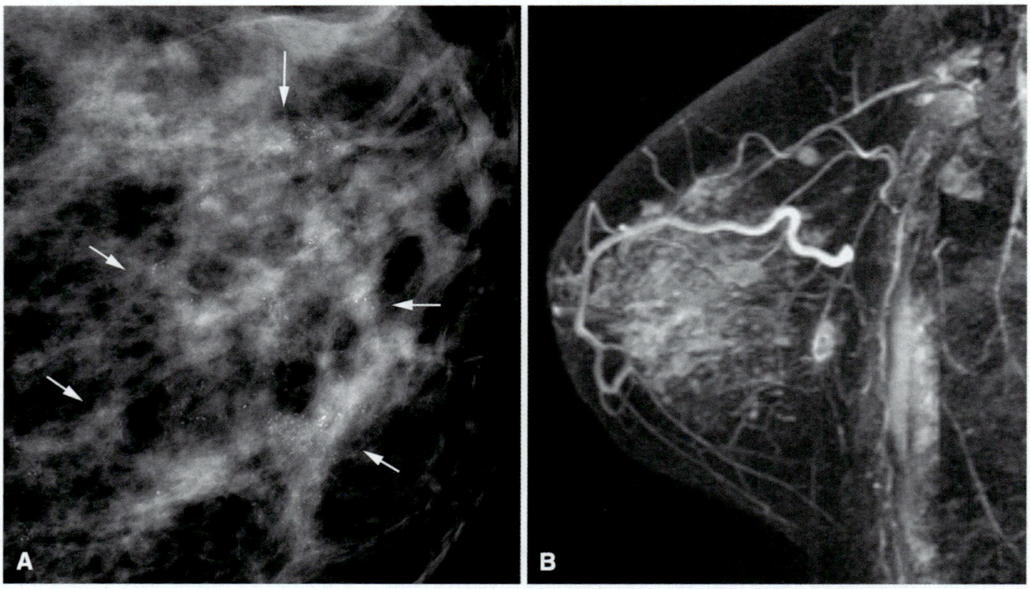

FIGURE 5-5: Left craniocaudal magnification views of a case of invasive carcinoma of NST showing extensive pleomorphic calcifications involving the medial left breast (*arrows*) (**A**). Maximum intensity projection MR image of the same case showing non–mass-like enhancement involving the superior and inferior aspects of the breast corresponding to the calcifications on mammography (**B**).

INVASIVE CARCINOMA OF NO SPECIAL TYPE, HISTOLOGY

The tumor can display variable amounts of glandular structures as well as solid, trabecular or syncytial growth patterns with variable amounts of stroma (Figures 5-6 to 5-10). The degree of glandular differentiation is one component of the grading system (see "Grading" section below). The cytoplasm is often eosinophilic, and the nuclei show variable degrees of pleomorphism. Foci of elastosis and necrosis (Figure 5-7) may be present.[2]

Also considered as invasive carcinoma of NST are tumors that contain a significant component of special type of invasive carcinoma (e.g., tubular, mucinous; see respective chapters) but less than what is required for actual designation as a special type of carcinoma. Although the actual percentage of tumor with the characteristic morphology to be classified as one of the special types

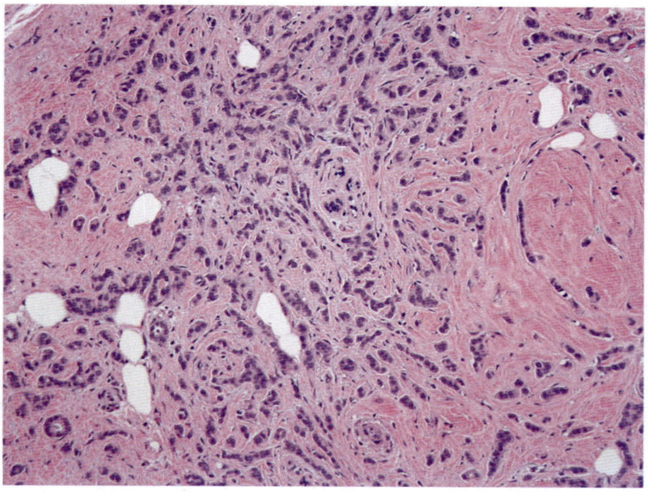

FIGURE 5-6: Intermediate-grade invasive carcinoma of NST exhibiting a lobular carcinoma–like growth pattern. However, the tumor lacks the characteristic cytomorphologic features of ILC. Notice the indistinct tubular formation with compressed lumina and invasion of adipose tissue.

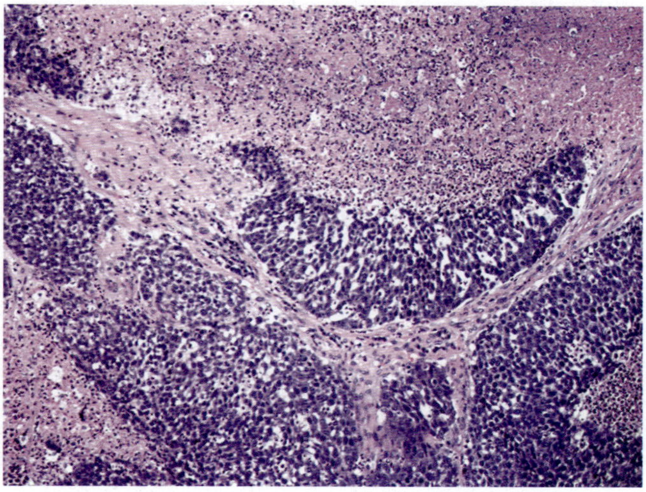

FIGURE 5-7: High-grade invasive carcinoma of NST in a patient with *BRCA-1* gene mutation. This grade is determined based on a score of 3 for tubules, 2 for nuclear pleomorphism, and 3 for mitotic activity. Notice extensive necrosis and stromal lymphocytic infiltration.

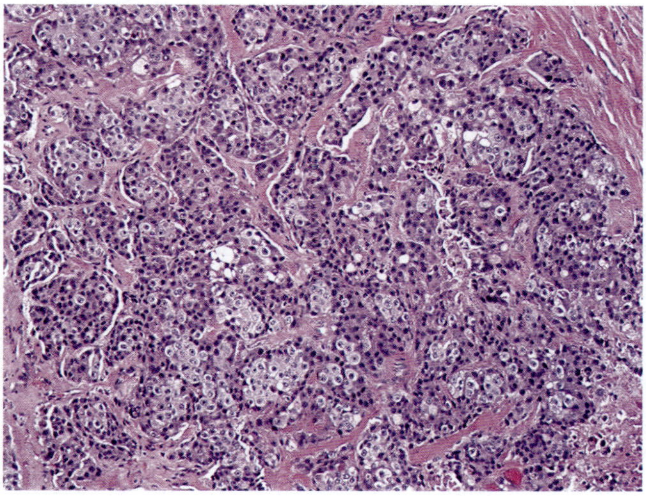

FIGURE 5-8: Intermediate-grade invasive carcinoma of NST. Tumor cells grow in solid pattern with indistinct tubule formation and clear cell changes. This field is best scored as 3 for tubules, 2 for nuclear pleomorphism, and 1 for mitotic activity.

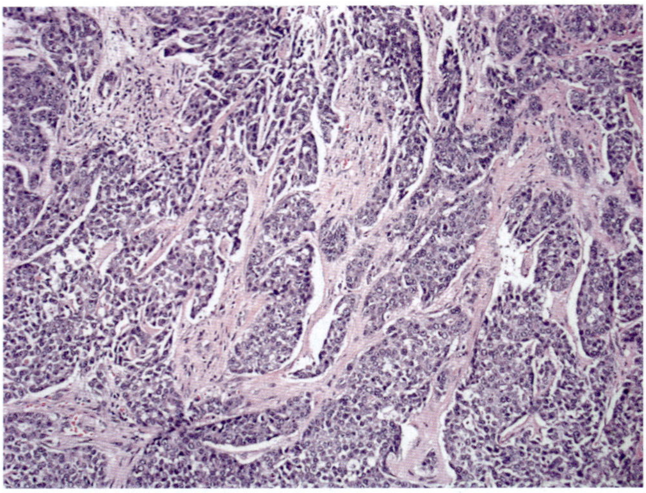

FIGURE 5-9: Intermediate-grade invasive carcinoma of NST. Tumor cells grow in solid pattern with some retraction around some tumor cell nests. The breakdown of scores in this case was 3 for tubules, 2 for nuclear pleomorphism, and 2 for mitotic activity.

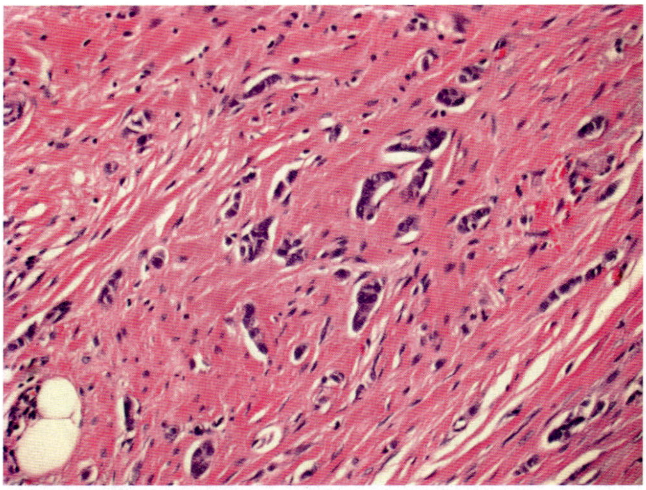

FIGURE 5-10: Low-grade invasive carcinoma of NST. Tumor cells grow in cords and solid nests within a cellular fibrotic stroma. The breakdown of scores in this case was 3 for tubules, 1 for nuclear pleomorphism, and 1 for mitotic activity.

of carcinoma is variable, if such morphology constitutes greater than 90%, the tumor is generally considered "pure" for that type; if between 50% and 90%, the tumor is considered mixed (or with the particular "special type" features); and if less, the tumor is considered of NST.[2] Many cases of invasive carcinoma have a variable extent of intermixed DCIS, the grade of which usually correlates well with the grade of the invasive carcinoma (Figure 5-11).

Recommended elements for reporting invasive carcinoma of the breast include clinical history, surgical procedure, lymph node sampling and status, specimen laterality, tumor focality, site and size, histologic type, presence of DCIS and/or LCIS, macroscopic and microscopic extent, microcalcifications, tumor grade, margin status, treatment effect, pathologic staging (pTNM), presence or absence of lymph–vascular invasion (Figure 5-12), and ancillary studies, including ER, PR, and HER2 status.[9]

Grading

Grading of invasive carcinoma of the breast is a universally accepted prognostic marker that is utilized in all tumors greater than 1 mm in extent. The original grading system was introduced in the 1950s,[10] and the Elston and Ellis or Nottingham grading system[11] in use today represents a modification of that. It is based on a semiquantitative evaluation of the

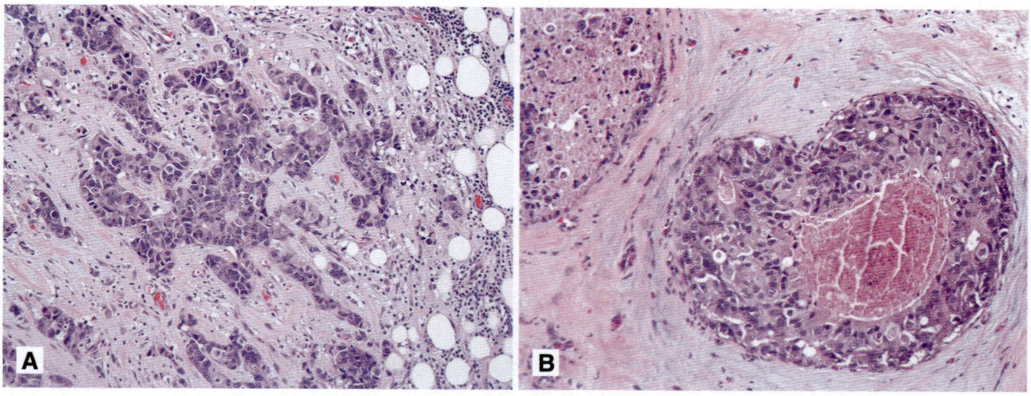

FIGURE 5-11: High-grade invasive carcinoma of NST (**A**) with adjacent high-grade cribriform DCIS with associated comedo (zonal) necrosis (**B**). In most cases of invasive carcinomas, the grade of the associated DCIS correlates with that of the invasive component.

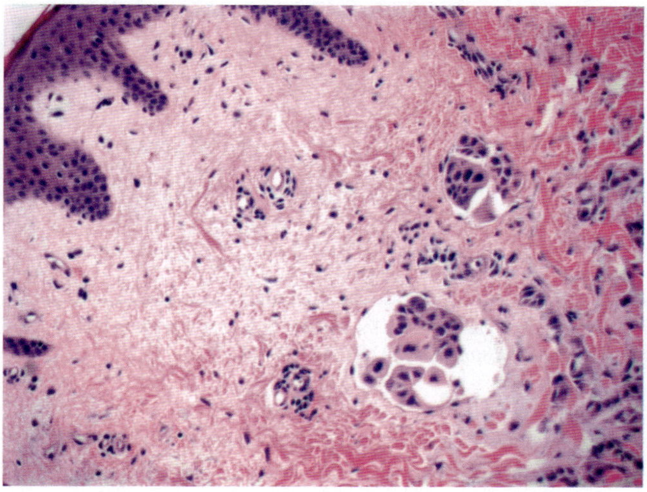

FIGURE 5-12: Lymphovascular space invasion. Section from the skin of the breast shows dilation and expansion of dermal lymphatics with tumor cells.

morphologic characteristics of the tumor, which include the degree of tubule/gland formation, the degree of nuclear pleomorphism, and the mitotic activity as displayed below and summarized in Table 5-1.

Glandular/Tubular Differentiation

Tubule/gland formation is a feature that reflects the degree of differentiation. Assessment of tubule/gland formation should be based on the entire tumor with consideration of structures in which there are clearly defined central lumina, surrounded by polarized tumor cells as well-formed glands. A score of 1, 2, or 3 is given when tubule/gland formation is evident in more than 75% (Figure 5-13), 10% to 75% (Figure 5-14), and less than 10% of the tumor (Figures 5-6 to 5-11), respectively.

Nuclear Pleomorphism

Nuclear pleomorphism is the most subjective element of tumor grade. The size and shape of normal epithelial cells (or lymphocyte) in the vicinity of the tumor is used as a reference to assign points for nuclear pleomorphism. Score 1 is given to tumors with small and regular nuclei showing little variation in size and shape (Figures 5-10, 5-13, and 5-14); score 2 when the nuclei are

Table 5-1 Method for Assessing Tumor Grade of Breast Carcinomas

Variable	Score
Glandular/Tubular Differentiation	
>75% tubule formation	1
10%–75% tubule formation	2
<10 tubule formation	3
Nuclear Pleomorphism	
Small, regular, little variation in size and shape	1
Large, open vesicular chromatin, moderate variation in size and shape	2
Marked variation in size and shape	3
Mitotic Count/10 HPF (depends on field area of the microscope)	
≤3 mitoses per mm^2	1
4–7 mitoses per mm^2	2
≥8 mitoses per mm^2	3
Overall Tumor Grade	**Total Score**
G1 (Low)	3–5
G2 (Intermediate)	6–7
G3 (High)	8–9

Data from Elston CW, Ellis IO. Pathological prognostic factors in breast cancer. I. The value of histological grade in breast cancer: experience from a large study with long-term follow-up. *Histopathology* 2002;41:154–161.

larger than normal and have a more open vesicular chromatin, with moderate variation in size and shape (Figures 5-6, 5-15, and 5-16); and score 3 for marked variation in size and shape, particularly when large and bizarre nuclei are present (Figures 5-11, 5-17, and 5-18). In both scores 2 and 3, nucleoli are usually easily identified.

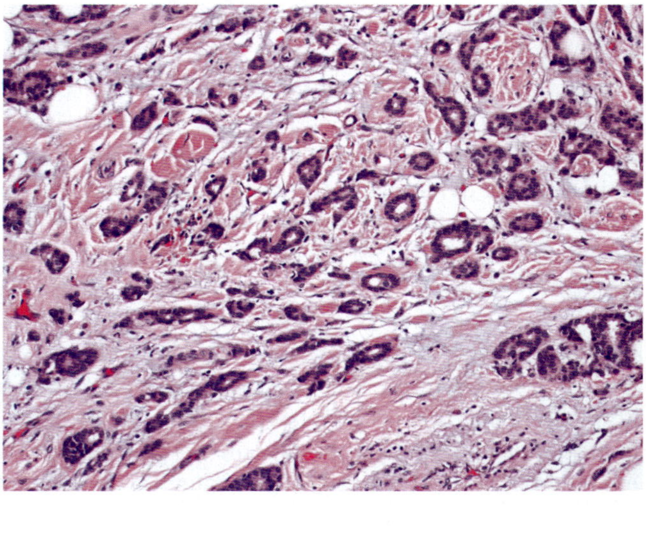

FIGURE 5-13: Low-grade invasive carcinoma of NST. Tumor composed predominantly of tubules and glands with central lumina and polarized one-cell layer. The breakdown of scores in this case was 1 for tubules, 1 for nuclear pleomorphism, and 1 for mitotic activity. Although there are some similarities, the tumor does not show the angulated glands and the desmoplastic stroma required for the diagnosis of "pure" invasive tubular carcinoma.

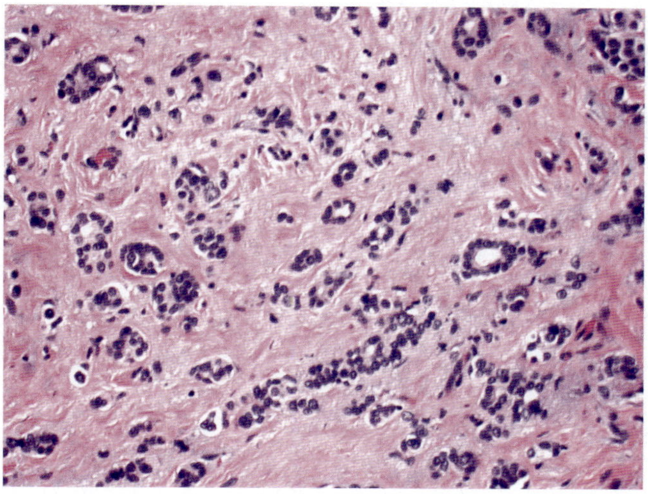

FIGURE 5-14: Low-grade invasive carcinoma of NST. Notice the fibrotic stroma surrounding the neoplastic tubules. The breakdown of scores in this case was 2 for tubules, 1 for nuclear pleomorphism, and 1 for mitotic activity.

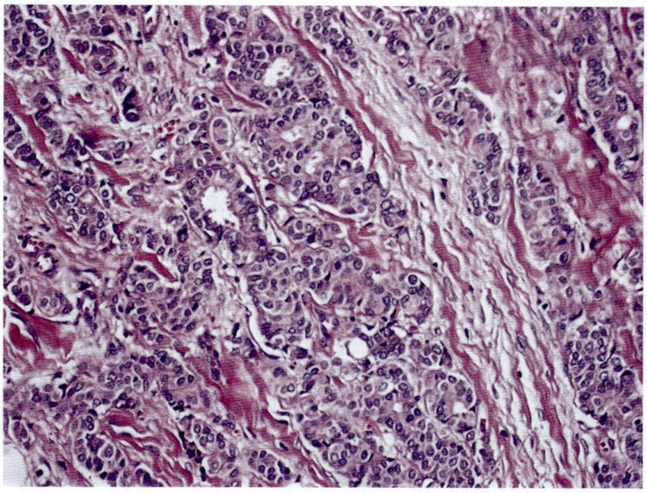

FIGURE 5-15: Intermediate-grade invasive carcinoma of NST. The overall breakdown of scores in this case was 3 for tubules, 2 for nuclear pleomorphism, and 1 for mitotic activity. A nuclear pleomorphism score of 2 is based on increased nuclear size with open vesicular structure and mild-to-moderate variation in size and shape.

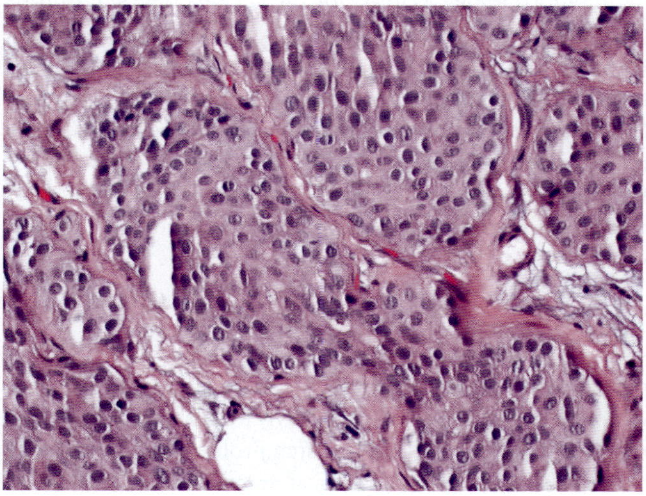

FIGURE 5-16: Intermediate-grade invasive carcinoma of NST with a score breakdown similar to the case in Figure 5-15. In this case, however, the tumor almost entirely displayed a solid growth pattern.

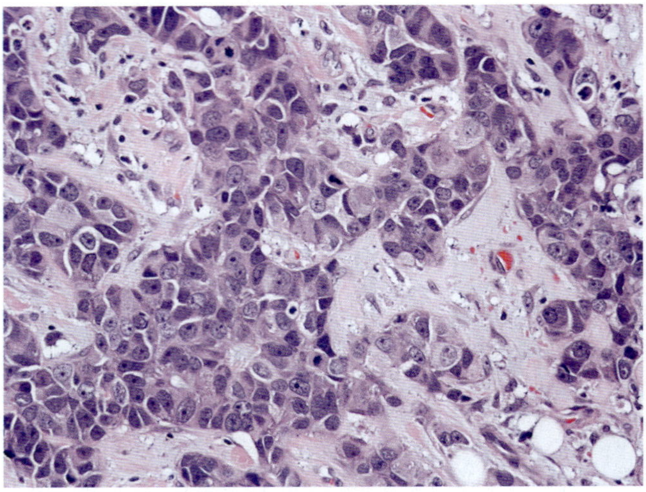

FIGURE 5-17: High-grade invasive carcinoma of NST with a solid growth pattern (score 3 for tubule formation), marked variation in size and shape of nuclei (score 3 for nuclear pleomorphism), and high mitotic count (score 3). Notice the desmoplastic stromal reaction around tumor cells.

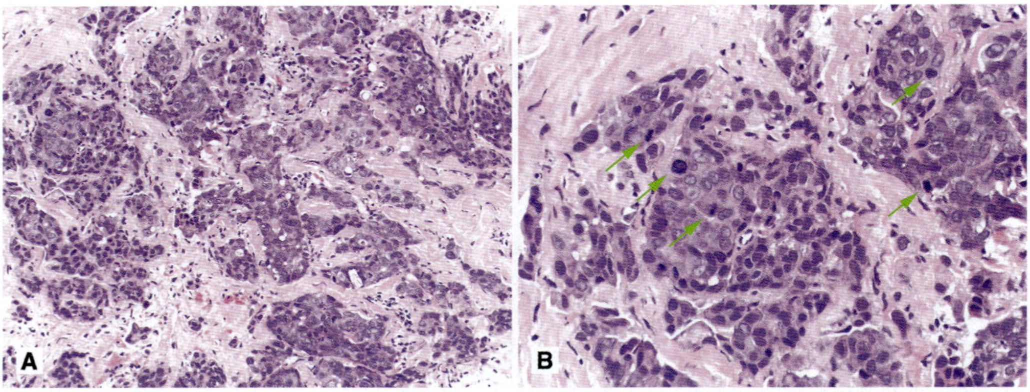

FIGURE 5-18: High-grade invasive carcinoma of NST. Notice the solid growth pattern with no tubule formation (score 3) (**A, B**), as well as the nuclear pleomorphism (score 3) (**B**) and the abundant mitotic activity (score 3) (**B**, *arrows*).

Mitotic Count

Only mitotic figures that clearly fulfill the morphologic criteria for the various stages of mitosis should be included. This is usually measured in 10 high-power fields (HPFs) with the greatest proliferative activity (usually referred to as "hot spots"[12]), often located at the periphery and/or least differentiated part of the tumor. It is important to be aware of the impact of HPF size variation of different microscopes (0.4–0.69 mm^2) on the mitotic rate cutoffs used to assign the mitotic score (1, 2, or 3), as that ultimately impacts the overall grade. Accordingly, the recommendation has been to use the number of mitoses per square millimeter (mm^2) for better standardization. Current data do not provide sufficient evidence to support the use of immunohistochemical stains for assessment of proliferative activity.

Expected Distribution of Tumor Grades in Invasive Carcinoma of NST

Published ratios for grades 1, 2, and 3 are approximately 2:3:5 in breast cancer.[13] There is greater interobserver variation in assigning grade 2, compared to grades 1 and 3. Attempts to further stratify grade 2 tumors include application of genomic grade index (GGI) to subclassify histologic grade 2 into two molecular subclasses (GGI1 and GGI3)[14] and by using proliferation biomarkers such as Ki-67.[15] None of these methods, however, are in use in clinical practice.

INVASIVE CARCINOMA OF NO SPECIAL TYPE, IMMUNOHISTOCHEMISTRY

Invasive carcinomas of NST are positive for luminal cytokeratins (e.g., CK18, CK8, CK7, and CK19) and epithelial membrane antigen (EMA). They are also frequently positive for lactalbumin (70%) and gross cystic disease fluid protein-15 (GCDFP-15) (~50%). Approximately 80% of NSTs are positive for estrogen receptor (ER) and androgen receptor (AR); approximately 70% are positive for progesterone receptor (PR); and approximately 20% show *HER2* overexpression or gene amplification. Basal keratins such as CK5, CK5/6, CK14, and CK17 are expressed in a small proportion of cases. Less than 10% of invasive carcinomas of NST are positive for neuroendocrine markers (synaptophysin and chromogranin-A). Positivity for neuroendocrine markers by itself, in the absence of supportive morphologic features, is not indicative of neuroendocrine carcinoma.[16]

INVASIVE CARCINOMA OF NO SPECIAL TYPE, DIFFERENTIAL DIAGNOSIS

As the name implies, NST carcinoma is a diagnosis of exclusion, and the distinction must be made between it and special types of carcinoma, especially those with an exceptionally favorable prognosis such as pure tubular carcinoma[17] (Chapter 7). As mentioned above, pure tubular carcinoma should be restricted to tumors with tubule formation in greater than 90% in addition to low-grade nuclei (Figure 5-19). Occasionally, invasive carcinoma of NST displays single-file or a targetoid pattern of infiltration that resembles ILC (Chapter 6); however, the cytomorphologic features of the latter are lacking, and close observation will reveal tubule formation with indistinct lumina (Figure 5-6). It is important to know that diagnosis of associated ILC component may have impact on the use of imaging in screening and follow-up of patients. The differentiation of invasive carcinoma of NST from other special types of carcinoma is discussed in subsequent chapters.[18] Some invasive tumors mimic solid or cribriform DCIS (Figure 5-20), and immunohistochemistry for myoepithelial markers may be helpful in such cases[11] (see Chapter 2 for more details).

Although uncommon, it is also important to consider metastatic tumors to the breast in the differential diagnosis (Figure 5-21). Features that favor primary versus metastatic tumors are associated DCIS and infiltrative pattern rather than displacement of normal-appearing breast parenchyma in primary tumors. Expression of GCDFP-15, mammoglobin, or GATA3 would also favor primary breast carcinoma.[19,20] Other markers may be helpful to delineate the primary site of metastatic carcinoma, for example, TTF1 for pulmonary, vimentin for endometrioid and renal

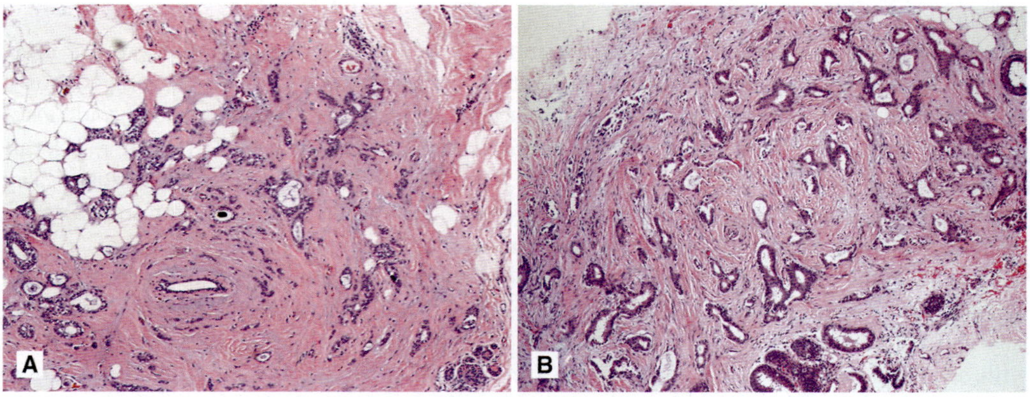

FIGURE 5-19: Low-grade invasive carcinoma of NST (**A**) and pure invasive tubular carcinoma (**B**). Notice the well-formed, mostly rounded, tubules with features of low-grade nuclei and inconspicuous nucleoli in carcinoma of NST (**A**) compared to angulated, haphazardly arranged tubules lined with one layer of bland-looking cells with little nuclear pleomorphism in pure tubular carcinoma.

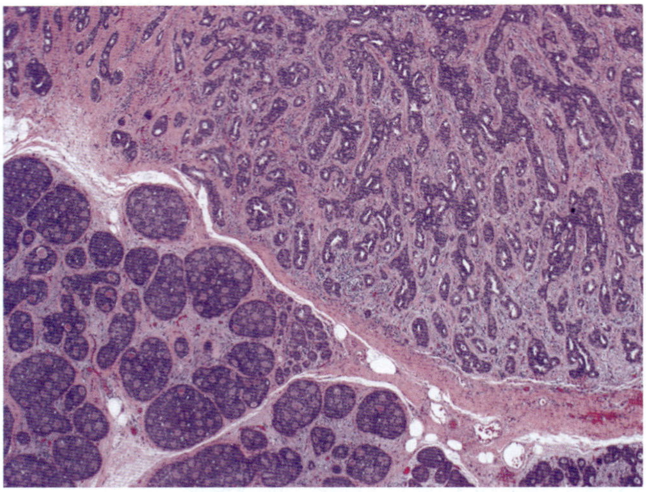

FIGURE 5-20: Moderately differentiated invasive carcinoma of NST with cribriform-like growth pattern (*upper half*), which could be mistaken for DCIS, similar to the adjacent cribriform DCIS with rounded counter (*lower half*).

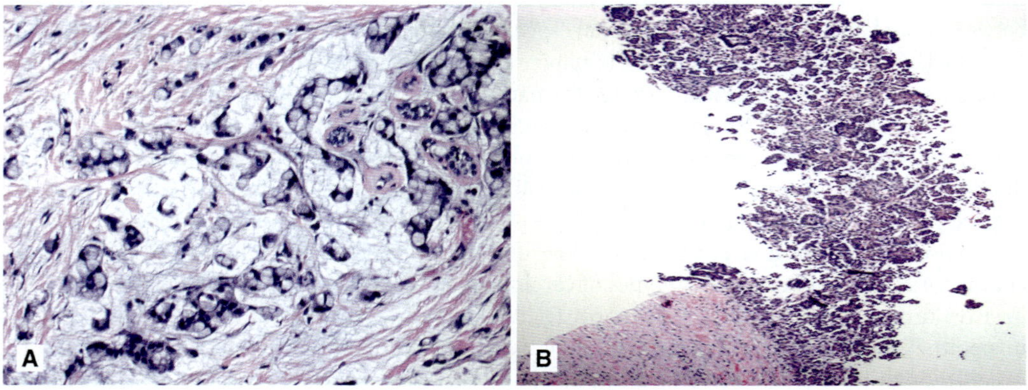

FIGURE 5-21: Metastatic carcinomas to the breast. Mucinous carcinoma of primary colonic origin (**A**). In contrast to most primary mucinous carcinomas of the breast, this tumor did not express estrogen or progesterone receptors by immunohistochemistry. Papillary serous carcinoma of primary ovarian origin (**B**). This tumor was also negative for estrogen and progesterone receptors but strongly expressed WT1.

cell carcinoma, WT1 for ovarian serous carcinoma, CDX2 for colorectal cancers, and PAX8 for primary müllerian tumors.[21]

The differential diagnosis of invasive carcinoma of NST (as well as many other types of invasive carcinoma) includes nonneoplastic infiltrative processes, for example, sclerosing adenosis, microglandular adenosis (MGA), and complex sclerosing lesion/radial scar. Sclerosing adenosis, especially when involved by intraductal neoplastic proliferations such as DCIS (Figure 5-22), can mimic invasive carcinoma. However, the lobulocentric distribution of sclerosing adenosis is key to reaching the correct diagnosis. Fortunately, myoepithelial markers are often prominent in sclerosing adenosis compared to complete absence in invasive carcinoma of the NST.[22]

MGA on the other hand does not have lobulocentric distribution and can infiltrate stroma and adipose tissue in random fashion (Figure 5-23). An added challenge is the lack of myoepithelial marker expression. At the architectural level, the glands in MGA are round and filled with secretion, whereas the glands in invasive carcinoma, NST, especially those with tubular features, are angulated and have open lumina. There is at least mild nuclear atypia and pleomorphism in carcinomas compared to the bland-looking ones in MGA. The stroma in MGA is relatively acellular compared to cellular and elastotic one in carcinomas. ER and EMA immunohistochemical stains may prove useful in this differential with both markers positive in

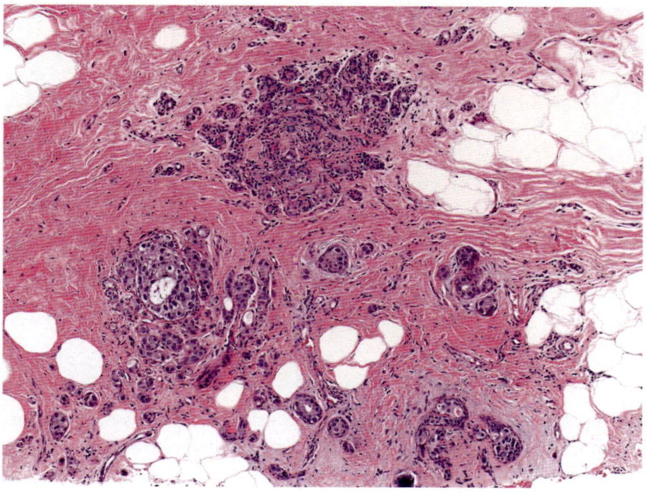

FIGURE 5-22: Sclerosing adenosis involved by DCIS, evident in the lower half of this figure, appears expanded by the eosinophilic neoplastic cells. Notice the smaller glandular aggregates in the lower left corner that resemble invasive ductal carcinoma of NST.

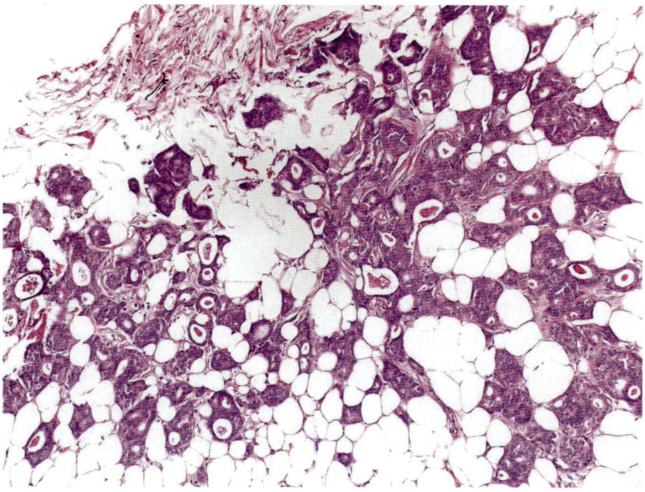

FIGURE 5-23: Microglandular adenosis. The eosinophilic luminal secretions characteristic of this lesion is one clue that helps in distinguishing it from invasive carcinoma.

most low-grade carcinomas compared to negativity in MGA lesions.[23,24] In addition, a *Periodic acid–Schiff* (PAS) stain or collagen type IV and laminin immunostains may also be useful as they have been found to highlight continuous basement membranes in MGA compared to absent to interrupted in invasive carcinomas.[25–27]

Complex sclerosing/radial scar lesions with their characteristic central fibrosis and elastosis with distorted tubular structures more prominent in the periphery also might be in the differential diagnosis. The glands at the periphery of radial scar show varying degree of dilation and usual hyperplasia. Myoepithelial markers are helpful in delineating myoepithelial cells in these lesions in contrast to complete absence in invasive carcinomas (Figure 5-24).

INVASIVE CARCINOMA OF NO SPECIAL TYPE, MOLECULAR GENETICS

Genetic alterations in intraductal and invasive components have shown similar patterns of loss of heterozygosity (LOH) in both components. This finding supports the hypothesis that DCIS is the precursor of invasive carcinoma of NST and that DCIS carry genetic signature of invasive

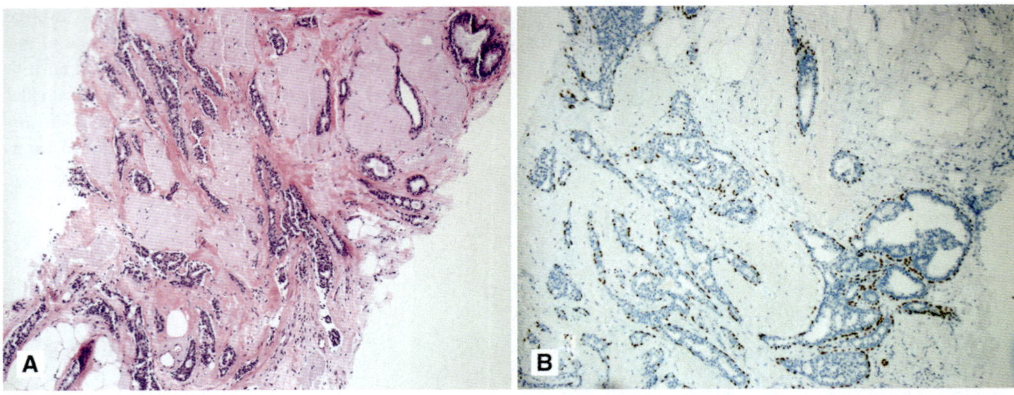

FIGURE 5-24: Radial scar. The lesion composed of acellular areas with collagen and elastic fibers with associated compressed tubules and epithelial proliferation simulating invasive carcinoma of NST (**A**). p63 immunohistochemical stain with nuclear positivity can be used confirm the diagnosis of benignity (**B**).

carcinoma even before invasion occurs in most cases.[28] Prognosis and clinical outcome of cases with invasive carcinoma on the basis of genetic differences were suggested by analysis of LOH in the primary tumor, lymph node metastasis, and recurrence. LOH studies identified that primary and recurrent tumor specimens are identical in a subset of patients. However, there is a significant increase in "total LOH" in recurrent tumors.[29] The impact of different mutations in genes such as BRCA1 and BRCA2 is the subject of multiple investigations. BRCA-associated breast carcinomas are more likely to be poorly differentiated and triple negative, exhibit prominent lymphocytic infiltrates and necrosis, and manifest high proliferative rate (Figure 5-7) especially in BRCA1 tumors compared to BRCA2-associated ones.[30] Increased frequency of p53 mutations and lower frequency of HER2 amplification in BRCA1 carcinomas compared to sporadic cases have been reported.[30] BRCA2-associated carcinomas have also been found to be of high grade and express luminal cytokeratins significantly more often and are less likely to overexpress HER2 protein.[31]

The presence of a germline BRCA mutation does not increase the risk of ipsilateral breast recurrence after breast conservation when compared to young women not known to have a germline BRCA mutation.[32] Patients with BRCA germline mutations had an increased 5-year (11.9%) and 10-year (37.6%) risk for contralateral carcinoma and 10% probability of ovarian carcinoma.[28] Family history of breast cancer in patients with BRCA mutation is the exception rather than the rule with 70% of BRCA1 carriers and 40% of BRCA2 carriers not having a family history in a first- or second-degree relative.[33] BRCA1-associated invasive carcinomas are reported to have a lower frequency of associated intraductal carcinoma compared to sporadic or nonhereditary carcinomas.[34] Additionally, the low frequency of pure intraductal carcinoma has been observed in studies of BRCA1-associated tumors compared to BRCA2-associated tumors, which do not have a different frequency of intraductal carcinoma compared to sporadic control cases.[4]

References

1. Li CI, Uribe DJ, Daling JR. Clinical characteristics of different histologic types of breast cancer. *Br J Cancer* 2005;93:1046–1052.
2. Ellis I, Collins L, Ichihara S, et al. Invasive carcinoma of no special type. In: Lakhani S, Ellis IO, Schnitt SJ, eds. *WHO Classification of Tumours of the Breast.* 4th ed. Lyon, France: International Agency for Research and Cancer (IARC); 2012:33–38.
3. Yoder BJ, Wilkinson EJ, Massoll NA. Molecular and morphologic distinctions between infiltrating ductal and lobular carcinoma of the breast. *Breast J* 2007;13:172–179.

4. Breast Cancer Linkage Consortium. Pathology of familial breast cancer: differences between breast cancers in carriers of BRCA1 or BRCA2 mutations and sporadic cases. *Lancet* 1997;349:1505–1510.
5. Arpino G, Bardou VJ, Clark GM, et al. Infiltrating lobular carcinoma of the breast: tumor characteristics and clinical outcome. *Breast Cancer Res* 2004;6:R149–R156.
6. Kocjan G. [Needle aspiration cytology of the breast: current perspective on the role in diagnosis and management]. *Acta Med Croatica* 2008;62:391–401.
7. Gruber IV, Rueckert M, Kagan KO, et al. Measurement of tumour size with mammography, sonography and magnetic resonance imaging as compared to histological tumour size in primary breast cancer. *BMC Cancer* 2013;13:328.
8. Anderson WF, Pfeiffer RM, Dores GM, et al. Comparison of age distribution patterns for different histopathologic types of breast carcinoma. *Cancer Epidemiol Biomarkers Prev* 2006;15:1899–1905.
9. Edge B, Byrd RD, Compton CC, et al. *AJCC Cancer Staging Manual*. 7th ed. New York: Springer; 2011.
10. Bloom HJ, Richardson WW. Histological grading and prognosis in breast cancer; a study of 1409 cases of which 359 have been followed for 15 years. *Br J Cancer* 1957;11:359–377.
11. Elston CW, Ellis IO. Pathological prognostic factors in breast cancer. I. The value of histological grade in breast cancer: experience from a large study with long-term follow-up. *Histopathology* 2002;41:154–161.
12. Pathology Reporting of Breast Disease. A Joint Document Incorporating the Third Edition of the NHS Breast Screening Programme's Guidelines for Pathology Reporting in Breast Cancer Screening and the Second Edition of The Royal College of Pathologists' Minimum Dataset for Breast Cancer Histopathology Published by the NHS Cancer Screening Programmes jointly with The Royal College of Pathologists. http://www.cancerscreening.nhs.uk/breastscreen/publications/nhsbsp58.html. January 2005.
13. Rakha EA, Ellis IO. Invasive ductal carcinoma of no special type and histologic grade. In: Dabbs D, ed. *Breast Pathology*. 1 Har/Psc edition. Saunders; 2012:429–445.
14. Sotiriou C, Wirapati P, Loi S, et al. Gene expression profiling in breast cancer: understanding the molecular basis of histologic grade to improve prognosis. *J Natl Cancer Inst* 2006;98:262–272.
15. Aleskandarany MA, Rakha EA, Macmillan RD, et al. MIB1/Ki-67 labelling index can classify grade 2 breast cancer into two clinically distinct subgroups. *Breast Cancer Res Treat* 2011;127:591–599.
16. Miremadi A, Pinder SE, Lee AH, et al. Neuroendocrine differentiation and prognosis in breast adenocarcinoma. *Histopathology* 2002;40:215–222.
17. Rakha EA, Lee AH, Evans AJ, et al. Tubular carcinoma of the breast: further evidence to support its excellent prognosis. *J Clin Oncol* 2010;28:99–104.
18. Damiani S, Eusebi V, Losi L, et al. Oncocytic carcinoma (malignant oncocytoma) of the breast. *Am J Surg Pathol* 1998;22:221–230.
19. Yan Z, Gidley J, Horton D, et al. Diagnostic utility of mammaglobin and GCDFP-15 in the identification of metastatic breast carcinoma in fluid specimens. *Diagn Cytopathol* 2009;37:475–478.
20. Liu H, Shi J, Prichard JW, et al. Immunohistochemical evaluation of GATA-3 expression in ER-negative breast carcinomas. *Am J Clin Pathol* 2014;141:648–655.
21. Zhou S, Yu B, Cheng Y, et al. [Metastases to the breast from non-mammary malignancies: a clinicopathologic study of 28 cases]. *Zhonghua Bing Li Xue Za Zhi* 2014;43:231–235.
22. Jao W, Recant W, Swerdlow MA. Comparative ultrastructure of tubular carcinoma and sclerosing adenosis of the breast. *Cancer* 1976;38:180–186.
23. Wen YH, Weigelt B, Reis-Filho JS. Microglandular adenosis: a non-obligate precursor of triple-negative breast cancer? *Histol Histopathol* 2013;28:1099–1108.
24. Eusebi V, Foschini MP, Betts CM, et al. Microglandular adenosis, apocrine adenosis, and tubular carcinoma of the breast. An immunohistochemical comparison. *Am J Surg Pathol* 1993;17:99–109.
25. Joshi MG, Lee AK, Pedersen CA, et al. The role of immunocytochemical markers in the differential diagnosis of proliferative and neoplastic lesions of the breast. *Mod Pathol* 1996;9:57–62.
26. Choi JE, Bae YK. Invasive breast carcinoma arising in microglandular adenosis: two case reports. *J Breast Cancer* 2013;16:432–437.
27. Shui RH, Cheng YF, Yang WT. [Invasive carcinoma arising in breast microglandular adenosis: a clinicopathologic study of three cases and review of the literature]. *Zhonghua Bing Li Xue Za Zhi* 2011;40:471–474.
28. Rosen P. *Rosen's Breast Pathology*. Philadelphia, PA: Lippincott Williams & Wilkins; 2008.
29. Regitnig P, Heckermann H, Moser R, et al. Molecular genetic comparison of primary and recurrent breast carcinoma? Significant increase of loss of heterozygosity (LOH) in the recurrence and specific LOH associated with early recurrence. *Mod Pathol* 2000:13:45A.

30. Honrado E, Benitez J, Palacios J. The molecular pathology of hereditary breast cancer: genetic testing and therapeutic implications. *Mod Pathol* 2005;18:1305–1320.
31. Bane AL, Beck JC, Bleiweiss I, et al. BRCA2 mutation-associated breast cancers exhibit a distinguishing phenotype based on morphology and molecular profiles from tissue microarrays. *Am J Surg Pathol* 2007;31:121–128.
32. Robson M, Svahn T, McCormick B, et al. Appropriateness of breast-conserving treatment of breast carcinoma in women with germline mutations in BRCA1 or BRCA2: a clinic-based series. *Cancer* 2005;103:44–51.
33. Armes JE, Egan AJ, Southey MC, et al. The histologic phenotypes of breast carcinoma occurring before age 40 years in women with and without BRCA1 or BRCA2 germline mutations: a population-based study. *Cancer* 1998;83:2335–2345.
34. Jacquemler J, Eisinger F, Guinebretiere JM, et al. Intraductal component and BRCA1-associated breast cancer. *Lancet* 1996;348:1098.

Invasive Lobular Carcinoma and Variants

6

Lobular lesions of the breast include atypical lobular hyperplasia, lobular carcinoma *in situ* (LCIS), and invasive lobular carcinoma (ILC). ILC represents 5% to 15% of all invasive breast cancers.[1] A number of distinct ILC subtypes are recognized with great diversity in morphology. Other than the classic ILC, these subtypes include solid, alveolar, pleomorphic, and tubulolobular. These variant subtypes have a worse prognosis than does the classic form[2,3] and are often associated with each other leading to the proposal of including a "mixed" subtype as well.

Unlike carcinoma of no special type (NST), ILC has continued to rise in incidence, especially in women aged greater than 50 years. This rise is thought to be unlikely secondary to increased mammographic screening alone.[4] The mean age of patients with ILC is 57 to 65, slightly higher than that of invasive carcinoma of NST.[5] In addition, contralateral carcinomas are about twice as frequent in ILC compared to invasive carcinoma of NST.[6] There is some controversy on whether the outcome of ILC is better, worse, or similar to invasive carcinoma of NST, which may be partly due to different outcomes among the variants of ILC.

INVASIVE LOBULAR CARCINOMA, CYTOLOGY

A diagnosis of ILC may be missed on fine needle aspiration (FNA) due to low cellularity. Characteristically, there is a monomorphic population of single cells or loosely cohesive clusters (Figure 6-1). The cytoplasm may be scant with well-defined borders, and intracytoplasmic spaces or "lumens" can be prominent and signet-ring cells may be evident. Nuclei are generally small (~1 to 2× the size of RBCs) and usually have fine and evenly distributed chromatin, mildly irregular nuclear membranes, and inconspicuous nucleoli. The degree of atypia is dependent on the variant of ILC (see below) with the pleomorphic variant exhibiting greater atypia.[7]

INVASIVE LOBULAR CARCINOMA, IMAGING AND GROSS FEATURES

The most common radiologic findings in ILC are spiculated mass or architectural distortion (Figure 6-2A). Calcification is less frequent compared to carcinoma of NST. Ultrasonography (Figure 6-2B) and magnetic resonance imaging (Figure 6-3) are often more sensitive than is mammogram in detecting ILC.[8] Grossly, ILCs usually appear as ill-defined, irregular tumors that may be difficult to identify or to accurately measure.[5]

INVASIVE LOBULAR CARCINOMA, HISTOLOGY

According to the World Health Organization (WHO), ILC is classified into classic, solid, pleomorphic, tubulolobular, and mixed types.[9] The nonclassic variants have also been classified into pleomorphic, signet-ring, histiocytoid, and apocrine subtypes.[10] Tumor grade of ILC is assessed

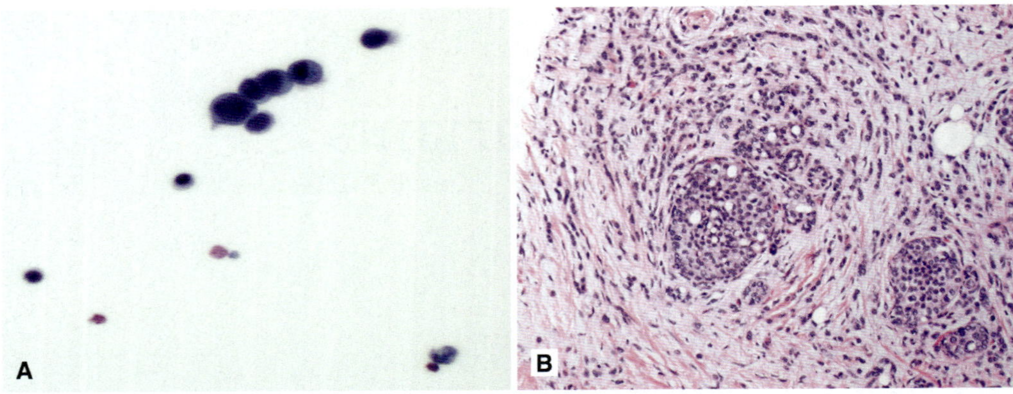

FIGURE 6-1: Fine-needle aspiration cytology showing low cellularity and scattered and small clusters of atypical cells with eccentric nuclei (plasmacytoid) (**A**). This case proved to be ILC (**B**). Notice the circumferential (targetoid) growth pattern of the invasive carcinoma around the breast lobules expanded by lobular neoplasia.

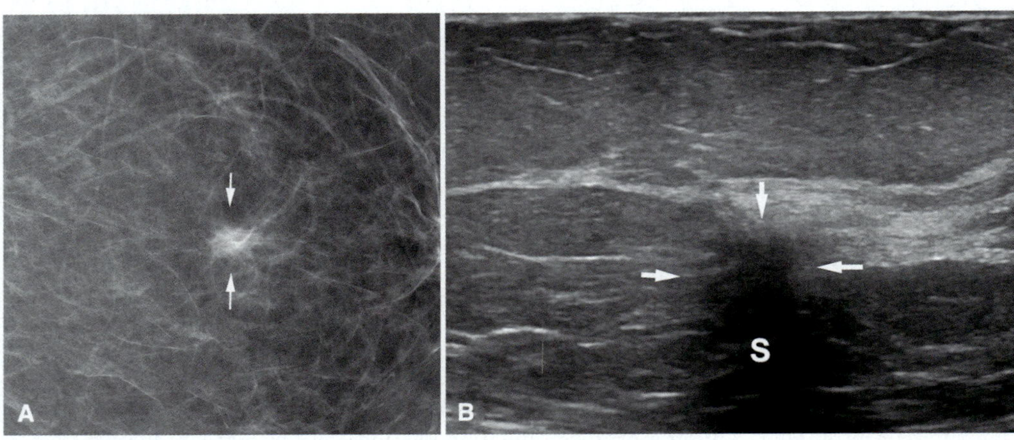

FIGURE 6-2: Left craniocaudal view shows an isodense irregular mass (*arrows*) with spiculated margins (**A**). Gray-scale US image confirms a hypoechoic irregular mass (*arrows*) with indistinct margins and posterior acoustic shadowing (*S*) (**B**). This lesion proved to be ILC.

FIGURE 6-3: Sagittal subtraction MR image reveals a new irregular area of non–mass-like enhancement (*arrows*) with rapid rise and washout kinetics in the left 12:00 breast of this patient undergoing high-risk screening for breast cancer. This lesion proved to be ILC.

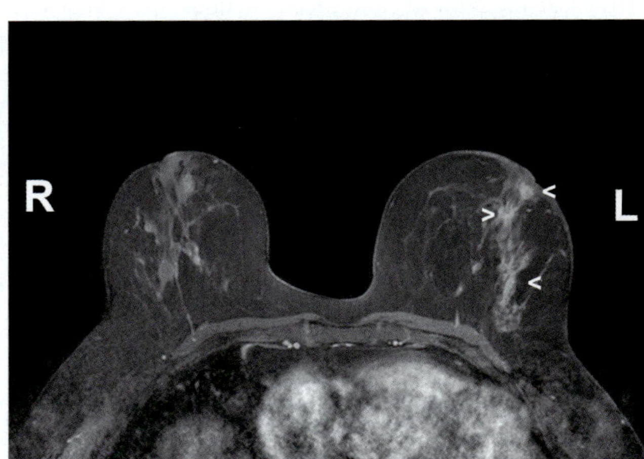

based on the same criteria as that of carcinoma of NST based on the combined assessment of tubule formation, nuclear grade, and mitotic activity.[11]

Invasive Lobular Carcinoma, Classic Type

The classic type is composed of small to medium-sized, uniform, dyshesive tumor cells usually with mild nuclear atypia and inconspicuous nucleoli. These cells usually infiltrate a dense fibrous stroma (Figures 6-4 to 6-8), as single cells, in linear files and sometimes grow around ducts and lobules in a concentric (targetoid) pattern.[12] As noted above, a signet-ring cell morphology may also be seen (Figure 6-9). Of note, however, such a morphology may be seen in other subtypes of ILC as well as other types of invasive carcinoma. Moreover, the term "signet-ring ILC" has been used to designate ILCs that are predominantly composed of such cells.[13] Skip lesions, where patches of tumor are seen separated from the main lesion by uninvolved breast tissue, are also common. Mitoses are sparse, and classic ILC is usually a low or intermediate-grade tumor.[14]

Invasive Lobular Carcinoma Variants

ILC, Pleomorphic Type

This type of ILC displays marked nuclear pleomorphism with higher mitotic index and thus more frequently grade 3[11] and associated with more aggressive outcomes. The growth pattern usually resembles that of the classic type but may also have a more solid pattern of growth (Figure 6-10).

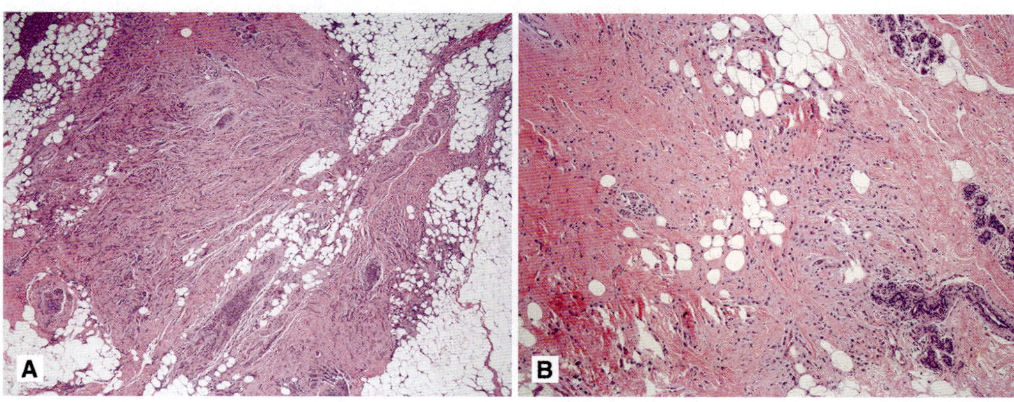

FIGURE 6-4: Low- and intermediate-power magnifications of ILC showing an irregular fibrotic lesion (**A**) with scattered single tumor cells (**B**).

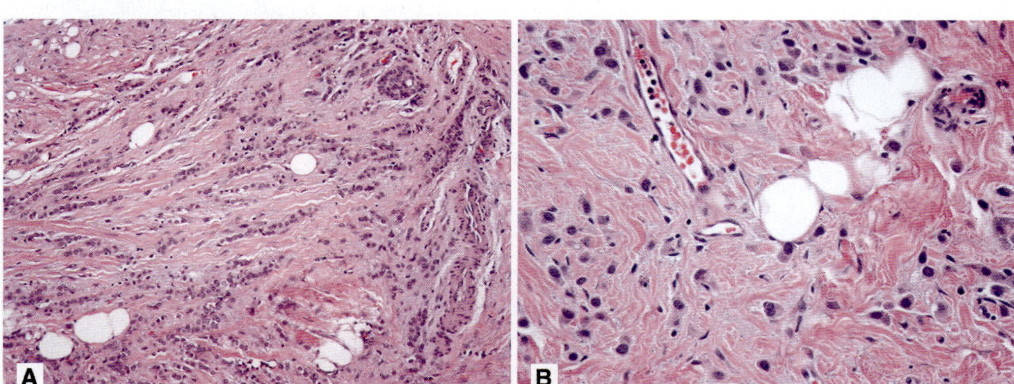

FIGURE 6-5: Intermediate power magnifications of ILC showing small to medium-sized, uniform, and dyshesive cells that arrange in linear strands (**A**) or individually infiltrate the stroma (**B**). Notice the slight hyperchromasia but otherwise minimal nuclear atypia.

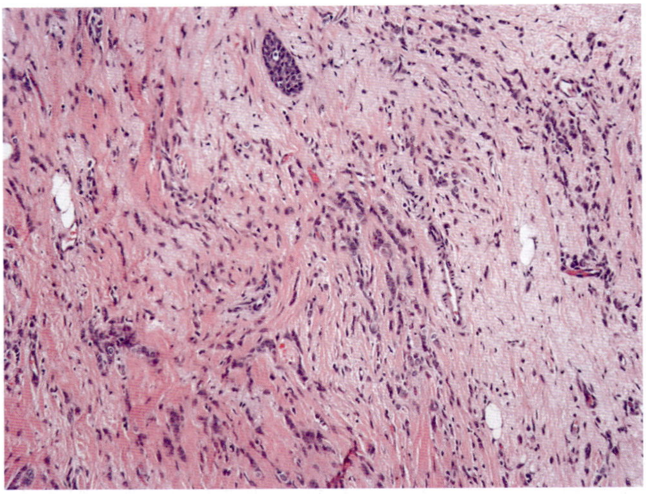

FIGURE 6-6: Invasive lobular carcinoma. Notice the diffuse infiltrative nature of relatively uniform neoplastic cells.

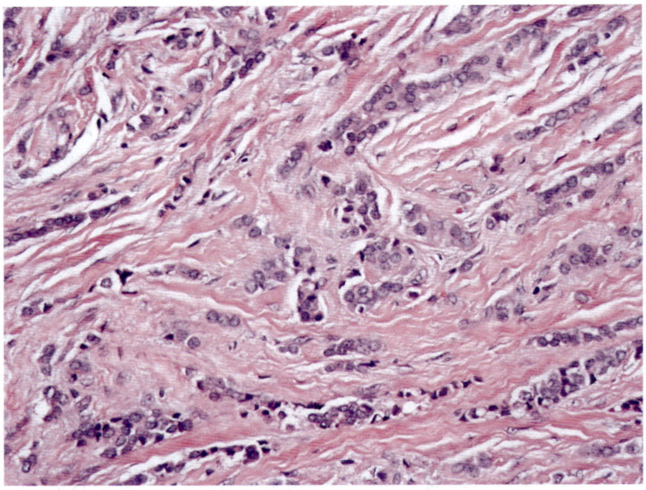

FIGURE 6-7: High-power view of ILC showing uniform small to medium-sized neoplastic cells arranged in linear strands.

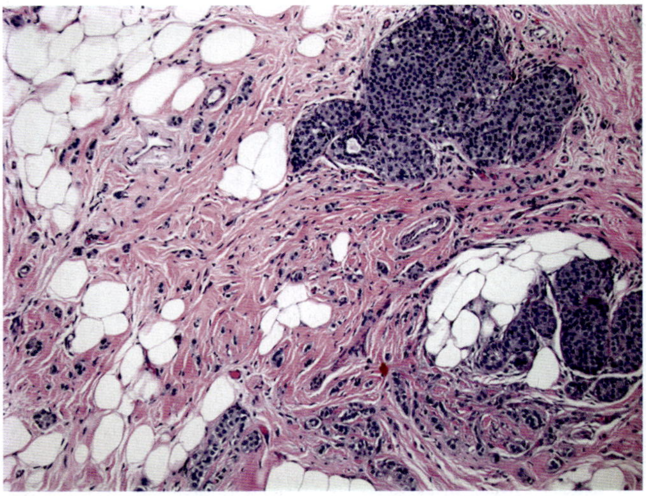

FIGURE 6-8: Invasive lobular carcinoma arising adjacent to breast lobules expanded by lobular neoplasia.

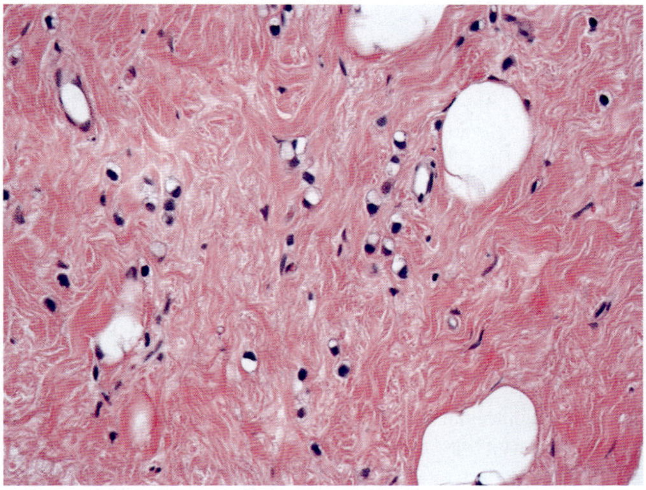

FIGURE 6-9: Invasive lobular carcinoma with signet-ring cell morphology.

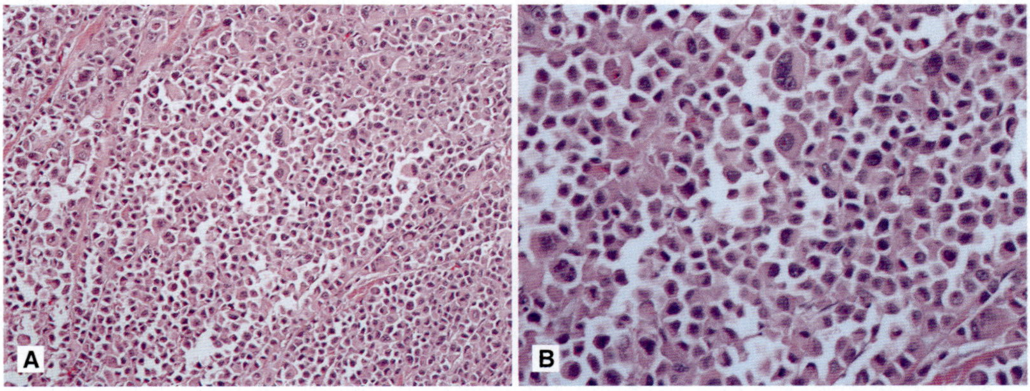

FIGURE 6-10: Invasive lobular carcinoma, pleomorphic type, medium (**A**) and higher (**B**) power magnifications. Notice marked nuclear pleomorphism. (Courtesy of Dr. T. Khoury, Buffalo, New York)

Apocrine/Histiocytoid Types

Cells within these tumors have large nuclei and copious cytoplasm resembling macrophages—hence the term "histiocytoid"[15] (Figure 6-11). Apocrine differentiation and histiocytoid-like appearance may be detected in ILC otherwise recapitulating the cytoarchitectural features of the pleomorphic type, but could represent the predominant cell populations of distinct tumors.

Alveolar Type

This pattern forms round aggregates of invasive neoplastic cells in a manner that mimics LCIS, but they lack myoepithelial cells and basement membrane at the periphery as detected by high molecular weight keratins, p63, smooth muscle myosin heavy chain, and other myoepithelial markers.[12] Tumor cells have the same uniform appearance as that in the classic type and usually cluster in aggregates of greater than 20 cells and separated by thin bands of fibrous stroma.[13]

Solid Type

In this variant, the neoplastic cells form sheets and can mimic other lesions, most notably lymphoma. Commonly, the lesion possesses high-grade nuclei. Close examination often reveals areas of classic ILC, usually at the margins of the lesion. The tumor cells of the solid type diffusely infiltrate the surrounding tissues in large solid sheets, with scarce intervening stroma.[12]

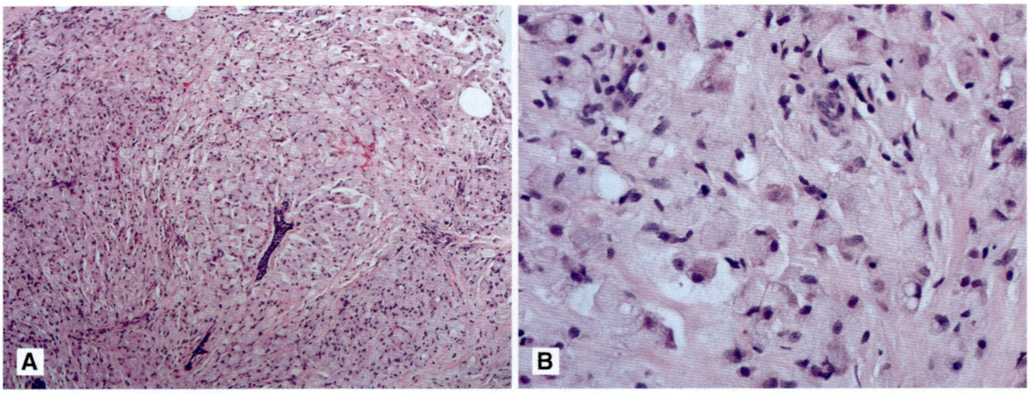

FIGURE 6-11: Invasive lobular carcinoma, histiocytoid type, medium (**A**) and higher (**B**) power magnifications. Neoplastic cells have large nuclei and copious cytoplasm resembling macrophages. (Courtesy of Dr. T. Khoury, Buffalo, New York)

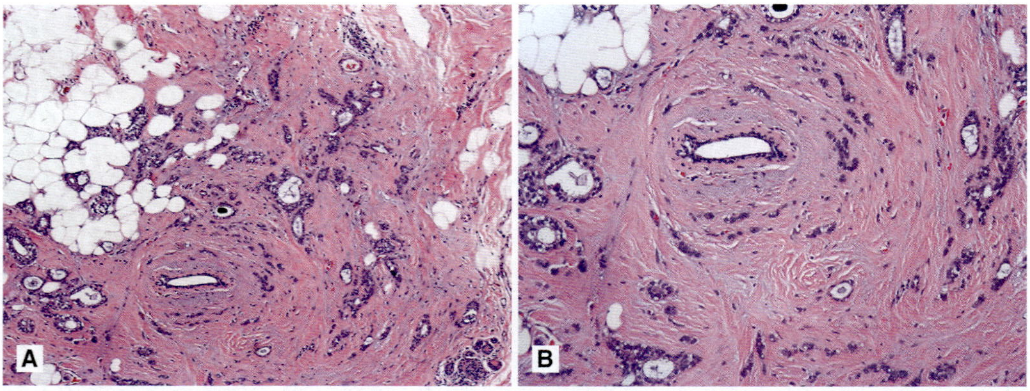

FIGURE 6-12: Tubulolobular carcinoma, medium (**A**) and higher (**B**) power magnifications. The tumor is characterized by classic ILC with tumor cells growing around ducts and lobules in a concentric (targetoid) pattern appearance and small tubules morphologically similar to tubular carcinoma.

Trabecular Type

This growth pattern is similar to classic ILCs but composed of broader bands of malignant cells instead of a single-file pattern.[12]

Tubulolobular Type

This tumor is characterized by the overall cytologic features of classic ILC, including single files and targetoid configurations, but differs by the presence of small tubules morphologically similar to invasive tubular carcinoma. Tubulolobular carcinoma showed a higher degree of crowding and architectural complexity[16] (Figure 6-12). Studies have shown that most tubulolobular carcinomas are positive for E-cadherin and have concluded that this tumor is more akin to carcinoma of NST rather than lobular carcinoma.[17] The observation that tubulolobular carcinoma is commonly accompanied by LCIS has led some authors to conclude that these lesions are truly lobular/NST hybrids[18]—not surprising in view of the cytogenetic similarity between low-grade carcinoma of NST and ILC,[12] while others categorize these lesions with carcinoma of NST.[19]

Grading of ILC

Pure ILCs usually receive a score of 3 for tubule formation; consequently, grading of ILC is significantly dependent on the nuclear grade.[20] Since the majority of ILCs display nuclear grade 2, most ILC are intermediate histologic grade. It has been reported that about 12% to 39%, 50% to 76%, and 11% to 12% of ILCs are grade 1, grade 2, and grade 3, respectively, and histologic grade was found to be an independent predictor of short-tern disease-free survival.[10,20]

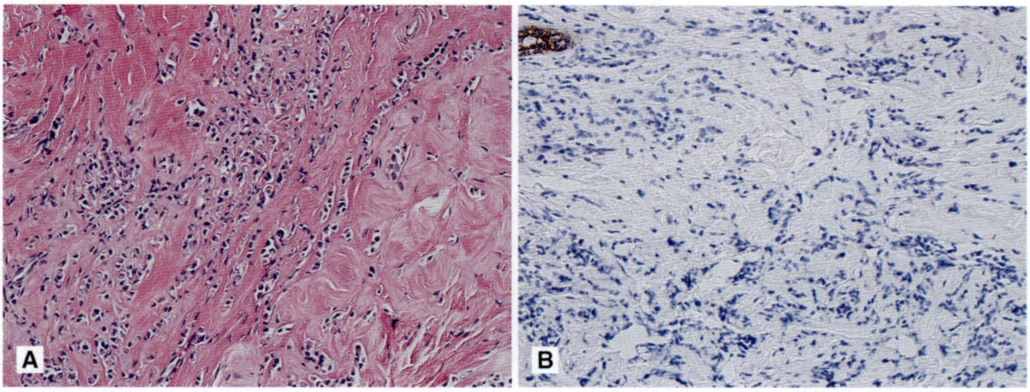

FIGURE 6-13: Invasive lobular carcinoma (**A**) with no E-cadherin expression by immunohistochemistry (**B**). Notice preserved expression in the benign duct at the left upper corner serving as an internal control.

INVASIVE LOBULAR CARCINOMA, IMMUNOHISTOCHEMISTRY

A characteristic feature of ILC is lack of membranous E-cadherin expression (Figure 6-13) and cytoplasmic (not membranous) expression of P120, which contrasts with most carcinomas of NST where both are expressed in a membranous fashion.[21–23] Given that some carcinoma of NST can also be E-cadherin negative,[5] the overall morphologic features need to be taken into account when immunohistochemistry is being used as adjunct to help confirm the diagnosis of ILC. ILC typically also expresses epidermal growth factor receptor 1 and high molecular weight cytokeratins, a finding shared with some carcinoma of NST.[17,24] Classic ILCs are almost all estrogen (ER) and progesterone (PR) receptor positive, lack HER2 protein overexpression/gene amplification, and have a low Ki-67 labeling index. On the other hand, pleomorphic ILC is often ER and PR negative, more frequently shows HER2 protein overexpression/gene amplification and a moderate-to-high Ki-67 labeling index, and is usually associated with p53 overexpression.

INVASIVE LOBULAR CARCINOMA, DIFFERENTIAL DIAGNOSIS

Invasive Carcinoma of NST

The growth pattern, cytologic features, and immunohistochemical profiles must be carefully assessed to reach a correct diagnosis. As mentioned above, carcinoma of NST in some cases displays a growth pattern similar to ILC with no tubule formation. Morphologically, carcinoma of NST does not show the typical cellular dyshesiveness of ILC. Intracytoplasmic vacuoles favor a lobular lesion. Immunohistochemistry with E-cadherin and p120 catenin is of help, but the staining pattern must be interpreted in the context of morphology.[22]

Hematolymphoid Lesions

Because many are composed of small dyshesive cells with minimal nuclear atypia, lymphomas and leukemias involving the breast can easily be confused with ILC. Careful attention to the clinical and morphologic findings as well as results of immunohistochemistry (e.g., lack of ER and PR expression among others) should point toward the correct diagnosis.

Stromal Proliferations

Due to the diffuse growth pattern of ILC, stromal proliferations rarely enter in the differential diagnosis. Nevertheless, epithelioid myofibroblastoma may mimic ILC in rare instances. The tumor is usually well circumscribed and lacks entrapped breast structures or associated LCIS.[25] Vimentin, smooth muscle actin, desmin, and CD34 expression correct diagnosis of myofibroblastoma in challenging cases.[26]

INVASIVE LOBULAR CARCINOMA, MOLECULAR GENETICS

The hallmark molecular feature of lobular tumors, as described previously, is the genetic abnormalities of CDH1 gene encoding E-cadherin.[27] Loss of expression at the protein level occurs by a combination of loss of heterozygosity and truncation mutations in E-cadherin gene (16q) or promoter silencing.[19] As a consequence of loss of E-cadherin, loss of adhesion of the cells with the morphologic appearance of single filing is apparent.

The classic cytogenetic changes of ILC are loss of 16q and gain of 1p, and in this regard and in terms of overall number of changes, ILC resembles low-grade carcinoma of NST.[28] In a study, pleomorphic ILC cases harbor more cytogenetic changes than in classic ILC, notably including amplification of c-myc and HER2. There are not, however, as many changes as seen in carcinoma of NST, and these changes, qualitatively, still resembled ILC more than high-grade carcinoma of NST.[29]

More recent studies have suggested that there are a number of other molecular changes, still shared by some carcinoma of NST phenotype and ILC as amplification of the fibroblast growth factor receptor 1 (FGFR1) gene at a complex locus 8p11.2, which may have therapeutic implications.[29,30] Interestingly, some rare families have been detected whose kindred have a heritable defect in the E-cadherin gene and who develop either lobular carcinoma or diffuse gastric carcinoma.[31]

References

1. Singletary SE, Patel-Parekh L, Bland KI. Treatment trends in early-stage invasive lobular carcinoma: a report from the National Cancer Data Base. *Ann Surg* 2005;242:281–289.
2. Jung SP, Lee SK, Kim S, et al. Invasive pleomorphic lobular carcinoma of the breast: clinicopathologic characteristics and prognosis compared with invasive ductal carcinoma. *J Breast Cancer* 2012;15:313–319.
3. Jacobs M, Fan F, Tawfik O. Clinicopathologic and biomarker analysis of invasive pleomorphic lobular carcinoma as compared with invasive classic lobular carcinoma: an experience in our institution and review of the literature. *Ann Diagn Pathol* 2012;16:185–189.
4. Li CI, Anderson BO, Daling JR, et al. Changing incidence of lobular carcinoma in situ of the breast. *Breast Cancer Res Treat* 2002;75:259–268.
5. Arpino G, Bardou VJ, Clark GM, et al. Infiltrating lobular carcinoma of the breast: tumor characteristics and clinical outcome. *Breast Cancer Res* 2004;6:R149–R156.
6. Arpino G, Allred DC, Mohsin SK, et al. Lobular neoplasia on core-needle biopsy—clinical significance. *Cancer* 2004;101:242–250.
7. Rajesh L, Dey P, Joshi K. Fine needle aspiration cytology of lobular breast carcinoma. Comparison with other breast lesions. *Acta Cytol* 2003;47:177–182.
8. Gruber IV, Rueckert M, Kagan KO, et al. Measurement of tumour size with mammography, sonography and magnetic resonance imaging as compared to histological tumour size in primary breast cancer. *BMC Cancer* 2013;13:328.
9. Lakhani S, Rakha E, Simpson PT. Invasive lobular carcinoma. In: Lakhani S, Ellis IO, Schnitt SJ, Tan PH, et al., ed. *WHO Classification of Tumours of the Breast*. Lyon, France: International Agency for Research and Cancer (IARC);2012:40–42.
10. Orvieto E, Maiorano E, Bottiglieri L, et al. Clinicopathologic characteristics of invasive lobular carcinoma of the breast: results of an analysis of 530 cases from a single institution. *Cancer* 2008;113;1511–1520.
11. Elston CW, Ellis IO. Pathological prognostic factors in breast cancer. I. The value of histological grade in breast cancer: experience from a large study with long-term follow-up. *Histopathology* 2002;41:154–161.

12. Martinez V, Azzopardi JG. Invasive lobular carcinoma of the breast: incidence and variants. *Histopathology* 1979;3:467–488.
13. Iorfida M, Maiorano E, Orvieto E, et al. Invasive lobular breast cancer: subtypes and outcome. *Breast Cancer Res Treat* 2012;133:713–723.
14. Nishizaki T, Chew K, Chu L, et al. Genetic alterations in lobular breast cancer by comparative genomic hybridization. *Int J Cancer* 1997;74:513–517.
15. Tan PH, Harada O, Thike AA, et al. Histiocytoid breast carcinoma: an enigmatic lobular entity. *J Clin Pathol* 2011;64:654–659.
16. Fisher ER, Gregorio RM, Redmond C, et al. Tubulolobular invasive breast cancer: a variant of lobular invasive cancer. *Hum Pathol* 1977;8:679–683.
17. Wheeler DT, Tai LH, Bratthauer GL, et al. Tubulolobular carcinoma of the breast: an analysis of 27 cases of a tumor with a hybrid morphology and immunoprofile. *Am J Surg Pathol* 2004;28:1587–1593.
18. Kuroda H, Tamaru J, Takeuchi I, et al. Expression of E-cadherin, alpha-catenin, and beta-catenin in tubulolobular carcinoma of the breast. *Virchows Arch* 2006;448:500–505.
19. O'Malley FP. Lobular neoplasia: morphology, biological potential and management in core biopsies. *Mod Pathol* 2010;23(suppl 2):S14–S25.
20. Rakha EA, El-Sayed ME, Menon S, et al. Histologic grading is an independent prognostic factor in invasive lobular carcinoma of the breast. *Breast Cancer Res Treat* 2008;111:121–127.
21. Goldstein NS, Bassi D, Watts JC, et al. E-cadherin reactivity of 95 noninvasive ductal and lobular lesions of the breast. Implications for the interpretation of problematic lesions. *Am J Clin Pathol* 2001;115:534–542.
22. Acs G, Lawton TJ, Rebbeck TR, et al. Differential expression of E-cadherin in lobular and ductal neoplasms of the breast and its biologic and diagnostic implications. *Am J Clin Pathol* 2001;115:85–98.
23. Dabbs DJ, Kaplai M, Chivukula M, et al. The spectrum of morphomolecular abnormalities of the E-cadherin/catenin complex in pleomorphic lobular carcinoma of the breast. *Appl Immunohistochem Mol Morphol* 2007;15:260–266.
24. Bratthauer GL, Moinfar F, Stamatakos MD, et al. Combined E-cadherin and high molecular weight cytokeratin immunoprofile differentiates lobular, ductal, and hybrid mammary intraepithelial neoplasias. *Hum Pathol* 2002;33:620–627.
25. Lakhani SR, Ellis IO, Schnitt SJ, et al. *WHO Classification of Tumours of the Breast*. Geneva, Switzerland: World Health Organization; 2012.
26. Magro G, Bisceglia M, Michal M, et al. Spindle cell lipoma-like tumor, solitary fibrous tumor and myofibroblastoma of the breast: a clinico-pathological analysis of 13 cases in favor of a unifying histogenetic concept. *Virchows Arch* 2002;440:249–260.
27. Salomon D, Sacco PA, Roy SG, et al. Regulation of beta-catenin levels and localization by overexpression of plakoglobin and inhibition of the ubiquitin-proteasome system. *J Cell Biol* 1997;139:1325–1335.
28. Reis-Filho JS, Simpson PT, Turner NC, et al. FGFR1 emerges as a potential therapeutic target for lobular breast carcinomas. *Clin Cancer Res* 2006;12:6652–6662.
29. Reis-Filho JS, Simpson PT, Jones C, et al. Pleomorphic lobular carcinoma of the breast: role of comprehensive molecular pathology in characterization of an entity. *J Pathol* 2005;207:1–13.
30. Elbauomy Elsheikh S, Green AR, Lambros MB, et al. FGFR1 amplification in breast carcinomas: a chromogenic in situ hybridisation analysis. *Breast Cancer Res* 2007;9:R23.
31. Keller G, Vogelsang H, Becker I, et al. Diffuse type gastric and lobular breast carcinoma in a familial gastric cancer patient with an E-cadherin germline mutation. *Am J Pathol* 1999;155:337–342.

7 Tubular Carcinoma and Cribriform Carcinoma

Tubular carcinoma and cribriform carcinoma are closely related well-differentiated neoplasms with excellent prognoses. They often coexist together within one invasive tumor, characteristically produce a prominent desmoplastic stromal reaction, and are frequently associated with the same group of low-grade precursor lesions.

TUBULAR CARCINOMA, CYTOLOGY

Cytologically, two characteristic but not entirely pathognomonic features are the presence of tubular structures and glands with an "arrowhead" outline (Figures 7-1 and 7-2). The lesional cells are typically bland with low- to intermediate-grade nuclei and minimal nuclear pleomorphism.

TUBULAR CARCINOMA, IMAGING AND GROSS FEATURES

On imaging, tubular carcinoma often presents as a small, irregular, or spiculated mass with associated calcifications (Figure 7-3).[1–3] Similarly, the gross appearance of tubular carcinoma is typically ill-defined, gray-white, firm, usually gritty, lesion. As such, the gross findings are indistinguishable from invasive ductal carcinoma of no special type. The lesion may be so small that it is discovered incidentally in needle biopsies for other reasons.

TUBULAR CARCINOMA, HISTOLOGY

The characteristic appearance of tubular carcinoma is that of haphazardly arranged, well-formed glands or tubules with a prominent infiltrative growth pattern. The variably sized neoplastic glands characteristically display angulated contours and tapering ends (Figure 7-4) and are composed of a single layer of cells with grade 1 or 2 nuclei. Apical cytoplasmic snouts are common (Figure 7-5) as is secretory material in glandular lumens, sometimes with associated calcifications (Figure 7-6).

More than 90% of the lesion should display the characteristic morphology to be classified as "pure" tubular carcinoma, while those showing tubular elements in 50% to 90% of the tumor classified as mixed [4] or "with tubular features." It is important to note that the presence of nuclear stratification, significant nuclear pleomorphism (grade 3 nuclei), or high mitotic index precludes a diagnosis of tubular carcinoma.[4]

Another important feature of tubular carcinoma is a prominent desmoplastic stromal response. Stromal elastosis may also be present. Finally, several lesions are commonly seen in association with tubular carcinoma, namely, flat epithelial atypia, low-grade ductal carcinoma *in situ* (DCIS), and, less frequently, lobular neoplasia.[5–7] The combination of tubular carcinoma, columnar cell lesions, and lobular carcinoma *in situ* (LCIS) has been termed "Rosen Triad."[8]

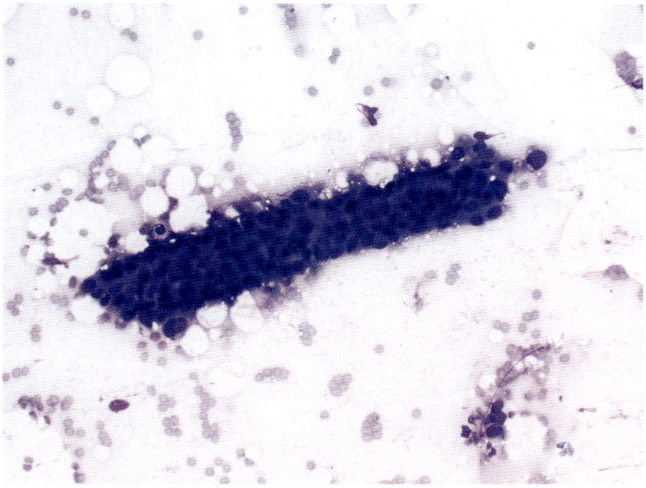

FIGURE 7-1: Tubular carcinoma. A scantly cellular specimen with a straight, open tubular structure with rigid-appearing borders. (Diff-Quik stain; Photomicrograph courtesy of Amberly L. Nunez, M.D.)

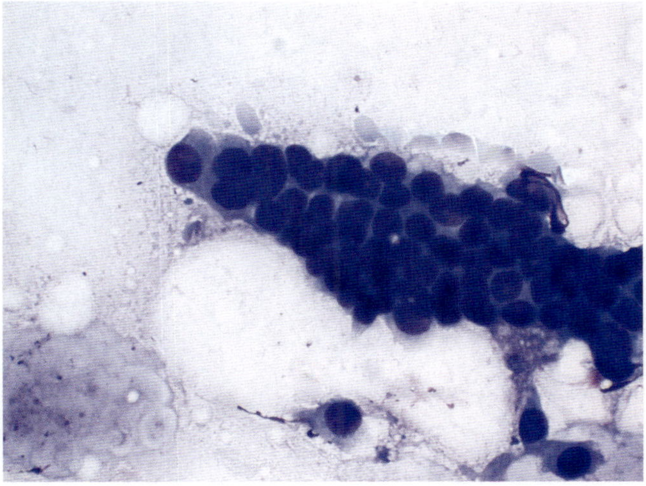

FIGURE 7-2: Tubular carcinoma. A group of ductal cells with an angulated, arrowhead appearance. The cells are fairly monotonous with minimal pleomorphism. (Diff-Quik stain; Photomicrograph courtesy of Amberly L. Nunez, M.D.)

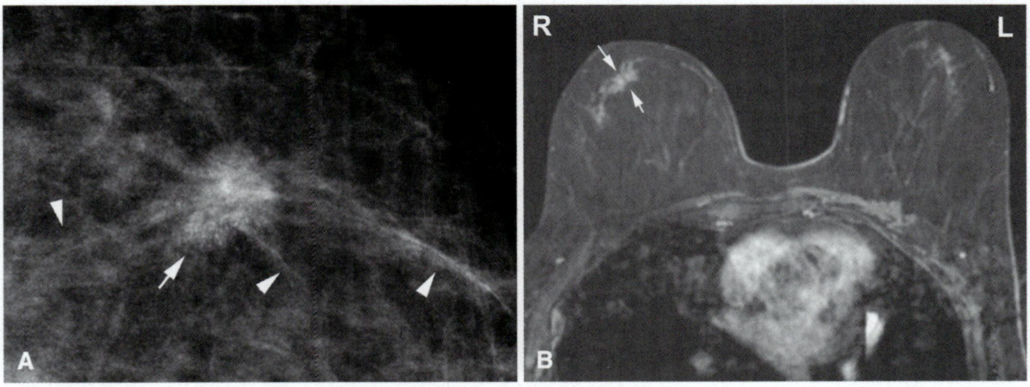

FIGURE 7-3: Imaging features of tubular carcinoma. A mammographic image demonstrates an irregular mass with spiculated margins and associated calcifications (*arrow*) (**A**). Note the long spicules (*arrowheads*). An axial T1 fat-saturated delayed postcontrast MR image reveals an enhancing irregular mass with spiculated margins (*arrows*) (**B**).

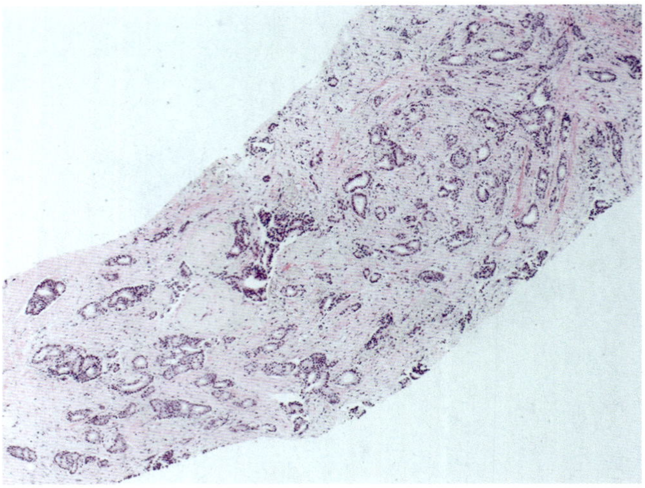

FIGURE 7-4: A low-power view of core needle biopsy demonstrates a tubular carcinoma with haphazardly distributed, angulated glands with open lumina.

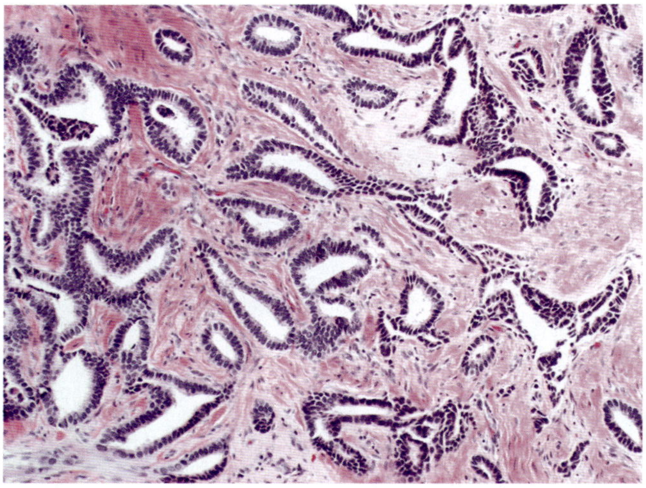

FIGURE 7-5: A higher magnification of tubular carcinoma. The tumor cells typically have grade 1 or 2 nucleus. Apical snouts are evident in this image.

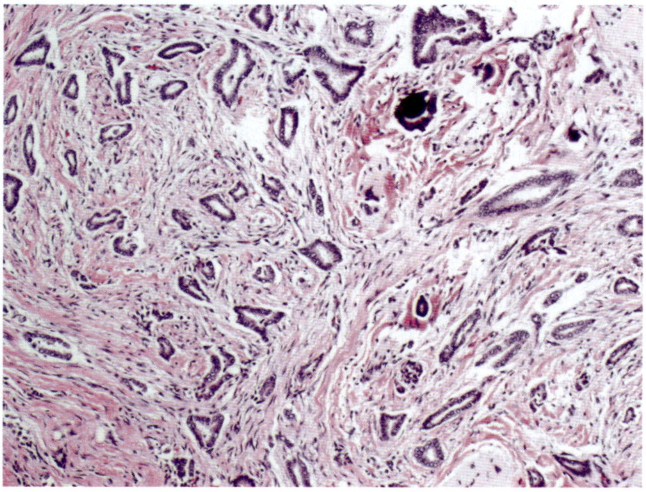

FIGURE 7-6: A tubular carcinoma with calcification of luminal secretion.

TUBULAR CARCINOMA, DIFFERENTIAL DIAGNOSIS

Although sclerosing adenosis can have a dense, fibrotic stroma and a focally infiltrative growth pattern, it typically maintains some lobular architecture (Figure 7-7) that helps in distinguishing it from tubular carcinoma. Other discriminatory features include compressed and distorted (rather than open angulated) glands, an intact myoepithelial cell layer, and typically discernible basement membrane (Figure 7-7 inset). When there is doubt, immunohistochemistry for myoepithelial marker expression can become very useful.

Microglandular adenosis usually has a nodular architecture but can show a haphazard, infiltrative pattern of growth and, since it lacks a myoepithelial cell layer, can be more challenging to differentiate from tubular carcinoma. In these situations, the rounded and regular glandular contours of microglandular adenosis as well as the presence of characteristic eosinophilic, colloid-like secretions (Figure 7-8) can become very useful in the distinction. Epithelial S100 protein expression is another distinguishing feature of microglandular adenosis, not present in tubular carcinoma.[9]

Radial scar/complex sclerosing lesions (Figure 7-9) and some sclerosed intraductal papillomas have fibrotic/elastotic stroma with entrapped glandular elements that can mimic tubular carcinoma. This stroma, however, is less cellular, and the compressed and distorted appearance of these entrapped ductal/tubular structures, as well as the presence of (sometimes attenuated) myoepithelial

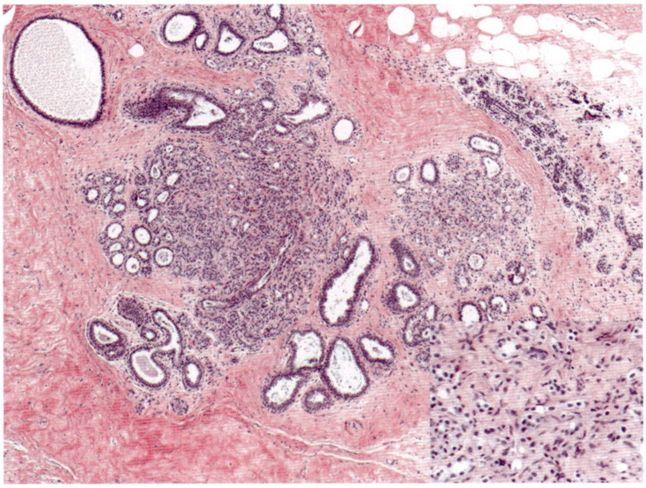

FIGURE 7-7: The lobulocentric architecture of sclerosing adenosis is best demonstrated at low-power view. The presence of myoepithelial cells and fully retained basement membrane is typically discernible at higher magnification (**inset**).

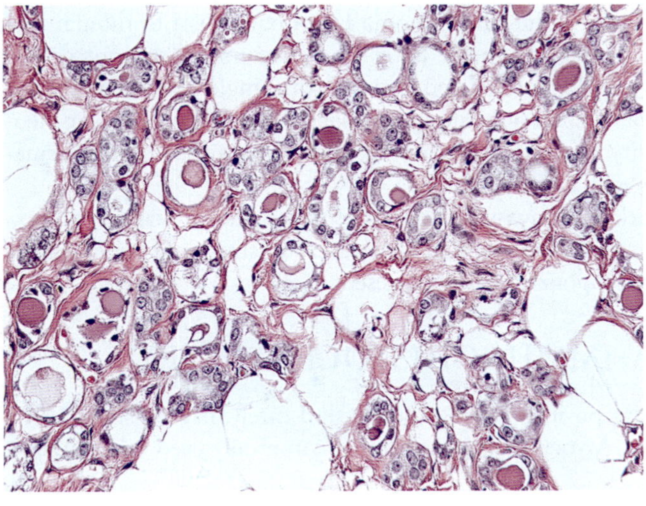

FIGURE 7-8: Microglandular adenosis typically consists of tubules with rounded and regular contours in contrast to the angular shapes in tubular carcinoma. The presence of eosinophilic, colloid-like secretions in lumens is a classic but not specific feature.

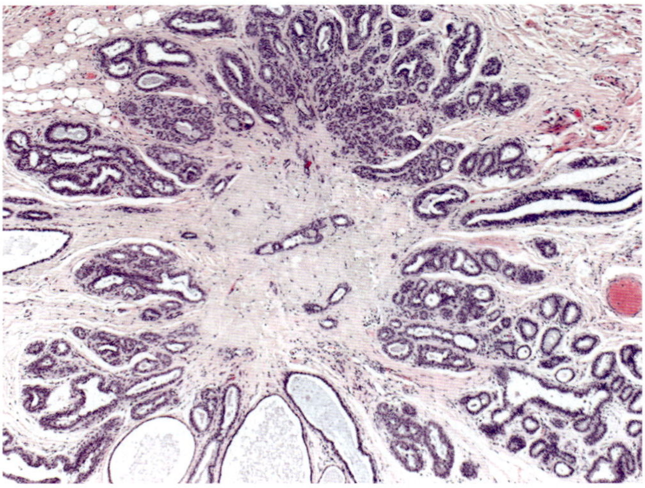

FIGURE 7-9: A radial scar demonstrates characteristic central fibrosis and elastosis, with varying degrees of duct dilatation and epithelial hyperplasia at the periphery.

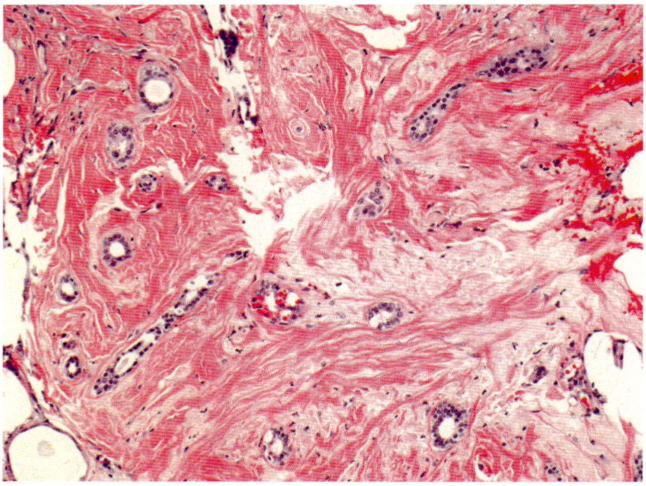

FIGURE 7-10: The entrapped ducts and tubules in the center of radial scars are often compressed and distorted and thus may closely mimic tubular carcinoma.

cells (Figure 7-10), should help make the distinction. This is especially important in needle biopsy material when other characteristic features of these mimickers are not readily evident.

Low-grade, well-differentiated invasive ductal carcinoma is not equivalent to tubular carcinoma and cannot be used synonymously, given the latter's superior prognostic outcomes.[7] The diagnosis of tubular carcinoma should be restricted to those with single-layered, angulated tubules composing greater than 90% of the lesion, along with lack of significant nuclear pleomorphism and marked mitotic activity. Low-grade carcinomas typically have less tubule formation and lack angular-shaped glands with atypical snouts.

Tubulolobular carcinoma is a variant of invasive lobular carcinoma characterized by admixture of tubular and linear growth patterns. The tubular structures are small and round rather than angulated, and a classic lobular component is always present.

TUBULAR CARCINOMA, IMMUNOHISTOCHEMISTRY

Tubular carcinomas are almost always positive for ER and PR and rarely, if ever, show HER2 overexpression or gene amplification.[10] Myoepithelial markers are commonly used to distinguish

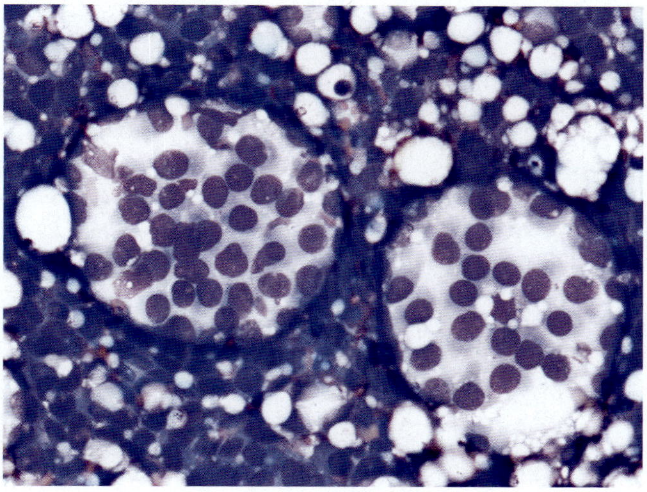

FIGURE 7-11: Cytologic features of cribriform carcinoma. A cohesive sheet of ductal cells with regular, punched-out spaces that are similar to the histomorphology. (Diff-Quik stain; photomicrograph courtesy of Amberly L. Nunez, M.D.)

tubular carcinoma from its benign mimickers. Immunostaining for S100 protein is the most helpful adjunct in distinction between tubular carcinoma and microglandular adenosis.

TUBULAR CARCINOMA, MOLECULAR GENETICS

As previously described, tubular carcinomas frequently occur in association with a spectrum of low-grade lesions, including flat epithelial atypia, low-grade DCIS, and LCIS. These lesions typically share similar immunophenotype (e.g., strong expression of ER and PR). They also share molecular genetic alterations, most frequently chromosomes 16q loss and 1q gain. Other less common alterations include 16p gain and loss of 8p, 3p, and 11q. Thus, a precursor role and biologic progression has been suggested.[7,11–15]

CRIBRIFORM CARCINOMA, CYTOLOGY

The fine needle aspiration biopsy of cribriform carcinoma typically shows cohesive sheets of ductal cells with regular, punched-out spaces (Figure 7-11).

CRIBRIFORM CARCINOMA, IMAGING AND GROSS FEATURES

There are no specific imaging and gross features to distinguish cribriform carcinoma from other types.

CRIBRIFORM CARCINOMA, HISTOLOGY

The diagnosis of cribriform carcinoma requires a cribriform growth pattern in greater than 90% of the lesion.[4] The tumor closely resembles cribriform DCIS but is different from the latter in that the islands of tumor cells often have irregular and angulated contours with an infiltrative pattern of growth (Figures 7-12 to 7-14). A prominent desmoplastic stromal reaction is a common association. A concurrent low-grade DCIS, generally of cribriform pattern, is frequently present. The tumor cells are typically small to intermediate in size, lack significant nuclear atypia, and have a low mitotic index, similar to tubular carcinoma. A component of tubular carcinoma (<50%) is frequently coexistent (Figure 7-15).[16]

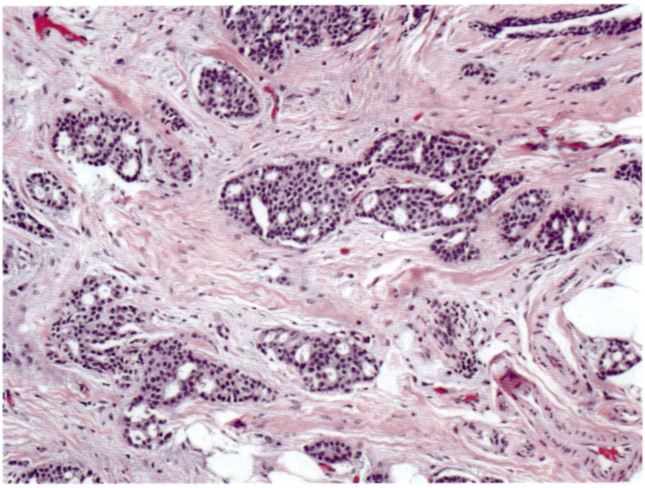

FIGURE 7-12: Invasive cribriform carcinoma differs from cribriform DCIS in that the islands of tumor cells often have irregular contours with an infiltrative growth pattern. The tumor cells typically show low to intermediate nuclear grade devoid of significant cytologic atypia.

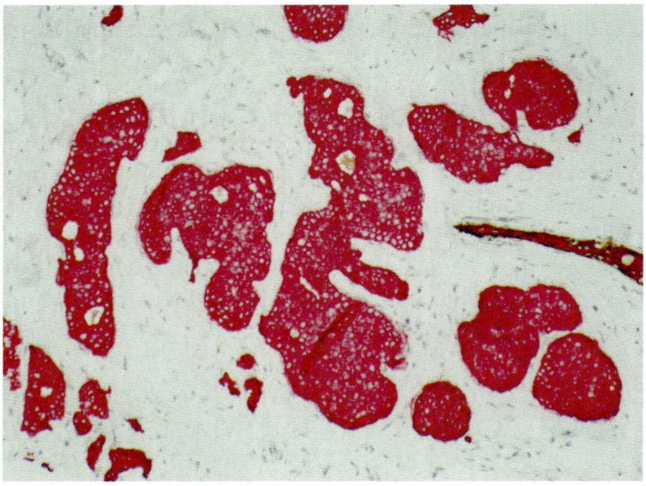

FIGURE 7-13: A cocktail immunostain in a cribriform carcinoma demonstrates the absence of p63/CK5/CK14-positive myoepithelial cells in the tumor islands, but clearly highlights the myoepithelial cell layer (*brown*) in a benign duct. The cocktail also highlights CK8/CK17-positive luminal epithelium (*red*).

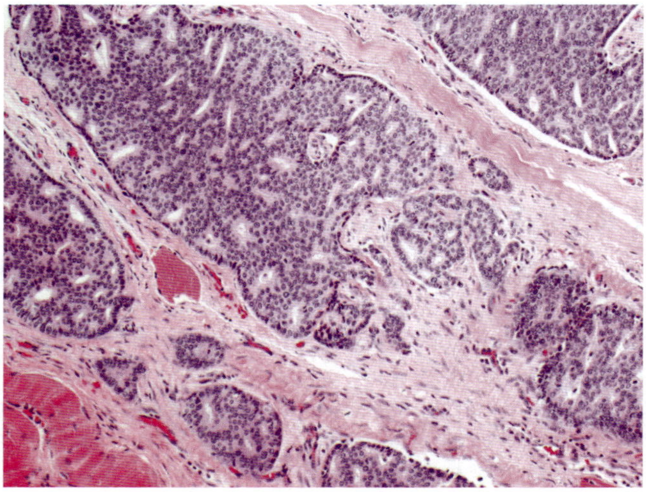

FIGURE 7-14: Another example of invasive cribriform carcinoma mimicking cribriform DCIS. The presence of infiltrative small glands and invasion into the chest wall skeletal muscle confirm its invasive nature.

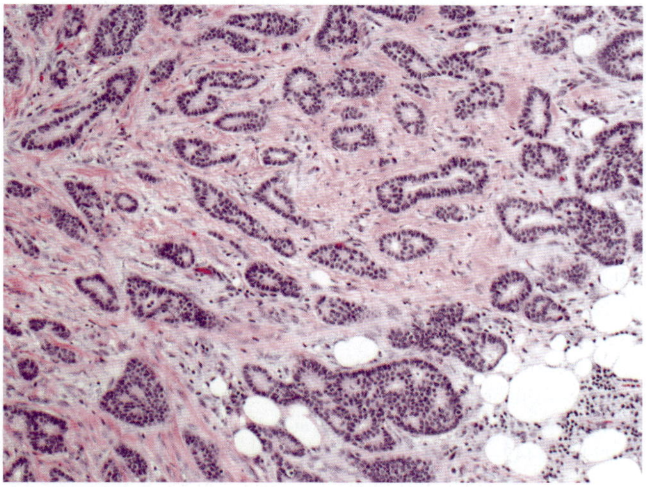

FIGURE 7-15: Coexistence of tubular carcinoma and cribriform carcinoma in one tumor.

CRIBRIFORM CARCINOMA, DIFFERENTIAL DIAGNOSIS

Cribriform DCIS, adenoid cystic carcinoma, and well-differentiated neuroendocrine carcinoma should be differentiated from cribriform carcinoma. Cribriform DCIS maintains the normal ductal and lobular architecture and shows a smooth and rounded contour, whereas invasive cribriform carcinoma typically exhibits, at least in areas, irregular configuration with a haphazard arrangement of tumoral islands. The presence or absence of myoepithelial cells at the periphery of glandular islands can be confirmed by immunostaining in cases of uncertainty.

In contrast to cribriform carcinoma, adenoid cystic carcinoma consists of a dual population of luminal and myoepithelial cells. The presence of intraluminal basement membrane–like material is an important clue. Adenoid cystic carcinoma is almost always negative for ER and PR, while cribriform carcinoma expresses ER in virtually all cases and is mostly positive for PR.

Well-differentiated neuroendocrine carcinoma is extremely rare in the breast. The tumor cells typically demonstrate low-grade nuclei with salt-and-pepper chromatin typically seen in neuroendocrine tumors of other organs.

CRIBRIFORM CARCINOMA, IMMUNOHISTOCHEMISTRY

Similar to tubular carcinoma, cribriform carcinoma typically shows high levels of ER expression in all cases and PR expression in more than two-thirds of cases.[17] The tumor typically lacks HER2 overexpression or gene amplification.

References

1. Sheppard DG, Whitman GJ, Huynh PT, et al. Tubular carcinoma of the breast: mammographic and sonographic features. *AJR Am J Roentgenol* 2000;174:253–257.
2. Feig SA, Shaber GS, Patchefsky AS, et al. Tubular carcinoma of the breast. Mammographic appearance and pathological correlation. *Radiology* 1978;129:311–314.
3. Elson BC, Helvie MA, Frank TS, et al. Tubular carcinoma of the breast: mode of presentation, mammographic appearance, and frequency of nodal metastases. *AJR Am J Roentgenol* 1993;161:1173–1176.

4. Rakha E, Pinder SE, Shin SJ, et al. Tubular carcinoma and cribriform carcinoma. In: Lakhani SR, Ellis IO, Schnitt SJ, et al., eds. *WHO Classification of Tumours of the Breast.* Lyon, France: IARC Press; 2012:43–45.
5. Fernandez-Aguilar S, Simon P, Buxant F, et al. Tubular carcinoma of the breast and associated intra-epithelial lesions: a comparative study with invasive low-grade ductal carcinomas. *Virchows Arch* 2005;447:683–687.
6. Goldstein NS, O'Malley BA. Cancerization of small ectatic ducts of the breast by ductal carcinoma in situ cells with apocrine snouts: a lesion associated with tubular carcinoma. *Am J Clin Pathol* 1997;107:561–566.
7. Rakha EA, Lee AH, Evans AJ, et al. Tubular carcinoma of the breast: further evidence to support its excellent prognosis. *J Clin Oncol* 2010;28:99–104.
8. Brandt SM, Young GQ, Hoda SA. The "Rosen Triad": tubular carcinoma, lobular carcinoma in situ, and columnar cell lesions. *Adv Anat Pathol* 2008;15:140–146.
9. Joshi MG, Lee AK, Pedersen CA, et al. The role of immunocytochemical markers in the differential diagnosis of proliferative and neoplastic lesions of the breast. *Mod Pathol* 1996;9:57–62.
10. Diab SG, Clark GM, Osborne CK, et al. Tumor characteristics and clinical outcome of tubular and mucinous breast carcinomas. *J Clin Oncol* 1999;17:1442–1448.
11. Abdel-Fatah TM, Powe DG, Hodi Z, et al. Morphologic and molecular evolutionary pathways of low nuclear grade invasive breast cancers and their putative precursor lesions: further evidence to support the concept of low nuclear grade breast neoplasia family. *Am J Surg Pathol* 2008;32:513–523.
12. Aulmann S, Elsawaf Z, Penzel R, et al. Invasive tubular carcinoma of the breast frequently is clonally related to flat epithelial atypia and low-grade ductal carcinoma in situ. *Am J Surg Pathol* 2009;33:1646–1653.
13. Man S, Ellis IO, Sibbering M, et al. High levels of allele loss at the FHIT and ATM genes in non-comedo ductal carcinoma in situ and grade I tubular invasive breast cancers. *Cancer Res* 1996;56:5484–5489.
14. Riener MO, Nikolopoulos E, Herr A, et al. Microarray comparative genomic hybridization analysis of tubular breast carcinoma shows recurrent loss of the CDH13 locus on 16q. *Hum Pathol* 2008;39:1621–1629.
15. Waldman FM, Hwang ES, Etzell J, et al. Genomic alterations in tubular breast carcinomas. *Hum Pathol* 2001;32:222–226.
16. Page DL, Dixon JM, Anderson TJ, et al. Invasive cribriform carcinoma of the breast. *Histopathology* 1983;7:525–536.
17. Venable JG, Schwartz AM, Silverberg SG. Infiltrating cribriform carcinoma of the breast: a distinctive clinicopathologic entity. *Hum Pathol* 1990;21:333–338.

Carcinomas with Medullary Features

8

CARCINOMAS WITH MEDULLARY FEATURES, CYTOLOGY

Cytologically, carcinoma with medullary features is composed of large, highly pleomorphic cells with no gland formation or mucin production. The cytoplasm is often delicate and easily strips off of the cells; thus, many naked nuclei are present. Small lymphocytes are interspersed among the tumor cells (Figure 8-1).

CARCINOMAS WITH MEDULLARY FEATURES, IMAGING AND GROSS FEATURES

Carcinomas with medullary features are round, oval, or lobular masses on mammography, MRI, and US with well-circumscribed, indistinct, or microlobulated margins (Figure 8-2).[1,2] Tumors usually have plateau or washout kinetics on MRI.[1] On gross examination, these tumors are typically well-circumscribed masses with soft to moderate consistency. Areas of necrosis and hemorrhage may be present and result in cystic degeneration.

CARCINOMAS WITH MEDULLARY FEATURES, HISTOLOGY

Historically, a diagnosis of medullary carcinoma is made when a tumor has the following morphologic traits: (a) syncytial architecture in greater than 75% of the tumor mass, (b) lack of glandular or tubular formation, (c) diffuse lymphoplasmacytic stromal infiltrate, (d) nuclear grade 2 or 3, and (e) complete histologic circumscription (Figure 8-3).[3–6] Tumors with some but not all features of medullary carcinoma have been classified as "atypical medullary carcinoma" or "invasive ductal carcinoma with medullary features." Medullary carcinomas, when strictly defined by morphologic criteria, reportedly have favorable prognosis. However, the variable stringency of the diagnostic criteria among different authorities rendered it difficult to apply, thus resulting in poor interobserver reproducibility. Therefore, the current WHO Classification recommends that classic medullary carcinoma, atypical medullary carcinoma, and invasive carcinoma with medullary features be grouped within the category of carcinomas with medullary features.[7]

The neoplastic cells are arranged in solid sheets or broad anastomosing bands. Areas of geographic necrosis are commonly present (Figure 8-4), and there is typically minimal collagenous stroma within the tumor. The characteristic lymphoplasmacytic infiltrate is most prominent at the interface of tumor and surrounding stroma (Figure 8-5). Tumor cells have abundant pale to eosinophilic cytoplasm and pleomorphic nuclei with one or more nucleoli (Figure 8-6). Numerous mitotic figures, including atypical forms, are frequently present. Variable metaplastic features may exist, most often being squamous differentiation (Figure 8-7). Multinucleated giant cells may also be seen. Rarely, a DCIS component is present.

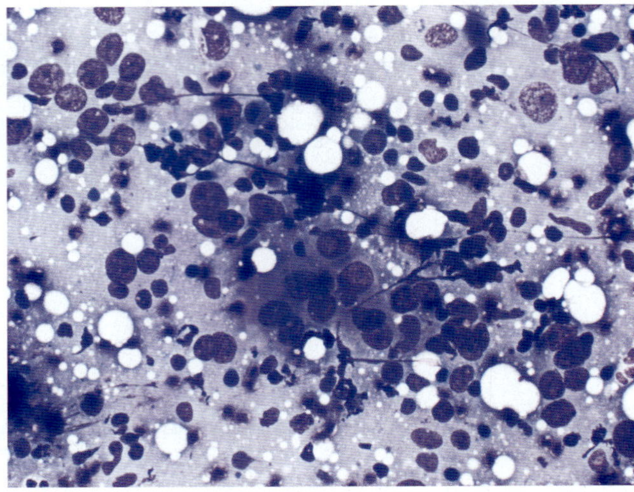

FIGURE 8-1: Carcinoma with medullary features. Diff-Quik stained fine needle aspiration shows discohesive, large, naked nuclei with significant nuclear pleomorphism including irregular nuclear membranes and prominent nucleoli. The cytoplasm is often delicate and easily strips off of the cells. Small lymphocytes are interspersed among the tumor cells. (Photomicrograph courtesy of Amberly L. Nunez, M.D.)

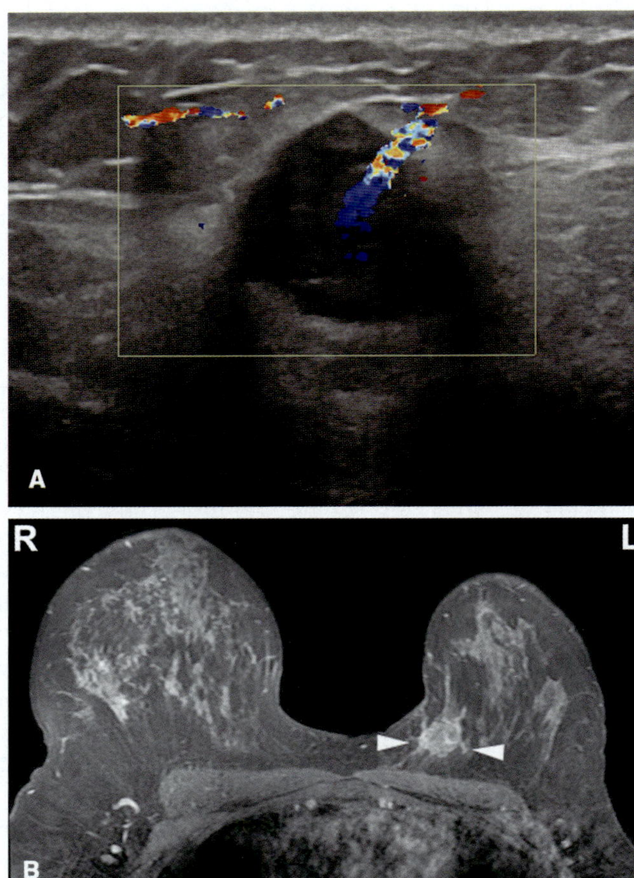

FIGURE 8-2: Imaging features of medullary carcinoma. Color Doppler US image reveals a round hypervascular hypoechoic mass with indistinct margins and posterior acoustic enhancement (**A**). Axial T1-delayed postcontrast fat-saturated image reveals a round mass with microlobulated margins (*arrowheads*) in the left upper inner breast with rim enhancement (**B**).

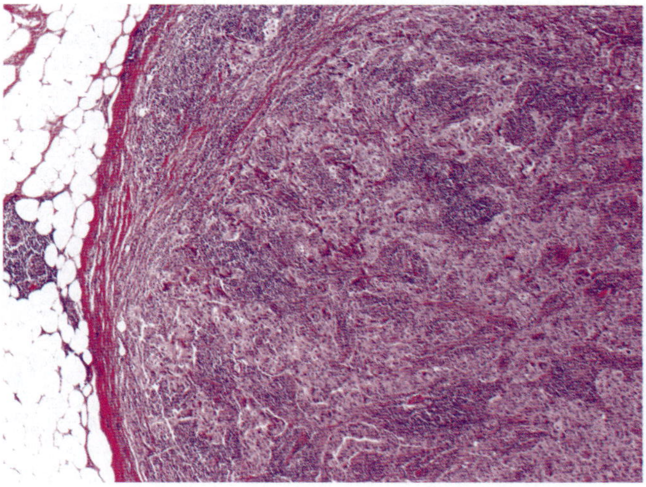

FIGURE 8-3: A low-power view shows a "typical" medullary carcinoma with complete circumscription and syncytial growth. Prominent lymphoplasmacytic infiltrate can also be appreciated at this magnification.

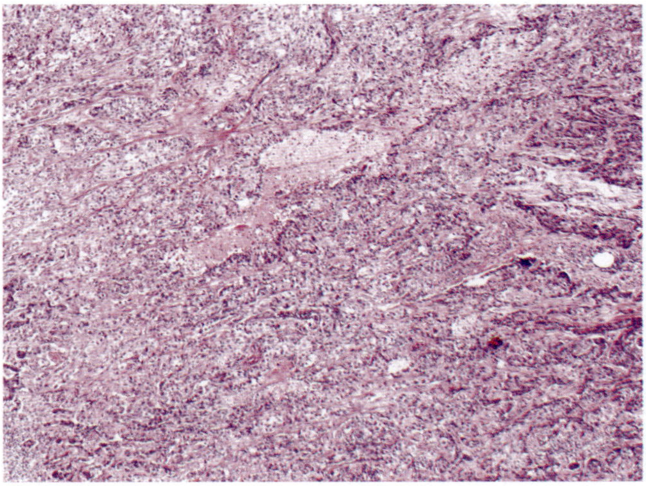

FIGURE 8-4: Medullary carcinoma showing solid growth, geographic necrosis, and cystic degeneration.

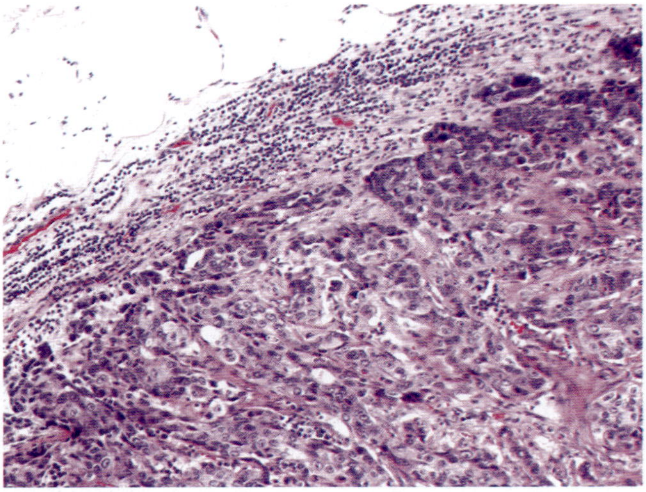

FIGURE 8-5: The lymphoplasmacytic infiltrate in medullary carcinomas is most prominent at the interface of tumor and surrounding stroma.

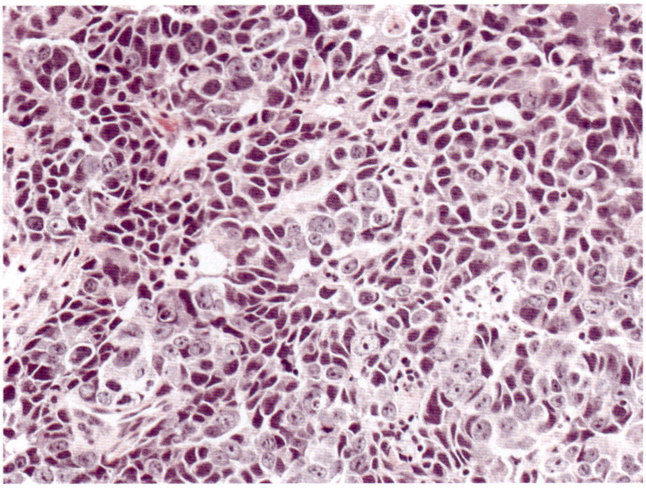

FIGURE 8-6: A high-power view of medullary carcinoma. The tumor invariably demonstrates high-grade, pleomorphic nuclei with one or more nucleoli and abundant pale to eosinophilic cytoplasm.

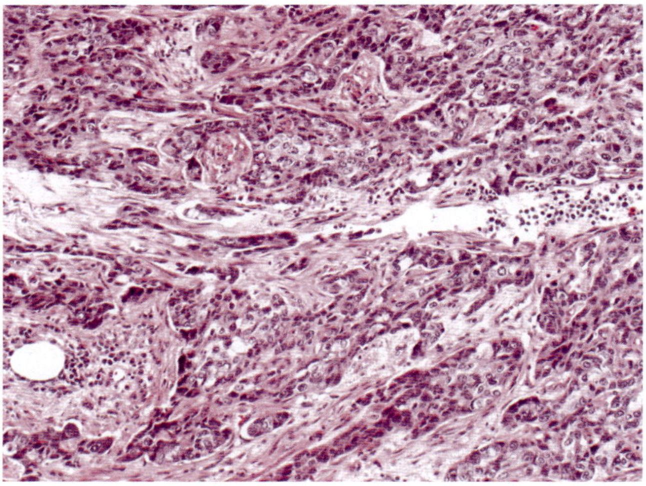

FIGURE 8-7: Medullary carcinoma showing squamous differentiation.

CARCINOMAS WITH MEDULLARY FEATURES, DIFFERENTIAL DIAGNOSIS

Cases with dense lymphoplasmacytic infiltrate obscuring the neoplastic epithelial cells can mimic lymphoma. Immunostains for epithelial and lymphoid markers may become necessary in such cases. In this context, it is preferable to use cytokeratin immunostains over epithelial membrane antigen (EMA) as anaplastic large cell lymphoma (Figure 8-8), increasingly reported in association with breast implants,[8] is usually positive for EMA.

The circumscription of the tumor along with the surrounding prominent lymphoplasmacytic infiltrate may lead to an erroneous impression of intramammary nodal metastasis (Figure 8-9). It is crucial to seek evidence of nodal structure including fibrous capsule and subcapsular sinuses. The presence of germinal centers is not helpful in distinguishing nodal metastasis from a carcinoma with medullar features, as germinal center formation can be associated with the latter.

Of note, the morphology of the exceedingly rare Epstein-Barr virus–associated lymphoepithelial-like carcinoma of the breast[9] is indistinguishable from other carcinomas with medullary features.

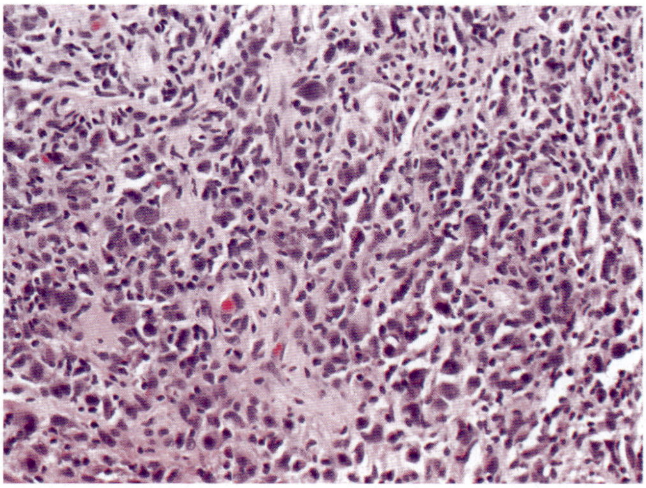

FIGURE 8-8: Anaplastic large cell lymphoma showing large and highly atypical cells in the background of small, reactive lymphocytes, thus representing a great mimicker of medullary carcinoma.

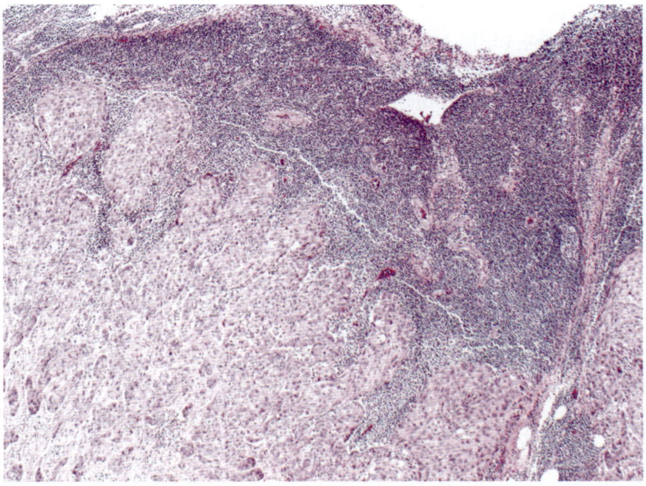

FIGURE 8-9: Metastasis to intramammary lymph node resembling medullary carcinoma. Note the presence of remaining nodal architecture including fibrous capsule and subcapsular sinuses.

CARCINOMAS WITH MEDULLARY FEATURES, IMMUNOHISTOCHEMISTRY

Tumors in this group are mostly "triple negative" (negative for ER, PR, and HER2). The neoplastic cells express luminal cytokeratins (CK8 and CK18), but also show variable expression of basal keratins (CK5/6 and CK14) and epidermal growth factor receptor (EGFR, HER1).

The tumor-infiltrating lymphocytes in medullary carcinomas consist predominantly of CD8+ cytotoxic T cells, consistent with a host immune response against tumor progression.[10,11] Interestingly, a recent study [12] found no significant survival differences between medullary carcinomas and other high-grade ductal carcinomas with prominent inflammation, which argues against separating classic and atypical medullary carcinomas. In addition, a 368-gene "medullary signature" has identified subgroups of basal-like carcinomas with prognostic value.[13] The finding of effective immune response in the good-prognosis subgroup by ontology analysis further supports the prognostic significance of lymphoplasmacytic infiltrate in carcinomas with medullary features.

CARCINOMAS WITH MEDULLARY FEATURES, MOLECULAR GENETICS

A significant proportion of tumors in this group are basal-like subtype by molecular profiling studies.[14] While only a small percentage of patients with carcinomas possessing medullary features were confirmed to have BRCA1 germline mutations,[15] most tumors from patients carrying BRCA1 mutations have medullary features.[16] A high level of BRCA1 promoter hypermethylation was detected in most tumors harboring medullary features without BRCA1 mutations, suggesting a possible role of this gene in the histomorphogenesis of these tumors.[17] TP53 mutations are the most common somatic alteration, disclosed in up to 80% of tumors with medullary features, although a prognostic significance has not been established.[18,19]

References

1. Jeong SJ, Lim HS, Lee JS, et al. Medullary carcinoma of the breast: MRI findings. *AJR Am J Roentgenol* 2012;198:W482–W487.
2. Meyer JE, Amin E, Lindfors KK, et al. Medullary carcinoma of the breast: mammographic and US appearance. *Radiology* 1989;170:79–82.
3. Ridolfi RL, Rosen PP, Port A, et al. Medullary carcinoma of the breast: a clinicopathologic study with 10 year follow-up. *Cancer* 1977;40:1365–1385.
4. Wargotz ES, Silverberg SG. Medullary carcinoma of the breast: a clinicopathologic study with appraisal of current diagnostic criteria. *Hum Pathol* 1988;19:1340–1346.
5. Pedersen L, Zedeler K, Holck S, et al. Medullary carcinoma of the breast, proposal for a new simplified histopathological definition. Based on prognostic observations and observations on inter- and intraobserver variability of 11 histopathological characteristics in 131 breast carcinomas with medullary features. *Br J Cancer* 1991;63:591–595.
6. Pedersen L, Holck S, Schiodt T, et al. Medullary carcinoma of the breast, prognostic importance of characteristic histopathological features evaluated in a multivariate Cox analysis. *Eur J Cancer* 1994;30A:1792–1797.
7. Jacquemier J, Reis-Fiho JS, Lakhani SR, et al. Carcinomas with medullary features. In: Lakhani SR, Ellis IO, Schnitt SJ, et al., eds. *WHO Classification of Tumours of the Breast*. Lyon, France: IARC Press; 2012:46–47.
8. Xu J, Wei S. Breast implant-associated anaplastic large cell lymphoma: review of a distinct clinicopathological entity. *Arch Pathol Lab Med* 2014;138(6):842–846.
9. Bonnet M, Guinebretiere JM, Kremmer E, et al. Detection of Epstein-Barr virus in invasive breast cancers. *J Natl Cancer Inst* 1999;91:1376–1381.
10. Guo X, Fan Y, Lang R, et al. Tumor infiltrating lymphocytes differ in invasive micropapillary carcinoma and medullary carcinoma of breast. *Mod Pathol* 2008;21:1101–1107.
11. Kuroda H, Tamaru J, Sakamoto G, et al. Immunophenotype of lymphocytic infiltration in medullary carcinoma of the breast. *Virchows Arch* 2005;446:10–14.
12. Rakha EA, Aleskandarany M, El-Sayed ME, et al. The prognostic significance of inflammation and medullary histological type in invasive carcinoma of the breast. *Eur J Cancer* 2009;45:1780–1787.
13. Sabatier R, Finetti P, Cervera N, et al. A gene expression signature identifies two prognostic subgroups of basal breast cancer. *Breast Cancer Res Treat* 2011;126:407–420.
14. Bertucci F, Finetti P, Cervera N, et al. Gene expression profiling shows medullary breast cancer is a subgroup of basal breast cancers. *Cancer Res* 2006;66:4636–4644.
15. Lakhani SR, Gusterson BA, Jacquemier J, et al. The pathology of familial breast cancer: histological features of cancers in families not attributable to mutations in BRCA1 or BRCA2. *Clin Cancer Res* 2000;6:782–789.
16. Eisinger F, Jacquemier J, Charpin C, et al. Mutations at BRCA1: the medullary breast carcinoma revisited. *Cancer Res* 1998;58:1588–1592.
17. Osin P, Lu YJ, Stone J, et al. Distinct genetic and epigenetic changes in medullary breast cancer. *Int J Surg Pathol* 2003;11:153–158.
18. Dendale R, Vincent-Salomon A, Mouret-Fourme E, et al. Medullary breast carcinoma: prognostic implications of p53 expression. *Int J Biol Markers* 2003;18:99–105.
19. Vincent-Salomon A, Gruel N, Lucchesi C, et al. Identification of typical medullary breast carcinoma as a genomic sub-group of basal-like carcinomas, a heterogeneous new molecular entity. *Breast Cancer Res* 2007;9:R24.

Metaplastic Carcinomas

9

Metaplastic carcinomas of the breast encompass a broad spectrum of tumors in which the neoplastic epithelium undergoes, at least in part, nonglandular differentiation. The metaplastic elements may have differentiation of another epithelial type (e.g., squamous metaplasia) but, more commonly, take on the appearance of differentiated or undifferentiated mesenchyme, including but not limited to spindled, chondroid, osseous, and rhabdomyoid cells. The metaplastic components, be they in pure form or mixed, may range from a small focus to completely comprising the tumor.

Surpluses of terminology have been used in the literature to describe subgroups of metaplastic carcinomas. In addition to those introduced in this chapter, other terms that have been coined include carcinosarcoma, sarcomatoid carcinoma, carcinoma with pseudosarcomatous metaplasia, and matrix-producing carcinoma.[1]

METAPLASTIC CARCINOMA, CYTOLOGY

The cytologic features of metaplastic carcinomas vary significantly among different histologic variants. Those with squamous differentiation are essentially indistinguishable from squamous cell carcinoma (Figures 9-1 and 9-2). Carcinomas with osseous or chondroid differentiation may exhibit osteoblasts, osteoclasts, chondrocytes, and/or extracellular bone or cartilage matrix (Figure 9-3). Alternatively, a high-grade metaplastic carcinoma may show frankly sarcomatoid features (Figure 9-4).

METAPLASTIC CARCINOMA, IMAGING AND GROSS FEATURES

There is no distinctive imaging or growth appearance of metaplastic carcinoma (Figure 9-5). The lesion can be well circumscribed or infiltrative. These tumors tend to be large (mean size of 3.9 cm; range, 1.2 to larger than 10 cm).[2,3] Cystic degeneration is frequent, particularly in those with squamous differentiation.

METAPLASTIC CARCINOMA, HISTOLOGIC VARIANTS

Low-Grade Adenosquamous Carcinoma

Low-grade adenosquamous carcinoma is a rare variant of metaplastic carcinoma. It comprises haphazardly arranged tumor nests with an infiltrative growth pattern in a spindle cell stroma (Figure 9-6). These nests of tumor cells are composed of admixture of well-formed glandular structures and solid cords of cells with squamous differentiation (Figure 9-7). The glandular elements are typically small and have rounded contours. They may be elongated but are not angulated. The solid epithelial nests contain squamous cells with occasional keratin pearls. Formation

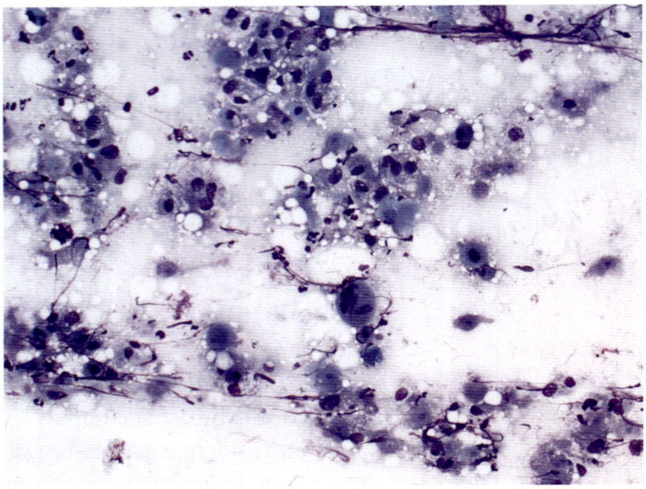

FIGURE 9-1: Metaplastic carcinoma (squamous cell carcinoma). Diff-Quik stained fine needle aspiration shows abundant single cells with irregular, smudgy nuclei, and dense blue cytoplasm, characteristic of keratinization by Romanowsky staining method. (Photomicrograph courtesy of Amberly L. Nunez, M.D.)

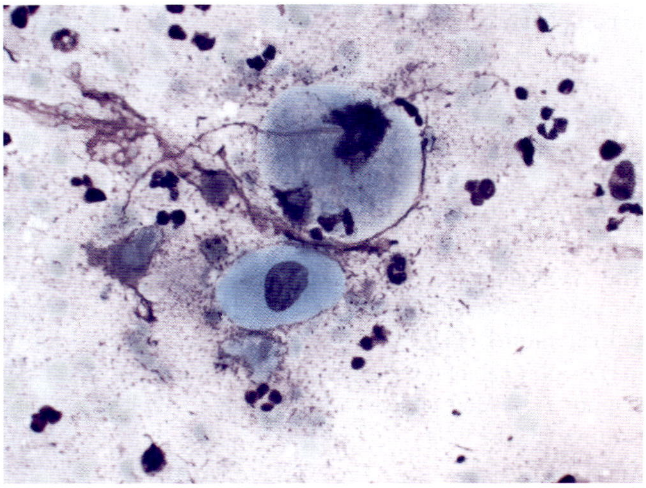

FIGURE 9-2: Metaplastic carcinoma (squamous cell carcinoma). A high-power view shows single cells with abundant "robin's egg blue" cytoplasm and sharp cytoplasmic membranes. Granular amorphous debris and inflammatory cells are present in the background. (Diff-Quik stain; photomicrograph courtesy of Amberly L. Nunez, M.D.)

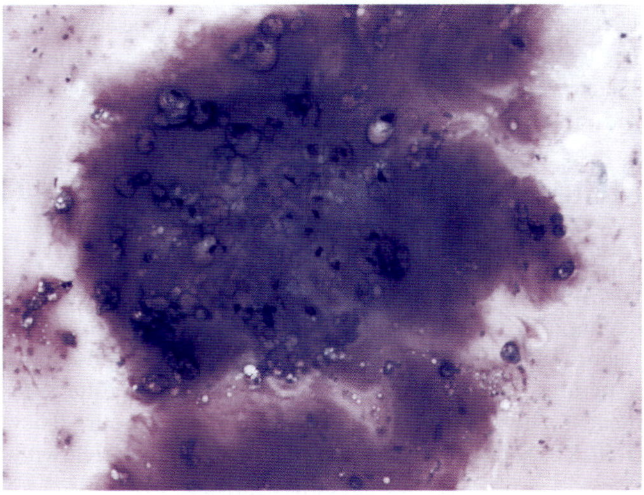

FIGURE 9-3: Metaplastic carcinoma with chondroid differentiation. Metachromatic cartilaginous matrix with numerous lacunae containing chondrocytes with small, round, condensed nuclei. (Diff-Quik stain; photomicrograph courtesy of Amberly L. Nunez, M.D.)

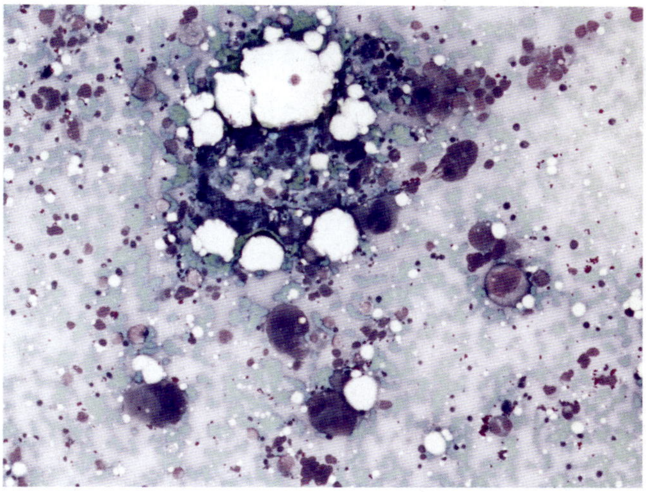

FIGURE 9-4: Metaplastic carcinoma with sarcomatoid features. Highly atypical cells containing bizarre, multiple nuclei and/or nuclear lobes with significant pleomorphism. Inflammatory cells are present within the background. (Diff-Quik stain; photomicrograph courtesy of Amberly L. Nunez, M.D.)

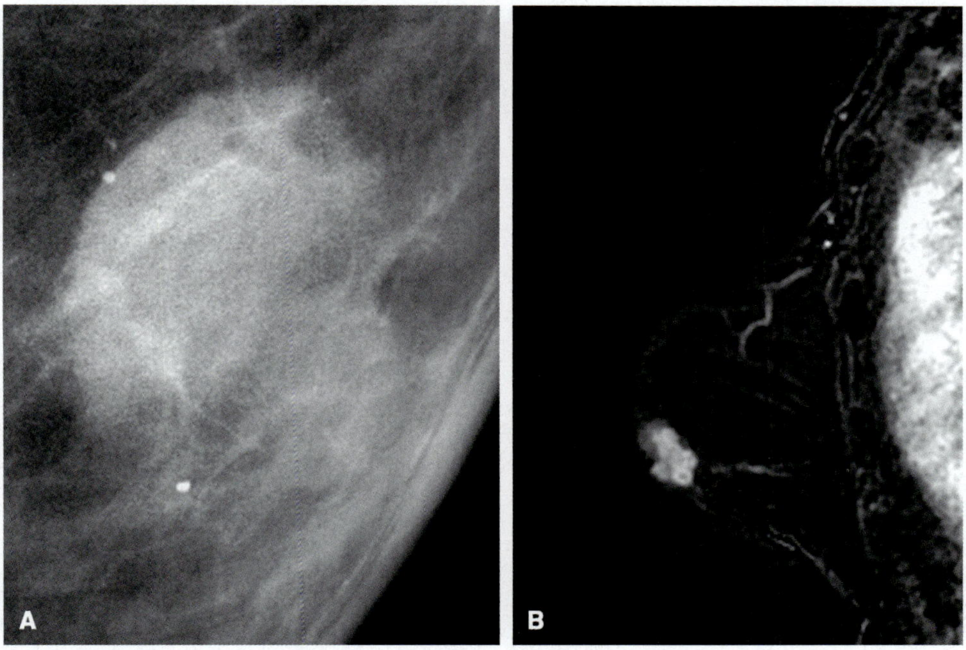

FIGURE 9-5: Imaging features of metaplastic carcinoma. A left craniocaudal mammographic view shows an oval hyperdense superficial mass with microlobulated margins (**A**). An MRI sagittal subtraction image reveals an enhancing oval mass in the left lower inner breast with irregular margins (**B**).

of microcysts filled with keratinaceous material is not uncommon (Figure 9-8). The spindle cells in the background stroma are typically cellular and may have a fibromatosis-like appearance. A possible association has been postulated between these tumors and benign proliferative sclerosing lesions as well as adenomyoepithelioma.[4–6]

Differential diagnostic considerations include syringomatous adenoma of the nipple and, less likely, tubular carcinoma in cases with prominent tubular formation.

Fibromatosis-like Metaplastic Carcinoma

Low-grade, fibromatosis-like metaplastic carcinoma is a peculiar variant of metaplastic carcinoma. It is so named because the tumor is predominantly or almost completely composed of

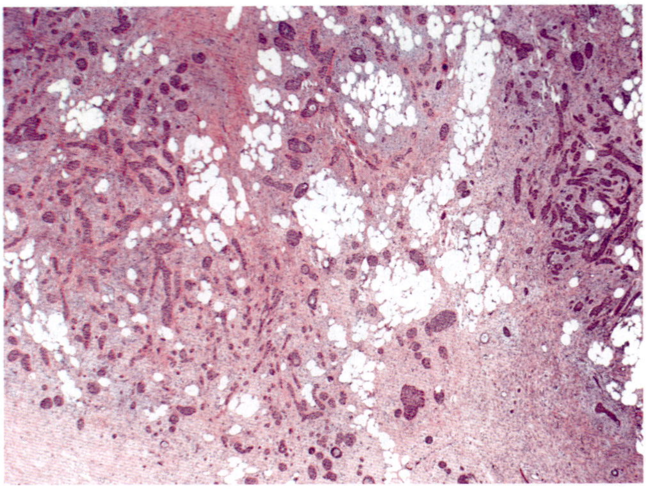

FIGURE 9-6: A low-power view of low-grade adenosquamous carcinoma shows haphazardly arranged tumor nests with an infiltrative growth pattern.

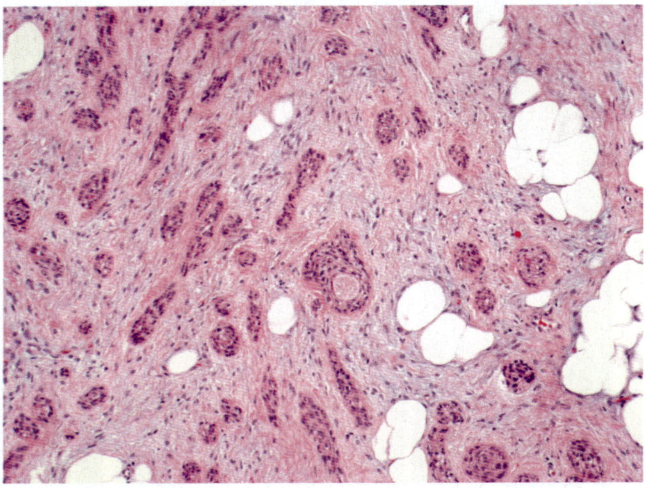

FIGURE 9-7: Low-grade adenosquamous carcinoma is composed of a variable admixture of glandular structures and squamous cell nests.

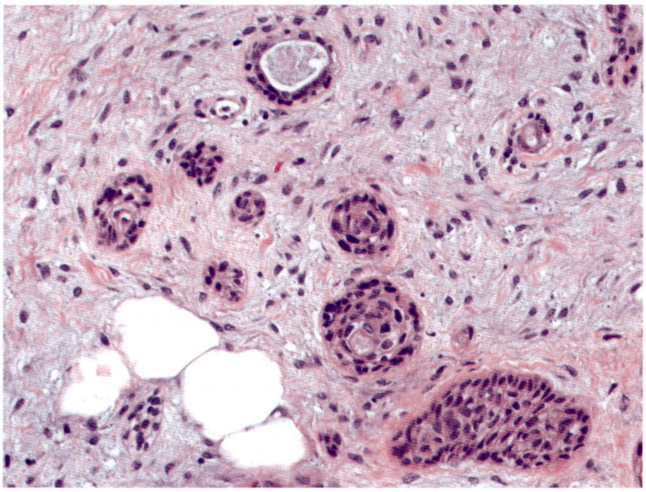

FIGURE 9-8: The glandular structures in low-grade adenosquamous carcinoma are typically small and rounded, while the squamous cell nests are usually solid and may contain occasional keratin pearls.

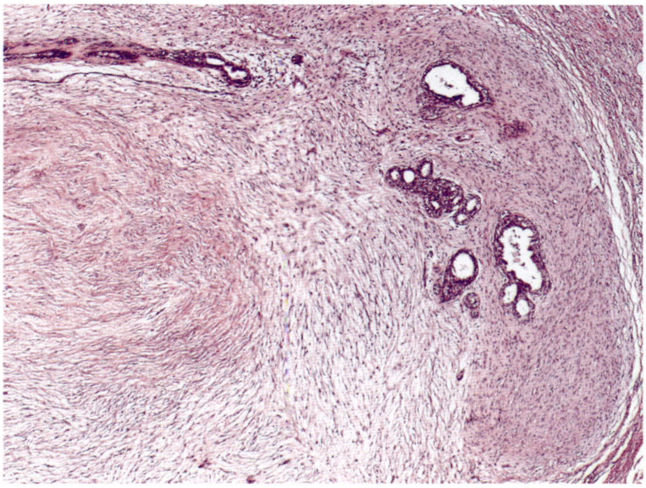

FIGURE 9-9: Fibromatosis-like metaplastic carcinoma. The tumor has an infiltrative growth pattern and is exclusively composed of bland spindle cells simulating those seen in fibromatosis.

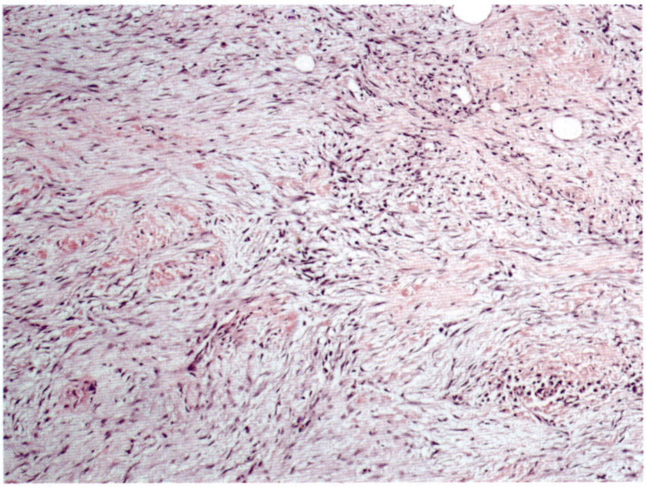

FIGURE 9-10: Fibromatosis-like metaplastic carcinoma showing bland spindle cells arranged in interlacing fascicles with a background of collagenized stroma.

bland spindle cells closely resembling those seen in fibromatosis or scar tissue (Figure 9-9).[7,8] The neoplastic cells are arranged in wavy, interlacing short fascicles or form long fascicles embedded in varying degrees of collagenized stroma (Figure 9-10). The lesion typically infiltrates normal glandular structures and adipose tissue, similar to fibromatosis. When involving deep dermis, the tumor may lead to an erroneous impression of a skin lesion (Figure 9-11). The cellularity varies from region to region. At higher magnification, the lesional cells exhibit pale eosinophilic cytoplasm and bland nuclei with tapered ends closely simulating reactive fibroblasts. Areas with plump spindled or epithelioid cells are frequently seen. Focal squamous differentiation in the epithelioid cell clusters may also be found.[1]

The diagnosis of fibromatosis-like metaplastic carcinoma invariably relies on the expression of epithelial markers, given that it is histologically indistinguishable from its benign mimickers. The intensity and proportion of lesional cells expressing cytokeratins varies significantly among these tumors. Like most other metaplastic carcinomas, p63 and high molecular weight cytokeratins (CK5/6 and CK903/34βE12) are more sensitive in diagnosing these tumors, although they may rarely express low molecular weight cytokeratins.

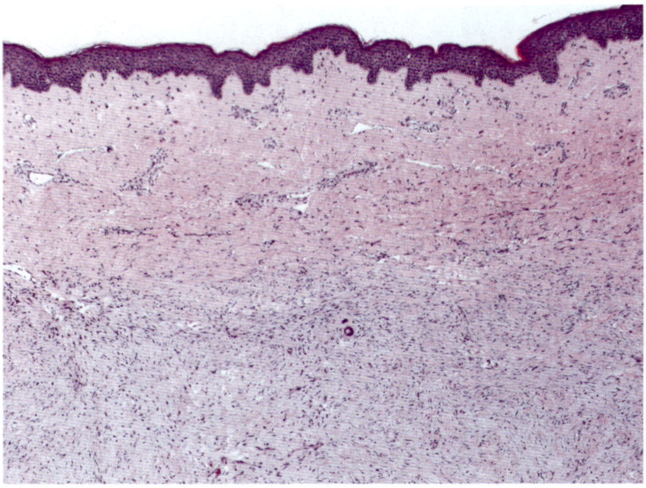

FIGURE 9-11: Fibromatosis-like metaplastic carcinoma involving the dermis closely mimics dermatofibroma.

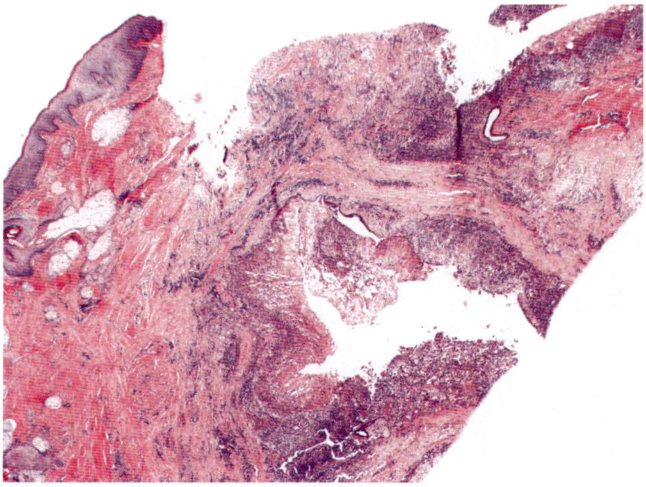

FIGURE 9-12: Carcinoma with squamous differentiation arising in the nipple–areolar region.

Squamous Cell Carcinoma

Although a pure form of squamous carcinoma of the breast does exist, it occurs more commonly in association with invasive carcinoma of no special type, or arises from glands with squamous metaplasia (Figure 9-12). Thus, a diagnosis of primary squamous cell carcinoma requires appropriate workup to rule out metastasis from other origin, especially skin.[9] Squamous cell carcinoma usually occurs adjacent to a cystic structure or exhibits prominent cystic degeneration (Figure 9-13).[9] A component of squamous cell carcinoma *in situ* may also be present in a cyst wall or duct (Figure 9-14). The squamous elements can vary from well to poorly differentiated and from keratinizing to nonkeratinizing. Extensive tumor necrosis is frequently seen, similar to squamous cell carcinomas of other organ systems. The cystic changes may become so pronounced that the tumor may partially present with squamous epithelium–lined cysts, thus mimicking infundibular cysts of skin (Figure 9-15). Rarely, the tumor may have an acantholytic growth pattern that forms pseudovascular spaces resembling angiosarcoma.[10]

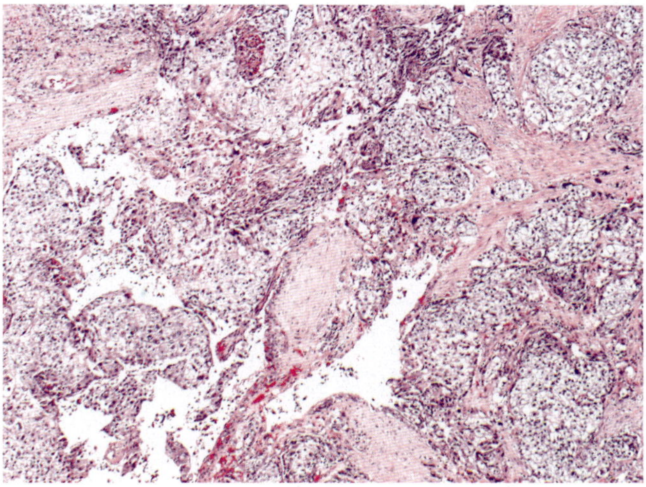

FIGURE 9-13: Squamous cell carcinoma exhibiting prominent cystic degeneration.

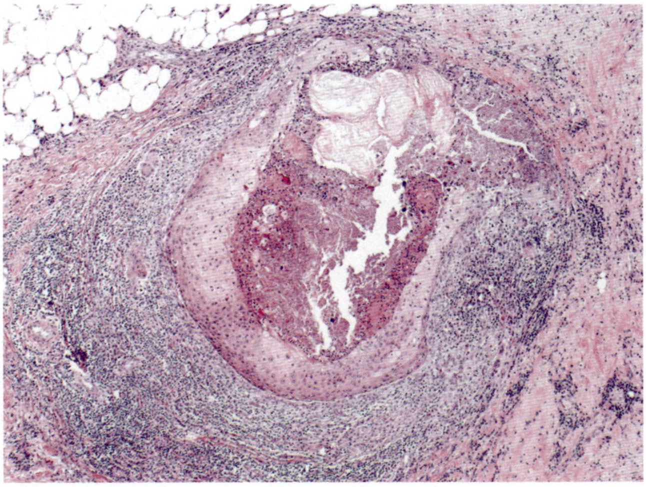

FIGURE 9-14: Squamous cell carcinoma *in situ* involving a large duct.

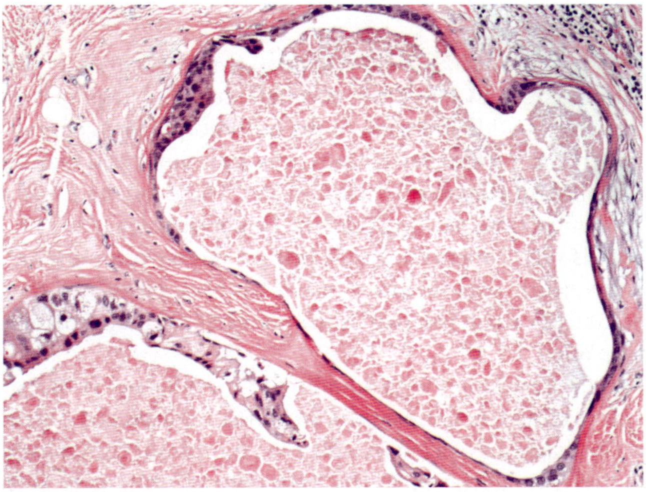

FIGURE 9-15: Squamous cell carcinoma shows extensive tumor necrosis and pronounced cystic changes, resulting in an architecture simulating infundibular cyst of skin.

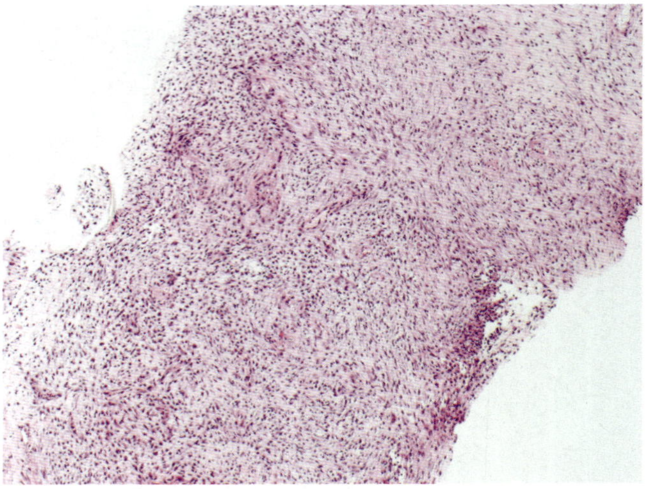

FIGURE 9-16: A low-power view of spindle cell carcinoma in a core needle biopsy.

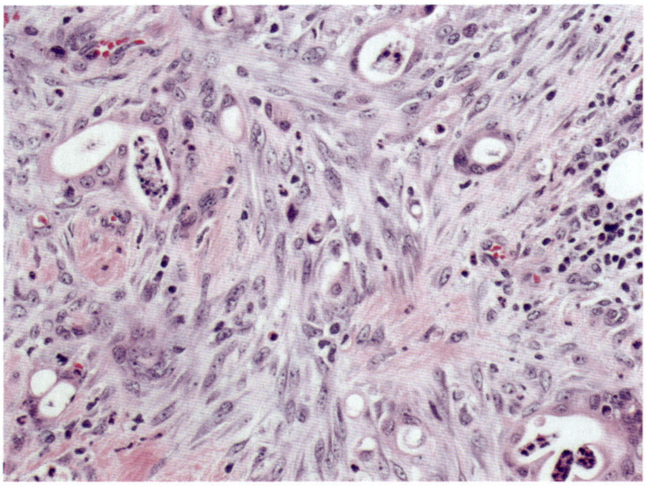

FIGURE 9-17: Spindle cell carcinoma showing admixture of spindle cells and glandular elements.

Spindle Cell Carcinoma

Spindle cell differentiation is commonly seen in metaplastic carcinomas. It may occur as a pure spindle cell carcinoma (Figure 9-16) or present as an admixture of spindle cells and glandular or heterologous elements (Figure 9-17). There is a wide spectrum in the histomorphologic appearances of spindle cell carcinoma.[11,12] The growth pattern varies from tumor to tumor and may be fascicular, storiform, fasciitis-like, or haphazard (Figures 9-18 and 9-19). These lesions usually have infiltrative margins but may also demonstrate pushing borders. Lymphoplasmacytic infiltrate is commonly present. The tumor cells vary from cytologically bland to highly pleomorphic. Focal squamous cell differentiation is frequently seen (Figure 9-20). It has been postulated that this group of tumors constitutes a spectrum of carcinomas, with squamous cell carcinoma on one end and myoepithelial carcinoma on the other.[13]

While the differential diagnosis of a breast lesion with spindle cell morphology is broad, any spindle cell proliferation should be regarded as spindle cell carcinoma until proved otherwise, especially on needle core biopsy. The diagnosis of a lesion with a carcinomatous component (also known as *carcinosarcoma*) is relatively straightforward. The "monophasic" tumors lacking an identifiable epithelial element typically require one or more epithelial markers, preferably p63

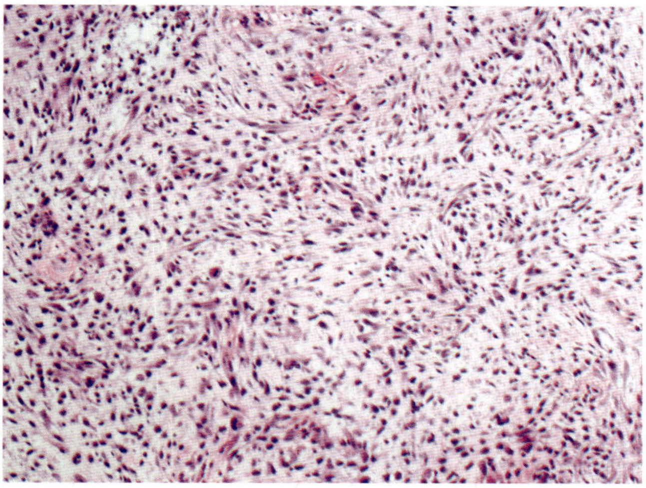

FIGURE 9-18: Spindle cell carcinoma with a storiform growth pattern.

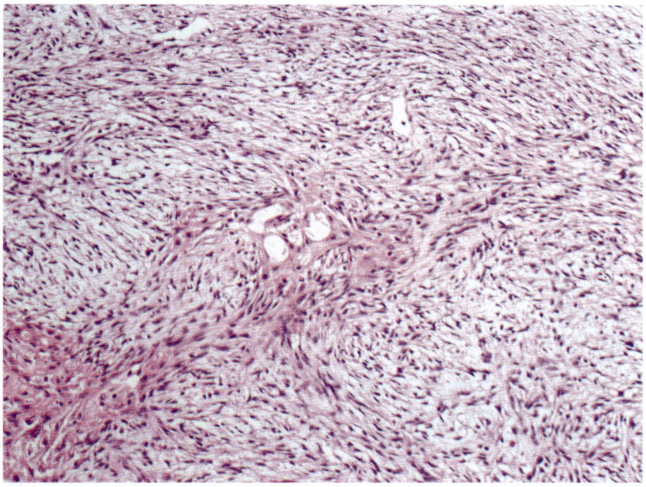

FIGURE 9-19: Fasciitis-like spindle cell carcinoma.

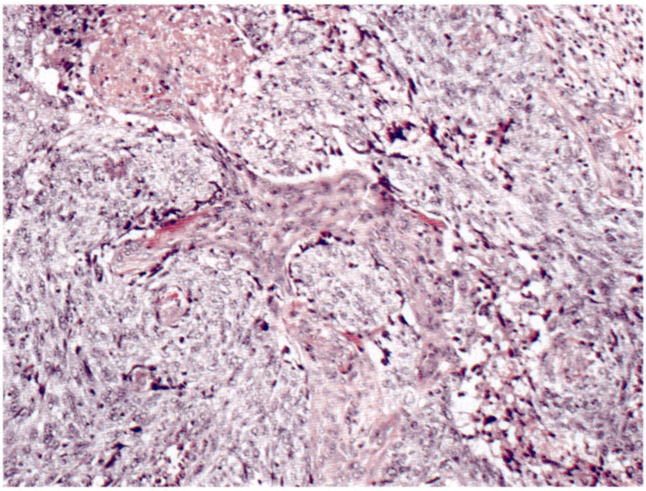

FIGURE 9-20: Areas of squamous cell differentiation are not uncommon in spindle cell carcinoma.

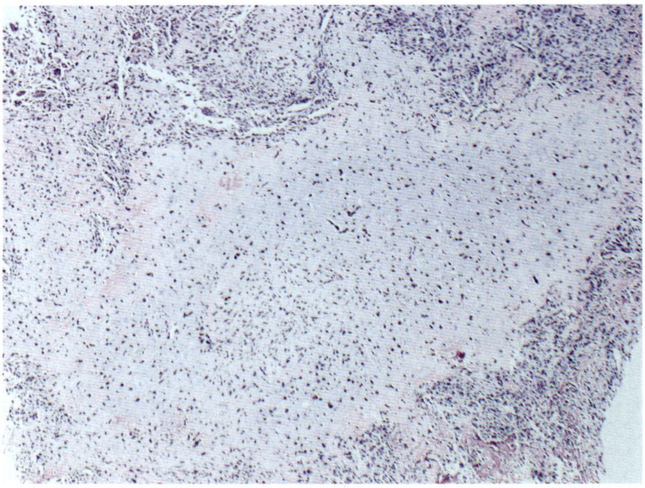

FIGURE 9-21: Matrix-producing carcinoma showing prominent chondroid differentiation.

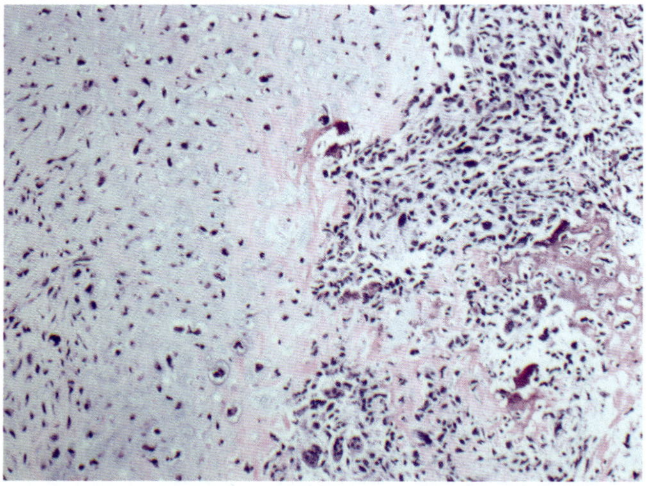

FIGURE 9-22: Matrix-producing carcinoma showing chondrosarcomatous and osteosarcomatous elements.

and high molecular weight cytokeratins, to demonstrate the epithelial nature. Furthermore, the presence of DCIS within the lesion or in the neighboring tissue should prompt the pathologist to render a diagnosis of spindle cell carcinoma. Once a spindle cell carcinoma is ruled out, other spindle cell malignancies such as malignant phyllodes tumor and primary sarcoma should be given serious diagnostic consideration.

Carcinoma with Mesenchymal Differentiation

Carcinoma with mesenchymal differentiation is the most common heterologous metaplastic carcinoma, frequently referred to as *matrix-producing carcinoma*.[14] In addition to a carcinomatous element, the admixed nonepithelial component may show a variety of mesenchymal differentiation, including cartilaginous, osseous, rhabdomyoid, or even neuroglial lineage (Figures 9-21 to 9-24).[15,16] The mesenchymal components, most frequently cartilage and bone, may range from normal appearing to frankly malignant, recapitulating high-grade chondrosarcoma and osteosarcoma, respectively. In cases with predominant heterologous metaplastic component, the epithelial element may be minimal or absent, thus necessitating a panel of immunohistochemical stains to document their epithelial nature. It should be noted that the expression of epithelial markers is typically focal and weak in these tumors; thus, extensive tissue sampling is required. The presence of DCIS in sarcomatous lesions, even in the absence of epithelial differentiation by histomorphology and immunophenotype, argues in favor of metaplastic carcinoma.

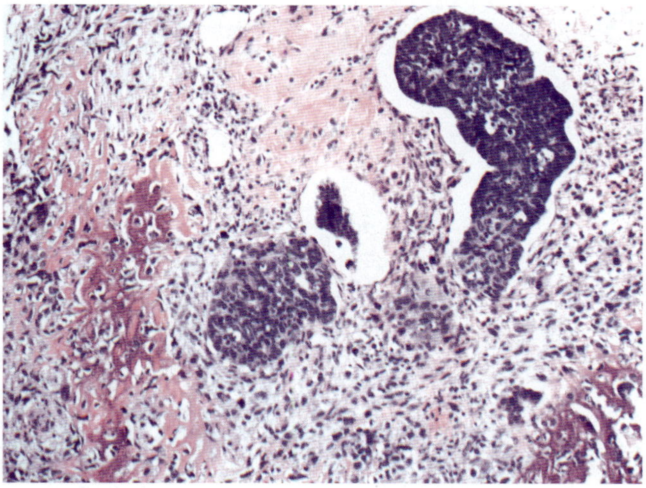

FIGURE 9-23: Matrix-producing carcinoma showing admixture of osseous elements and obvious high-grade carcinoma.

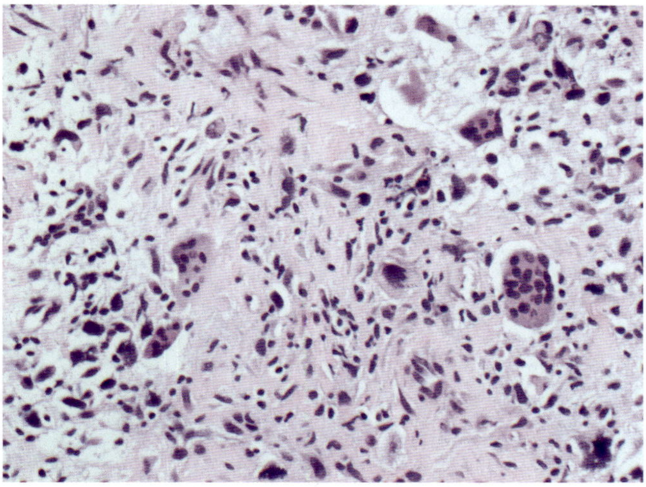

FIGURE 9-24: Matrix-producing carcinoma showing abundant osteoclasts and subtle osteoid production.

METAPLASTIC CARCINOMA, DIFFERENTIAL DIAGNOSIS

A carcinoma with squamous differentiation warrants further workup to rule out cutaneous primary. A spindle cell or sarcomatous lesion of breast should be regarded as metaplastic carcinoma until proved otherwise. Once the diagnosis of metaplastic carcinoma is completely excluded, the differential diagnostic consideration includes phyllodes tumor and primary or metastatic sarcoma. While a number of specific types of primary sarcoma have been documented in the breast, angiosarcoma is the most common primary mammary sarcoma, which more commonly occurs in the site of prior radiation.

METAPLASTIC CARCINOMA, IMMUNOHISTOCHEMISTRY

Given the absence, or only focal presence, of morphologic evidence of epithelial differentiation in some cases of metaplastic carcinoma, the immunoexpression of one or more epithelial markers is often needed for the diagnosis. In practice, a panel of immunohistochemical stains is typically performed as the commonly used antibodies have variable sensitivities for identification of epithelial differentiation. In this regard, metaplastic carcinomas may only demonstrate focal (or no) immunoreactivity with antibodies directed against broad-spectrum (AE1/AE3) and low molecular weight cytokeratins (e.g., CAM5.2), and antibodies directed against high molecular weight cytokeratins (such as CK 5/6, CK903/34βE12, and CK14) are often more sensitive in this setting

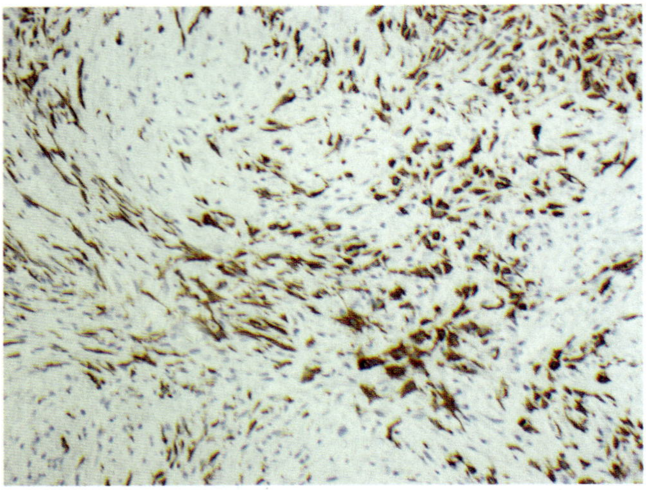

FIGURE 9-25: A CK5/6 immunostain in a spindle cell carcinoma. Note that only a subset of tumor cells express the epithelial marker.

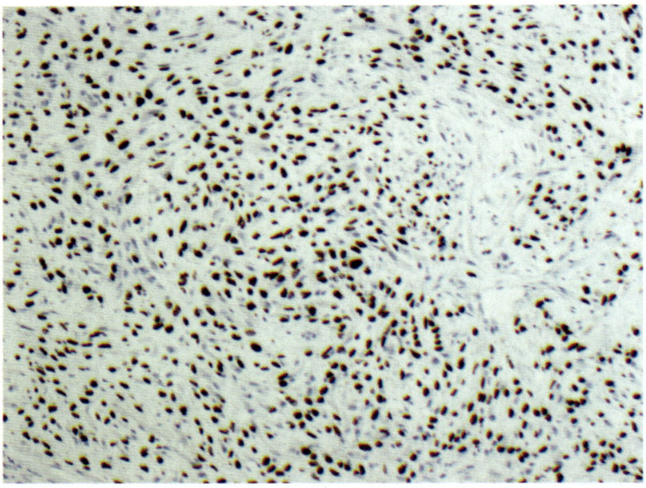

FIGURE 9-26: A p63 stain in the spindle cell carcinoma seen in Figure 9-25 labels more lesional cells than does CK5/6.

(Figure 9-25).[15,17] p63, a member of the p53 family of transcription factors, is expressed in both squamous cells and myoepithelial cells. Expression of p63 has been reportedly seen in greater than 90% of metaplastic carcinomas, rendering it a superior marker in this setting (Figure 9-26).[1,15,18,19] Further, p63 is typically negative in stromal fibroblasts/myofibroblasts and phyllodes tumor and thus is most advantageous in differentiating metaplastic carcinoma from phyllodes tumor with stromal overgrowth.[20] Additional useful markers in this scenario include CD34 and BCL2, which are both negative in metaplastic carcinomas but frequently expressed in phyllodes tumors.[20] One should also note that, in addition to epithelial markers, metaplastic carcinomas often express one or more mesenchymal markers such as vimentin and smooth muscle actin.

The vast majority (>90%) of metaplastic carcinomas are negative for ER, PR, and HER2.[1]

METAPLASTIC CARCINOMA, HISTOGENESIS

The histogenesis of metaplastic carcinoma remains controversial. These tumors mostly arise *de novo,* but an association with a variety of benign fibrosclerotic lesions has also been reported, including papillomas, complex sclerosing lesions, and nipple adenomas.[6] Recent immunohistochemical and gene expression profiling studies indicate that many of these tumors, particularly those with spindle cell morphology, are part of the spectrum of basal-like carcinomas and display a myoepithelial or epithelial to mesenchymal transition-like molecular makeup.[21–23]

References

1. Reis-Fiho JS, Lakhani SR, Gobbi D, et al. Metaplastic carcinomas. In: Lakhani SR, Ellis IO, Schnitt SJ, et al., eds. *WHO Classification of Tumours of the Breast.* Lyon, France: IARC Press; 2012:45–52.
2. Pezzi CM, Patel-Parekh L, Cole K, et al. Characteristics and treatment of metaplastic breast cancer: analysis of 892 cases from the National Cancer Data Base. *Ann Surg Oncol* 2007;14:166–173.
3. Chhieng C, Cranor M, Lesser ME, et al. Metaplastic carcinoma of the breast with osteocartilaginous heterologous elements. *Am J Surg Pathol* 1998;22:188–194.
4. Van Hoeven KH, Drudis T, Cranor ML, et al. Low-grade adenosquamous carcinoma of the breast. A clinicopathologic study of 32 cases with ultrastructural analysis. *Am J Surg Pathol* 1993;17:248–258.
5. Foschini MP, Pizzicannella G, Peterse JL, et al. Adenomyoepithelioma of the breast associated with low-grade adenosquamous and sarcomatoid carcinomas. *Virchows Arch* 1995;427:243–250.
6. Gobbi H, Simpson JF, Jensen RA, et al. Metaplastic spindle cell breast tumors arising within papillomas, complex sclerosing lesions, and nipple adenomas. *Mod Pathol* 2003;16:893–901.
7. Gobbi H, Simpson JF, Borowsky A, et al. Metaplastic breast tumors with a dominant fibromatosis-like phenotype have a high risk of local recurrence. *Cancer* 1999;85:2170–2182.
8. Sneige N, Yaziji H, Mandavilli SR, et al. Low-grade (fibromatosis-like) spindle cell carcinoma of the breast. *Am J Surg Pathol* 2001;25:1009–1016.
9. Wargotz ES, Norris HJ. Metaplastic carcinomas of the breast. IV. Squamous cell carcinoma of ductal origin. *Cancer* 1990;65:272–276.
10. Eusebi V, Lamovec J, Cattani MG, et al. Acantholytic variant of squamous-cell carcinoma of the breast. *Am J Surg Pathol* 1986;10:855–861.
11. Wargotz ES, Deos PH, Norris HJ. Metaplastic carcinomas of the breast. II. Spindle cell carcinoma. *Hum Pathol* 1989;20:732–740.
12. Wargotz ES, Norris HJ. Metaplastic carcinomas of the breast. III. Carcinosarcoma. *Cancer* 1989;64:1490–1499.
13. Hungermann D, Buerger H, Oehlschlegel C, et al. Adenomyoepithelial tumours and myoepithelial carcinomas of the breast—a spectrum of monophasic and biphasic tumours dominated by immature myoepithelial cells. *BMC Cancer* 2005;5:92.
14. Wargotz ES, Norris HJ. Metaplastic carcinomas of the breast. I. Matrix-producing carcinoma. *Hum Pathol* 1989;20:628–635.
15. Carter MR, Hornick JL, Lester S, et al. Spindle cell (sarcomatoid) carcinoma of the breast: a clinicopathologic and immunohistochemical analysis of 29 cases. *Am J Surg Pathol* 2006;30:300–309.
16. Downs-Kelly E, Nayeemuddin KM, Albarracin C, et al. Matrix-producing carcinoma of the breast: an aggressive subtype of metaplastic carcinoma. *Am J Surg Pathol* 2009;33:534–541.
17. Adem C, Reynolds C, Adlakha H, et al. Wide spectrum screening keratin as a marker of metaplastic spindle cell carcinoma of the breast: an immunohistochemical study of 24 patients. *Histopathology* 2002;40:556–562.
18. Koker MM, Kleer CG. p63 expression in breast cancer: a highly sensitive and specific marker of metaplastic carcinoma. *Am J Surg Pathol* 2004;28:1506–1512.
19. Reis-Filho JS, Schmitt FC. p63 expression in sarcomatoid/metaplastic carcinomas of the breast. *Histopathology* 2003;42:94–95.
20. Dunne B, Lee AH, Pinder SE, et al. An immunohistochemical study of metaplastic spindle cell carcinoma, phyllodes tumor and fibromatosis of the breast. *Hum Pathol* 2003;34:1009–1015.
21. Leibl S, Gogg-Kammerer M, Sommersacher A, et al. Metaplastic breast carcinomas: are they of myoepithelial differentiation? Immunohistochemical profile of the sarcomatoid subtype using novel myoepithelial markers. *Am J Surg Pathol* 2005;29:347–353.
22. Reis-Filho JS, Milanezi F, Steele D, et al. Metaplastic breast carcinomas are basal-like tumours. *Histopathology* 2006;49:10–21.
23. Weigelt B, Kreike B, Reis-Filho JS. Metaplastic breast carcinomas are basal-like breast cancers: a genomic profiling analysis. *Breast Cancer Res Treat* 2009;117:273–280.

10 Carcinomas with Apocrine Differentiation

Apocrine metaplasia, characterized by morphologic appearance resembling apocrine sweat glands, is a fairly common finding in normal mammary glands. Similarly, apocrine differentiation is not uncommon in invasive and *in situ* carcinomas. However, carcinomas with exclusive apocrine differentiation are rare, constituting only 1% to 4% of invasive carcinomas.[1,2] Apocrine carcinoma has been previously defined as a tumor where greater than 90% of tumor cells display cytologic and immunohistochemical features of apocrine cells. As such, "apocrine carcinoma" includes a heterogeneous group of neoplasms rather than a distinct clinicopathologic entity. Thus, tumors with apocrine differentiation are still characterized based on their underlying histologic pattern.[2–5]

CARCINOMA WITH APOCRINE DIFFERENTIATION, CYTOLOGY

Cytologically, the cells of carcinomas with apocrine differentiation typically have abundant, fine granular cytoplasm and enlarged nuclei with coarsely clumped chromatin and prominent nucleoli (Figures 10-1 and 10-2). The cytoplasm may stain variably gray purple in Diff-Quik stain and pink to blue gray in Papanicolaou stain. Binucleation can be occasionally seen (Figure 10-3).

CARCINOMA WITH APOCRINE DIFFERENTIATION, IMAGING AND GROSS FEATURES

The radiologic appearance of carcinomas with apocrine differentiation is variable. These lesions may present as a well-circumscribed mass or irregular, non–mass-like enhancement (Figures 10-4 and 10-5). Similarly, there are no distinct macroscopic features for carcinomas with apocrine differentiation.

CARCINOMA WITH APOCRINE DIFFERENTIATION, HISTOLOGY

Carcinomas with apocrine differentiation may have various histologic patterns, mostly showing that of no special type but can also be tubular, lobular, micropapillary, and medullary.[5] The tumor cells are typically large in size with abundant acidophilic cytoplasm with eosinophilic granules (Figure 10-6). The cells characteristically have large, round, central, or eccentric vesicular nuclei with one or more prominent nucleoli, but may also show nuclear hyperchromasia (Figure 10-7). The cytoplasm of the constituent cells varies from intensely eosinophilic showing diastase-resistant periodic acid–Schiff positivity (so-called type A cells; Figure 10-8) to foamy, vacuolated

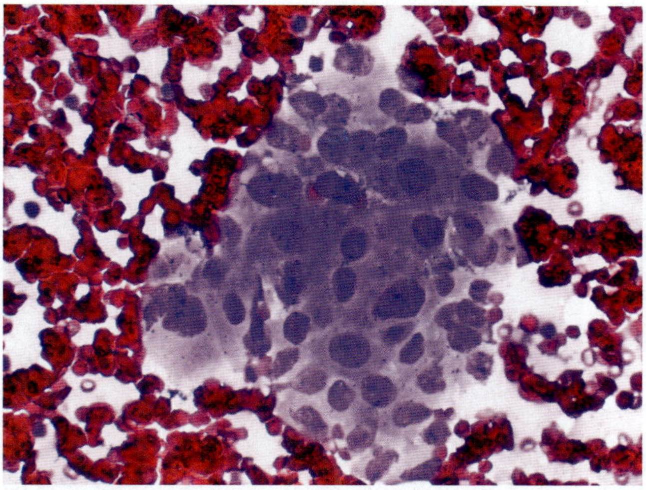

FIGURE 10-1: Apocrine carcinoma. Diff-Quik stained fine needle aspiration shows a sheet of epithelial cells with apocrine features characterized by abundant, finely granular cytoplasm. The cells demonstrate marked atypia including overlapping, enlarged nuclei, and irregular nuclear membranes. (Photomicrograph courtesy of Amberly L. Nunez, M.D.)

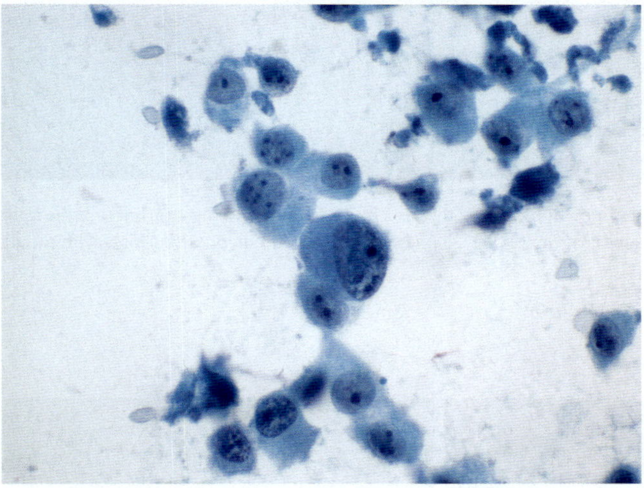

FIGURE 10-2: Apocrine carcinoma. Papanicolaou stain shows discohesive, plasmacytoid cells with nuclear pleomorphism, prominent nucleoli, and coarsely clumped chromatin. The cytoplasm is relatively abundant and finely granular. (Photomicrograph courtesy of Amberly L. Nunez, M.D.)

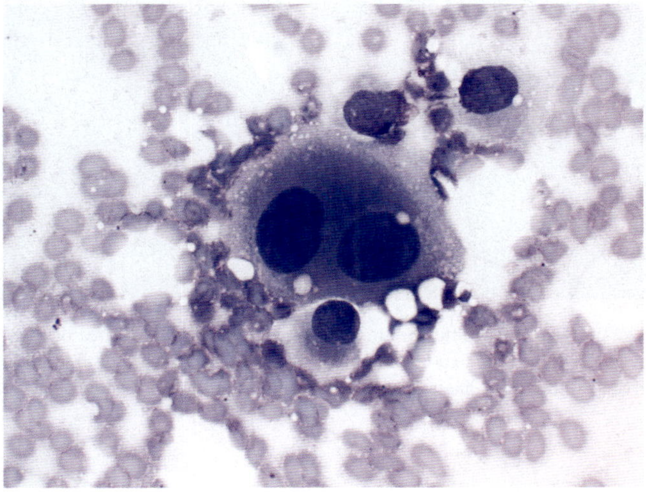

FIGURE 10-3: A binucleated cell in apocrine carcinoma. (Diff-Quik stain; photomicrograph courtesy of Amberly L. Nunez, M.D.)

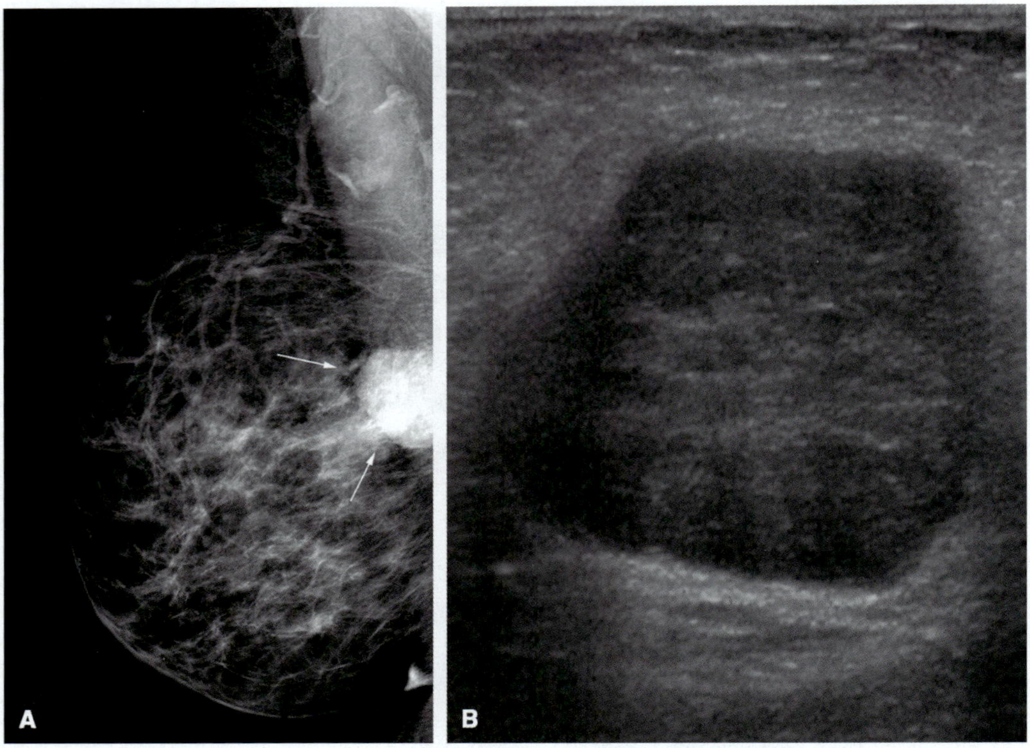

FIGURE 10-4: Right mediolateral oblique mammographic image reveals a hyperdense round mass (*arrows*) in the right posterior breast with well-circumscribed margins (**A**). Gray-scale US image reveals a round hypoechoic mass with focally indistinct margins (**B**).

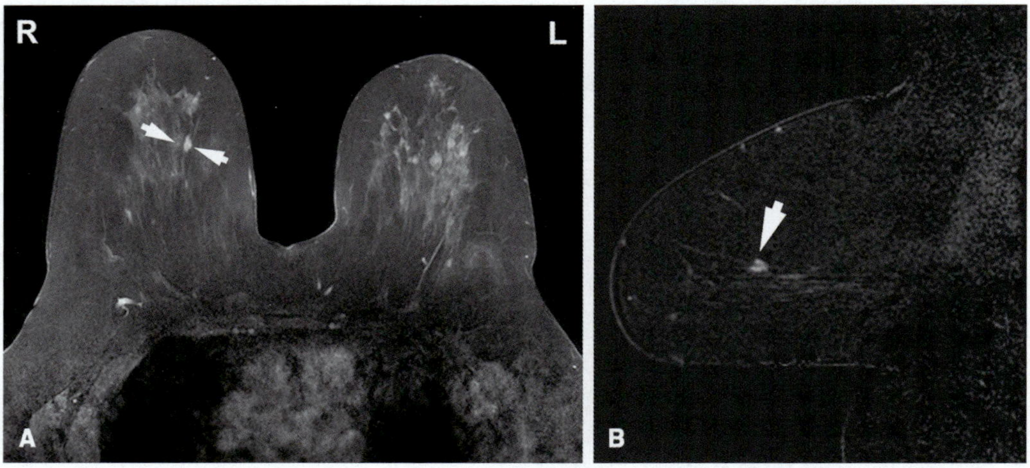

FIGURE 10-5: An axial T1 fat-saturated image post–contrast administration reveals an 8-mm irregular area of non–mass-like enhancement (*arrows*) that was new in this patient undergoing high-risk screening (**A**). A sagittal subtraction image confirms the homogeneous area of irregular non–mass-like enhancement (*arrow*) with rapid rise and plateau kinetics (**B**).

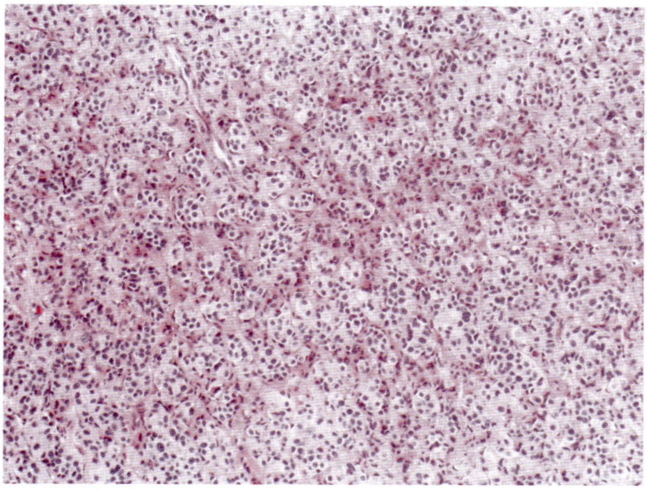

FIGURE 10-6: Apocrine carcinoma with a solid growth pattern showing large tumor cells with abundant eosinophilic cytoplasm.

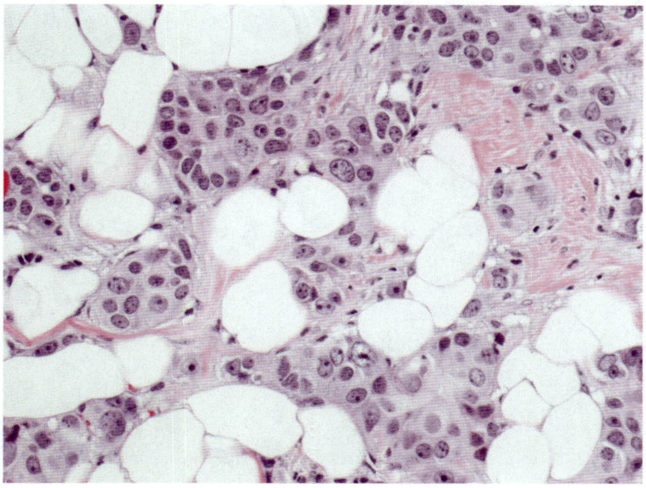

FIGURE 10-7: The constituent cells in apocrine carcinoma typically have large, round, vesicular nuclei with one or more nucleoli and finely granular cytoplasm.

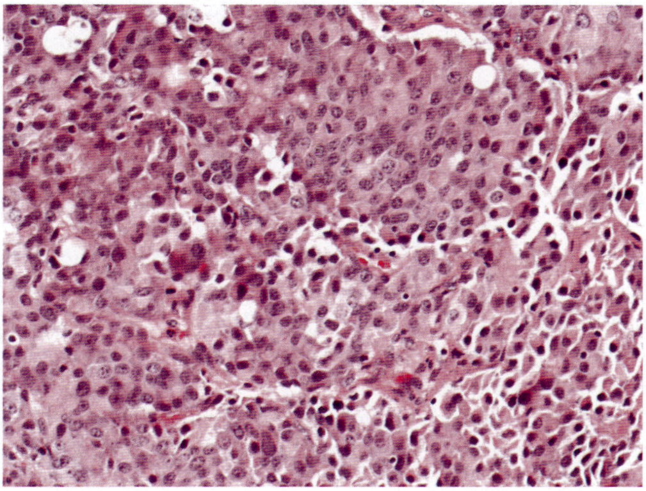

FIGURE 10-8: Apocrine carcinoma with intensely eosinophilic cytoplasm (so-called type A cells).

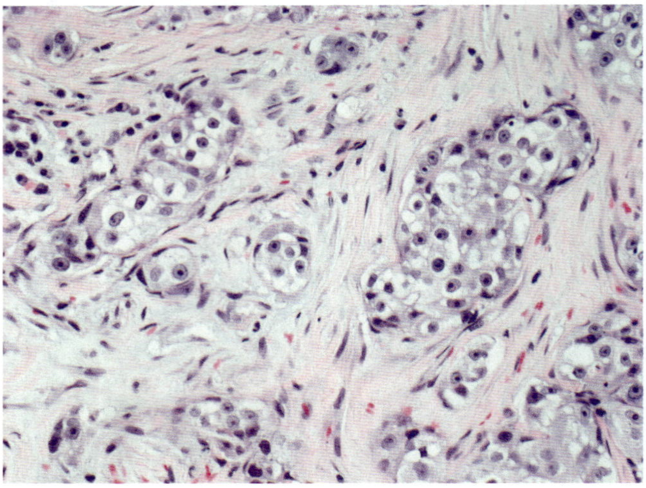

FIGURE 10-9: Apocrine carcinoma with foamy, vacuolated cytoplasm (so-called type B cells). Note the well-defined cell borders.

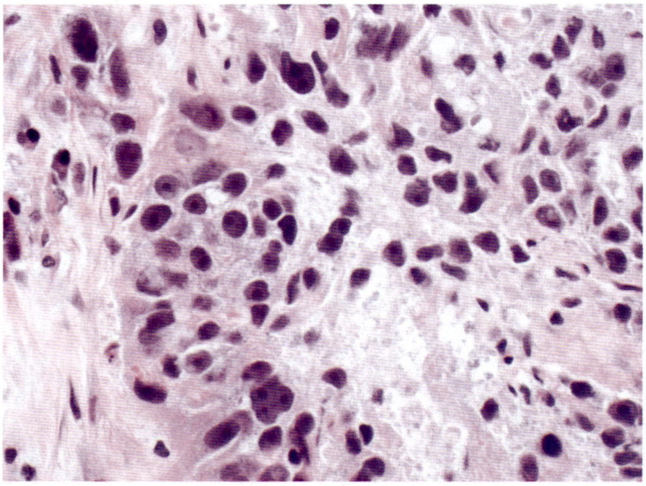

FIGURE 10-10: Apocrine carcinoma showing highly pleomorphic nuclei and inconspicuous cell borders.

appearance simulating histiocytes (type B cells; Figure 10-9). Intracytoplasmic lipid accumulation has also been demonstrated.[2,6] The cell borders are typically well defined but are sometimes inconspicuous (Figure 10-10). Associated carcinoma *in situ* is not uncommon in these tumors and usually shows apocrine differentiation as well.

CARCINOMA WITH APOCRINE DIFFERENTIATION, DIFFERENTIAL DIAGNOSIS

Granular cell tumor can occur primarily in the breast and typically has an infiltrating growth pattern, thus a great mimicker of apocrine carcinoma. The cells of granular cell tumor have abundant granular eosinophilic cytoplasm, well-defined cell borders, and round to oval nuclei, but lack significant nuclear pleomorphism (Figures 10-11 and 10-12). Granular cell tumor characteristically expresses S100 protein but is negative for cytokeratin.

Other less common differential diagnostic considerations include prominent histiocytic reaction, DCIS arising in a background of sclerosing adenosis, and sweat gland carcinoma of the skin.

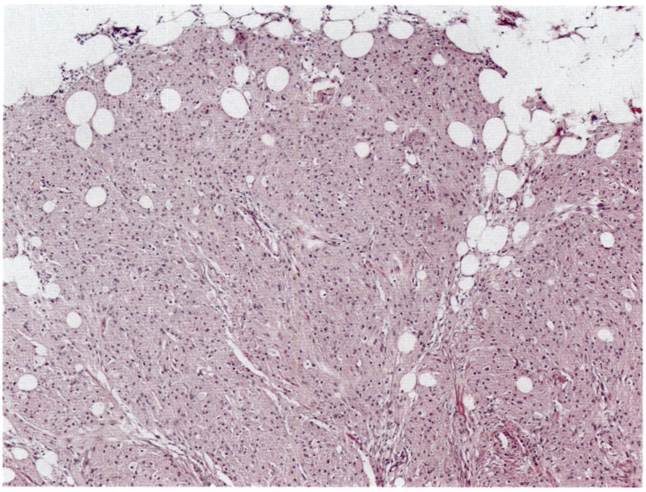

FIGURE 10-11: Granular cell tumor typically shows an infiltrating growth pattern. The tumor cells have abundant granular cytoplasm, thus mimicking apocrine carcinoma.

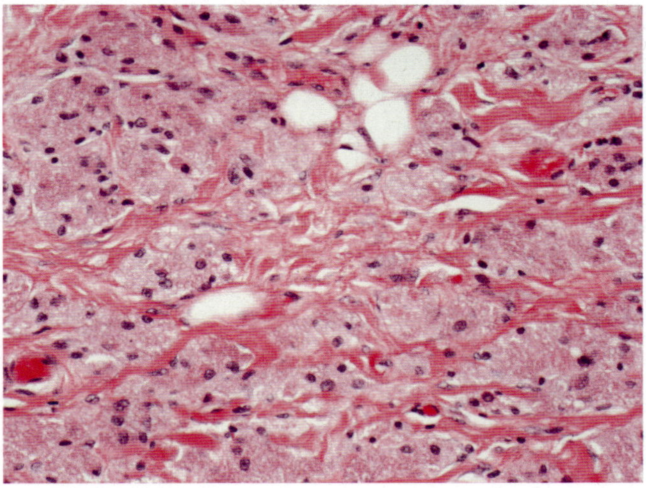

FIGURE 10-12: At higher magnification, the cells of granular cell tumor have abundant granular eosinophilic cytoplasm but lack significant nuclear pleomorphism such as large nuclei and prominent nucleoli characteristic of apocrine carcinoma.

CARCINOMA WITH APOCRINE DIFFERENTIATION, IMMUNOHISTOCHEMISTRY

Carcinomas with apocrine differentiation are usually negative for ER and PR, and show HER2 overexpression or gene amplification in up to 50% of cases. These tumors can be further corroborated by the immunoexpression of androgen receptor (56% to 100%) and gross cystic disease fluid protein-15 (GCDFP-15) (Figure 10-13).[7–11] The combination of these markers may characteristically define the group of tumors with "apocrine phenotype."

CARCINOMA WITH APOCRINE DIFFERENTIATION, MOLECULAR GENETICS

Gene expression microarray analysis has identified a group of breast carcinomas with "apocrine molecular signature," which is largely driven by increased androgen signaling.[12] These "molecular apocrine tumors" contain all of the ER-negative and non–basal-like carcinomas,

FIGURE 10-13: Carcinomas with apocrine differentiation frequently express GCDFP-15 (as illustrated in this image) and androgen receptor (56% to 100%).

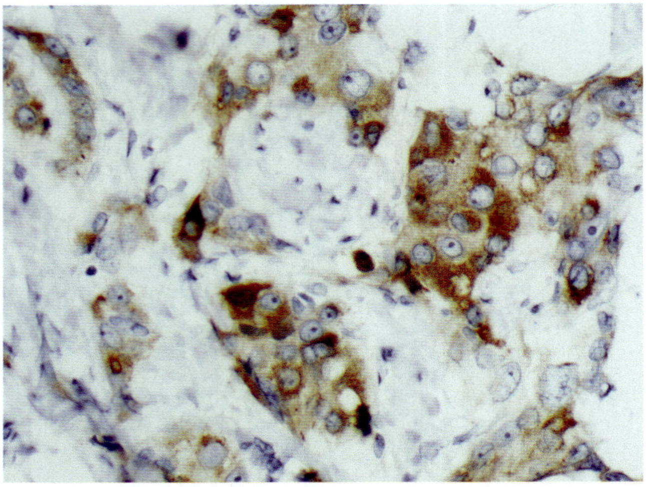

demonstrate strong apocrine features on histologic examination, and show androgen receptor immunoexpression. However, only about half of carcinomas with apocrine differentiation show this molecular signature. In addition, comparative genomic hybridization analysis has revealed a number of chromosomal alterations in carcinomas with apocrine differentiation that are commonly seen in breast carcinomas in general, including gains of 1p, 1q, and 2q and losses of 1p, 12q, 16q, 17q, and 22q.[13] Taken together, the data support that carcinomas with apocrine differentiation represent a heterogeneous group of tumors with common cytomorphology and immunophenotype. Thus, "apocrine carcinoma" is not regarded as a distinct pathologic entity by the current WHO classification.[5]

References

1. Mossler JA, Barton TK, Brinkhous AD, et al. Apocrine differentiation in human mammary carcinoma. *Cancer* 1980;46:2463–2471.
2. Eusebi V, Millis RR, Cattani MG, et al. Apocrine carcinoma of the breast. A morphologic and immunocytochemical study. *Am J Pathol* 1986;123:532–541.
3. Abati AD, Kimmel M, Rosen PP. Apocrine mammary carcinoma. A clinicopathologic study of 72 cases. *Am J Clin Pathol* 1990;94:371–377.
4. Eusebi V, Magalhaes F, Azzopardi JG. Pleomorphic lobular carcinoma of the breast: an aggressive tumor showing apocrine differentiation. *Hum Pathol* 1992;23:655–662.
5. O'Malley F, Eusebi V, Lakhani SR. Carcinomas with apocrine differentiation. In: Lakhani SR, Ellis IO, Schnitt SJ, et al., eds. *WHO Classification of Tumours of the Breast*. Lyon, France: IARC Press; 2012:53–54.
6. Moritani S, Ichihara S, Hasegawa M, et al. Intracytoplasmic lipid accumulation in apocrine carcinoma of the breast evaluated with adipophilin immunoreactivity: a possible link between apocrine carcinoma and lipid-rich carcinoma. *Am J Surg Pathol* 2011;35:861–867.
7. Gatalica Z. Immunohistochemical analysis of apocrine breast lesions. Consistent over-expression of androgen receptor accompanied by the loss of estrogen and progesterone receptors in apocrine metaplasia and apocrine carcinoma in situ. *Pathol Res Pract* 1997;193:753–758.
8. Bhargava R, Beriwal S, Striebel JM, et al. Breast cancer molecular class ERBB2: preponderance of tumors with apocrine differentiation and expression of basal phenotype markers CK5, CK5/6, and EGFR. *Appl Immunohistochem Mol Morphol* 2010;18:113–118.

9. Niemeier LA, Dabbs DJ, Beriwal S, et al. Androgen receptor in breast cancer: expression in estrogen receptor-positive tumors and in estrogen receptor-negative tumors with apocrine differentiation. *Mod Pathol* 2010;23:205–212.
10. Suzuki T, Miki Y, Takagi K, et al. Androgens in human breast carcinoma. *Med Mol Morphol* 2010;43:75–81.
11. O'Malley FP, Bane A. An update on apocrine lesions of the breast. *Histopathology* 2008;52:3–10.
12. Farmer P, Bonnefoi H, Becette V, et al. Identification of molecular apocrine breast tumours by microarray analysis. *Oncogene* 2005;24:4660–4671.
13. Jones C, Damiani S, Wells D, et al. Molecular cytogenetic comparison of apocrine hyperplasia and apocrine carcinoma of the breast. *Am J Pathol* 2001;158:207–214.

11 Adenoid Cystic Carcinoma

Adenoid cystic carcinoma of the breast is rare, accounting for less than 0.1% of all breast cancers.[1] The tumor is histologically indistinguishable from its counterpart in the salivary gland. Unlike the latter, adenoid cystic carcinoma of the breast is associated with an excellent prognosis paradoxical to its unfavorable, triple-negative hormonal receptor profile and gene expression recurrence score.[1,2] Thus, recognizing this rare entity is important to prevent overtreatment.

ADENOID CYSTIC CARCINOMA, CYTOLOGY

Adenoid cystic carcinoma is composed of small, uniform, basaloid cells with bland nuclei. The presence of intensely metachromatic, basement membrane–like material in the form of hyaline globules is highly characteristic of this tumor. The extracellular hyaline globules are bright magenta by Diff-Quik stain (Figure 11-1) and pale blue or pink by Papanicolaou stain. The differential diagnosis includes collagenous spherulosis; however, the hyaline globules of collagenous spherulosis are not intensely metachromatic.

ADENOID CYSTIC CARCINOMA, IMAGING AND GROSS FEATURES

The subareolar region is the most common location for adenoid cystic carcinoma.[1] Imaging findings are fairly nonspecific but can include developing asymmetries or irregular masses at mammography and irregular heterogeneous or hypoechoic masses at ultrasound (Figure 11-2).[3] The tumor is usually circumscribed and variable in size.[4]

ADENOID CYSTIC CARCINOMA, HISTOLOGY

Microscopically, adenoid cystic carcinoma commonly takes on the appearance of a nodular growth pattern but may also be infiltrative (Figures 11-3 and 11-4). The histologic hallmark is that the tumors consist of two main cell types: ductal epithelial and modified myoepithelial cells. Similar to that arising in salivary gland, mammary adenoid cystic carcinoma demonstrates three defined architectural configurations: tubular, cribriform, and solid. In the tubular form, tumor cells are arranged in conspicuous ducts and tubules with true glandular lumina lined by inner luminal cells and outer myoepithelial cells (Figure 11-5A–C). The luminal secretions are PAS-positive, diastase-resistant mucin (Figure 11-5D).[5–7] The cribriform pattern is characterized by fenestrated nests of cells forming cylindromatous microcystic spaces that give rise to a "Swiss cheese" appearance (Figure 11-6A). These basal–myoepithelial cell–lined pseudolumina contain mucoid or basement membrane–like material positive for Alcian blue and immunoreactive for type IV collagen (Figure 11-6B–D). The cells in the uncommon solid variant are typically

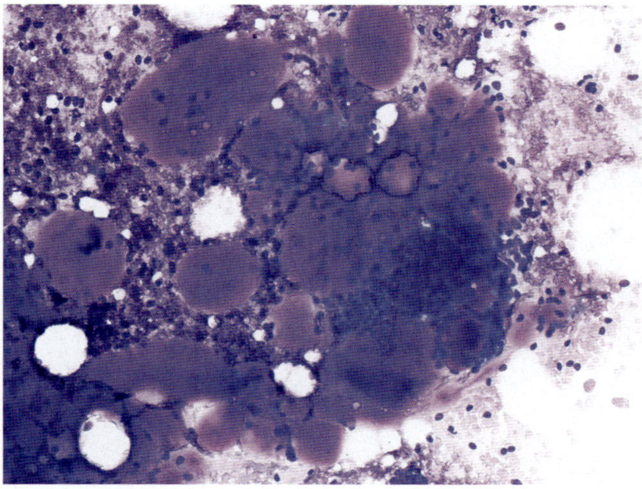

FIGURE 11-1: Adenoid cystic carcinoma. Diff-Quik–stained fine needle aspiration shows variably sized, metachromatic extracellular hyaline globules highly characteristic of this tumor. The interspersed small, basaloid cells are uniform, with high nuclear-to-cytoplasmic ratio, round to oval nuclei, and scant cytoplasm. (Photomicrograph courtesy of Amberly L. Nunez, M.D.)

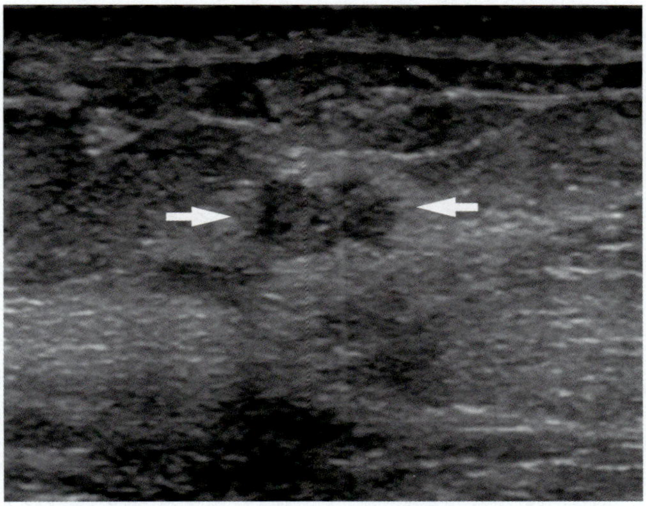

FIGURE 11-2: Adenoid cystic carcinoma. Ultrasound image shows an irregular hypoechoic mass.

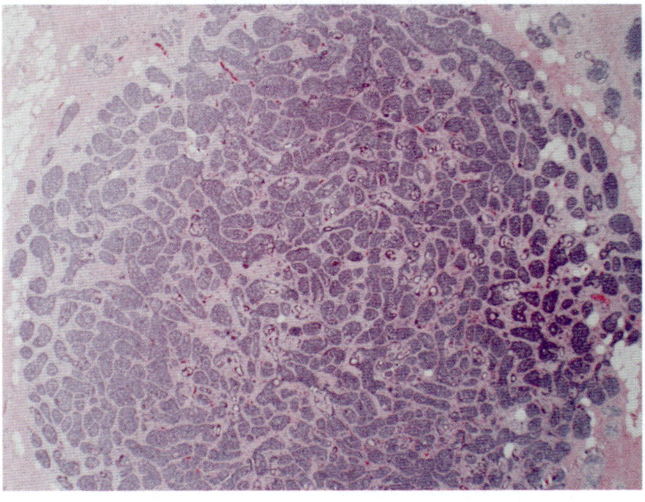

FIGURE 11-3: Adenoid cystic carcinoma with a nodular growth pattern.

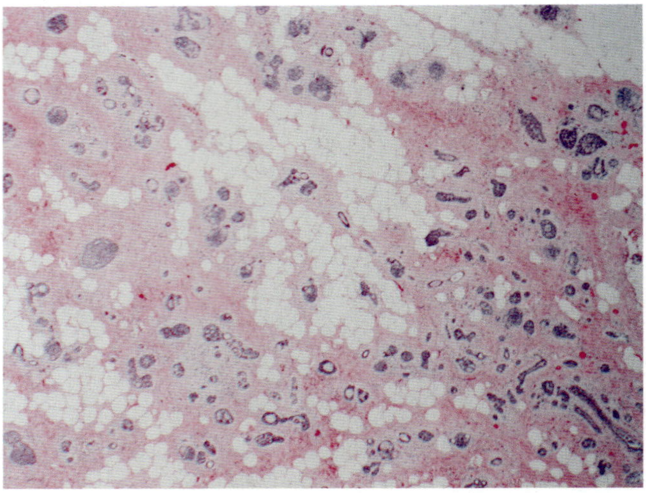

FIGURE 11-4: Adenoid cystic carcinoma with an infiltrative growth pattern.

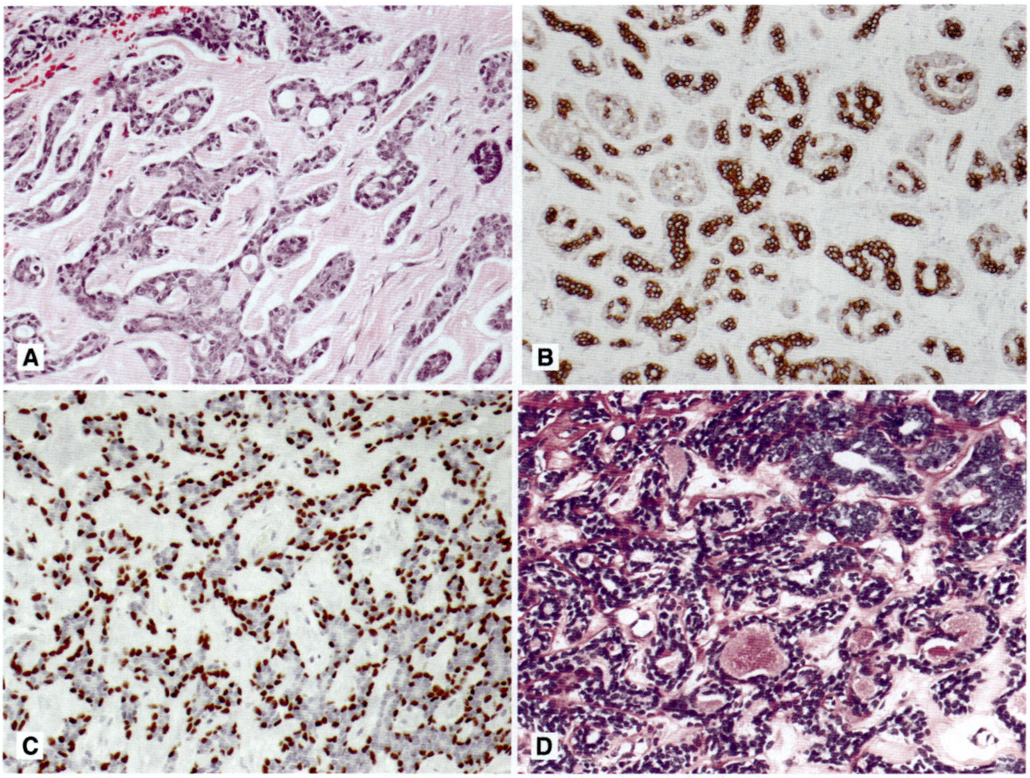

FIGURE 11-5: Tubular pattern of adenoid cystic carcinoma. The glandular spaces are lined by inner luminal cells and outer myoepithelial cells (**A**). The luminal epithelial cells are strongly immunoreactive for CAM5.2 (**B**), whereas an immunostain for p63 highlighted the outer myoepithelial cells (**C**). The luminal secretions in the tubular pattern are PAS-positive, diastase-resistant mucin (**D**).

basaloid (Figure 11-7).[8–10] Any of these histologic patterns can be the dominant form but is more commonly present as a component in a composite tumor. Associated ductal carcinoma *in situ* (DCIS) may be present but is difficult to distinct from the invasive component.[4]

Unusual metaplastic changes, such as squamous metaplasia and stromal myxoid pseudocartilaginous foci, may be observed in adenoid cystic carcinoma of the breast, in contrast to that in

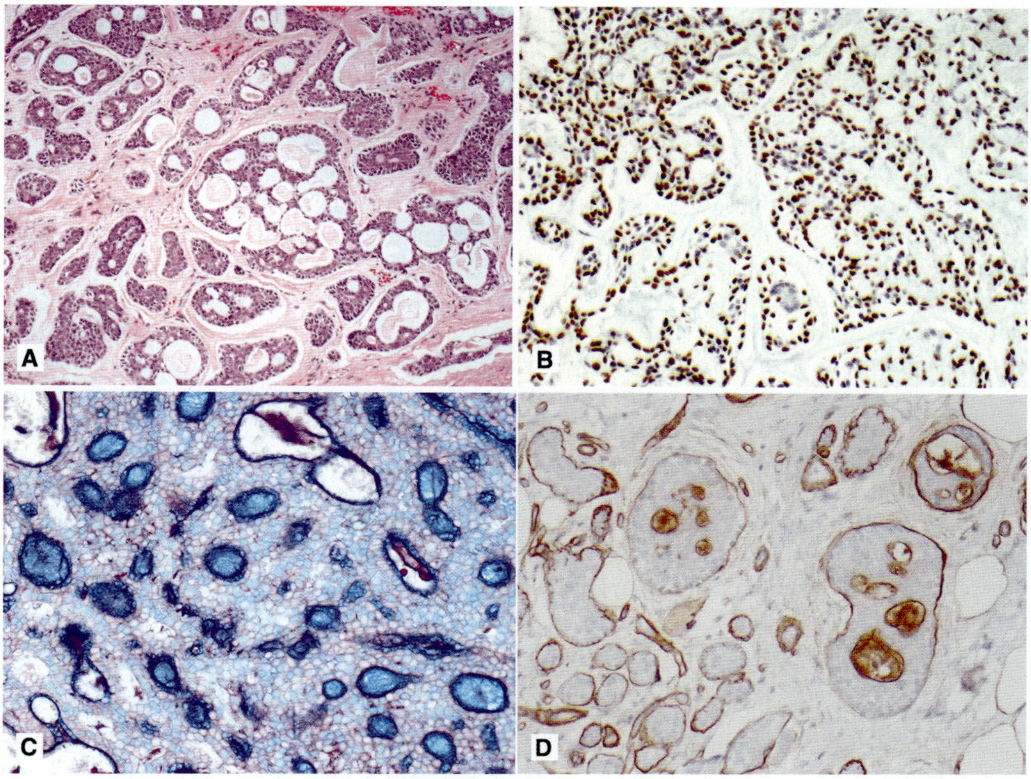

FIGURE 11-6: The cribriform pattern of adenoid cystic carcinoma with a characteristic "Swiss cheese" appearance (**A**). The pseudolumina in the cribriform pattern are lined by myoepithelial cells, as demonstrated by the p63 immunostain (**B**). The basement membrane–like material in the pseudolumina is positive for Alcian blue (**C**) and is outlined by an immunostain for collagen IV (**D**).

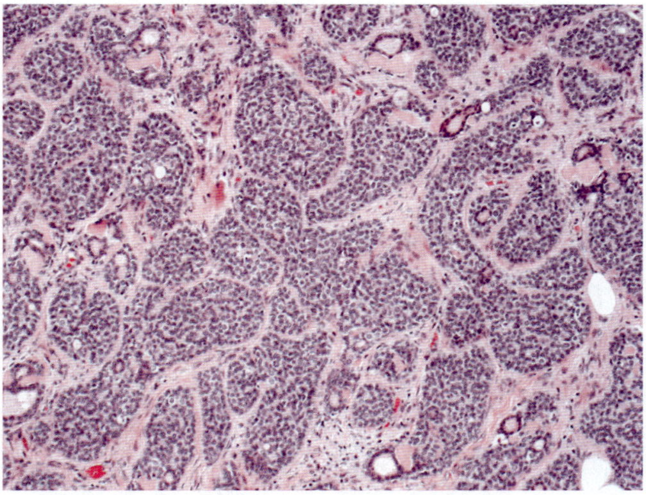

FIGURE 11-7: Adenoid cystic carcinoma with a predominantly solid growth pattern.

salivary gland.[7] Association with other adenomyoepithelial-type lesions has been seen, including tubular adenosis, adenomyoepithelioma, and low-grade syringomatous carcinoma, suggesting a possible relationship among this group of lesions.[11–13] The stroma is usually densely fibrotic or hyalinized.

ADENOID CYSTIC CARCINOMA, DIFFERENTIAL DIAGNOSIS

The cribriform variant of adenoid cystic carcinoma may be mistaken for invasive cribriform carcinoma. The empty spaces in the latter are surrounded by luminal epithelial cells and are devoid of mucoid or basement membrane–like material. Almost all cribriform carcinomas are positive for ER and PR in contrast to adenoid cystic carcinomas, which are usually ER and PR negative. Cribriform-type DCIS may also be encountered in the differential diagnosis in this regard. The myoepithelial cells in cribriform DCIS are only present at the periphery of the cellular nests but not around the empty spaces.

Collagenous spherulosis also shows rounded myoepithelial cell–lined spaces that often contain basement membrane–like material. However, collagenous spherulosis is usually small and found incidentally and is more commonly associated with other benign proliferative lesions such as usual ductal hyperplasia, sclerosing adenosis, and intraductal papilloma but, rarely, lobular carcinoma *in situ*.[14]

The solid variant of adenoid cystic carcinoma is a mimicker of small cell carcinoma given its prominent basaloid appearance. Thus, appropriate immunohistochemical workup may become necessary to reach the correct diagnosis. Adenoid cystic carcinoma typically shows expression of both low and high molecular weight cytokeratins and is negative for neuroendocrine markers, whereas small cell carcinoma has an opposite immunoprofile.

ADENOID CYSTIC CARCINOMA, IMMUNOHISTOCHEMISTRY

The luminal epithelial cells are positive for low molecular weight cytokeratins (e.g., CK7, AE1, and CAM5.2) and EMA. Myoepithelial cells can be highlighted by high molecular weight cytokeratins (e.g., CK5/6, 34βE12), p63, S100 protein, calponin, and SMA. CD117 (c-Kit) expression in mammary adenoid cystic carcinoma is also recognized, as in its salivary counterpart (Figure 11-8).[15]

Adenoid cystic carcinoma of the breast is typically negative for ER, PR, and HER2. Overexpression of EGFR protein has been frequently detected without EGFR gene amplification.[16]

ADENOID CYSTIC CARCINOMA: MOLECULAR GENETICS

Similar to that in salivary gland, the recurrent chromosomal translocation t(6;9)(q22-23;p23-24) is also observed in mammary adenoid cystic carcinoma, which results in fusion transcripts of MYB and NFIB genes.[17] Thus, overexpression of MYB–NFIB transcripts may be a genetic hallmark and play a key role in the pathogenesis of adenoid cystic carcinoma.

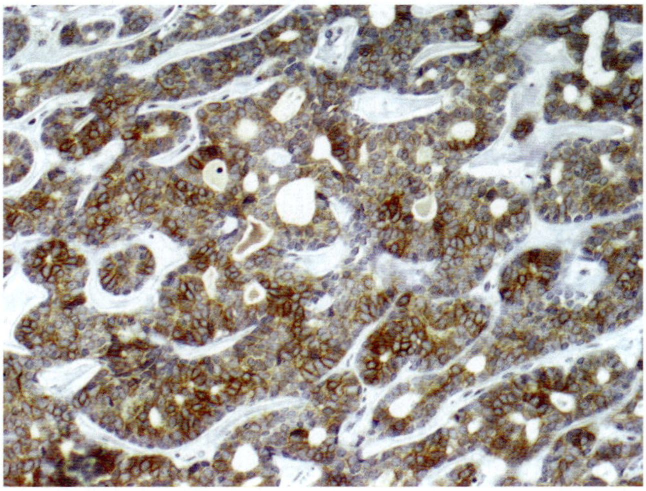

FIGURE 11-8: C-Kit expression in mammary adenoid cystic carcinoma.

References

1. Ghabach B, Anderson WF, Curtis RE, et al. Adenoid cystic carcinoma of the breast in the United States (1977 to 2006): a population-based cohort study. *Breast Cancer Res* 2010;12:R54.
2. Weigelt B, Horlings HM, Kreike B, et al. Refinement of breast cancer classification by molecular characterization of histological special types. *J Pathol* 2008;216:141–150.
3. Glazebrook KN, Reynolds C, Smith RL, et al. Adenoid cystic carcinoma of the breast. *AJR Am J Roentgenol* 2010;194:1391–1396.
4. Sapino A, Sneige N, Eusebi V. Adenoid cystic carcinoma. In: Lakhani SR, Ellis IO, Schnitt SJ, et al., eds. *WHO Classification of Tumours of the Breast.* Lyon, France: IARC Press; 2012:56–57.
5. Ro JY, Silva EG, Gallager HS. Adenoid cystic carcinoma of the breast. *Hum Pathol* 1987;18: 1276–1281.
6. Kleer CG, Oberman HA. Adenoid cystic carcinoma of the breast: value of histologic grading and proliferative activity. *Am J Surg Pathol* 1998;22:569–575.
7. Lamovec J, Us-Krasovec M, Zidar A, et al. Adenoid cystic carcinoma of the breast: a histologic, cytologic, and immunohistochemical study. *Semin Diagn Pathol* 1989;6:153–164.
8. Shin SJ, Rosen PP. Solid variant of mammary adenoid cystic carcinoma with basaloid features: a study of nine cases. *Am J Surg Pathol* 2002;26:413–420.
9. Cabibi D, Cipolla C, Maria Florena A, et al. Solid variant of mammary "adenoid cystic carcinoma with basaloid features" merging with "small cell carcinoma". *Pathol Res Pract* 2005;201:705–711.
10. Zhou RJ, Hu CY, Yu L, et al. Solid variant of mammary adenoid cystic carcinoma with basaloid features: a clinicopathologic and immunohistochemical study. *Zhonghua Bing Li Xue Za Zhi* 2012;41: 803–807.
11. Da Silva L, Buck L, Simpson PT, et al. Molecular and morphological analysis of adenoid cystic carcinoma of the breast with synchronous tubular adenosis. *Virchows Arch* 2009;454:107–114.
12. Van Dorpe J, De Pauw A, Moerman P. Adenoid cystic carcinoma arising in an adenomyoepithelioma of the breast. *Virchows Arch* 1998;432:119–122.
13. Rosen PP. Adenoid cystic carcinoma of the breast. A morphologically heterogeneous neoplasm. *Pathology Annual* 1989;24 (Pt) 2:237–254.
14. Sgroi D, Koerner FC. Involvement of collagenous spherulosis by lobular carcinoma in situ. Potential confusion with cribriform ductal carcinoma in situ. *Am J Surg Pathol* 1995;19:1366–1370.
15. Arpino G, Clark GM, Mohsin S, et al. Adenoid cystic carcinoma of the breast: molecular markers, treatment, and clinical outcome. *Cancer* 2002;94:2119–2127.
16. Vranic S, Frkovic-Grazio S, Lamovec J, et al. Adenoid cystic carcinomas of the breast have low Topo IIalpha expression but frequently overexpress EGFR protein without EGFR gene amplification. *Hum Pathol* 2010;41:1617–1623.
17. Persson M, Andren Y, Mark J, et al. Recurrent fusion of MYB and NFIB transcription factor genes in carcinomas of the breast and head and neck. *Proc Natl Acad Sci U S A* 2009;106:18740–18744.

12 Mucinous Carcinoma and Carcinomas with Signet-Ring Cell Differentiation

Mucinous carcinoma, also known as *colloid carcinoma*, is characterized by small clusters of uniform cells dispersed in abundant extracellular pools of stromal mucin. It occurs over a wide age range, but is more commonly seen in patients older than 55 years, with the mean age in the seventh decade.[1] Pure mucinous carcinoma is rare, accounting for about 2% of all breast carcinomas in most series.[2]

MUCINOUS CARCINOMA, CYTOLOGY

The cytologic hallmark of mucinous carcinoma is the presence of variably sized clusters or islands of tumor cells floating in a sea of pale pink mucin by Diff-Quik stain (Figure 12-1). Numerous single cells are also typically present. The cells are fairly bland with round nuclei and smooth nuclear membranes.

MUCINOUS CARCINOMA, IMAGING AND GROSS FEATURES

On imaging, the most common appearance of mucinous carcinoma is a mass on mammography and a hypoechoic mass on sonography (Figure 12-2).[3] Grossly, the tumor typically shows a well-circumscribed mass with pushing margins. Upon sectioning, the lesion is readily recognized by its soft consistency with a glistening and gelatinous cut surface. The tumor size varies from less than 1 cm to greater than 20 cm.[1]

MUCINOUS CARCINOMA, HISTOLOGY

Microscopically, the presence of abundant extracellular mucin production is the hallmark of mucinous carcinoma. The extent of stromal mucin varies from region to region and from tumor to tumor (Figures 12-3 to 12-6). The pools or lakes of mucin are typically transversed by delicate fibrous septa and divided into compartments. The periphery of the lesion is usually circumscribed without an infiltrative growth pattern. The clusters of neoplastic cells are variable in size and shape and may be solid and sheet-like or form tubular, cribriform, or micropapillary structures (Figure 12-7). For a diagnosis of mucinous carcinoma, nuclei should be low to intermediate grade; those with high-grade features (Figure 12-8) are classified as carcinomas of no special type with mucinous features. Tumor necrosis may also be seen in such high-grade lesions. Neuroendocrine differentiation, as demonstrated by the presence of cytoplasmic argyrophilic granules or immunoexpression of neuroendocrine markers, can be frequently seen in the hypercellular variant that is subclassified as *type B mucinous carcinoma* by some authorities. This is in contrast to the classic, paucicellular variant (also called "*type A*") in which neuroendocrine

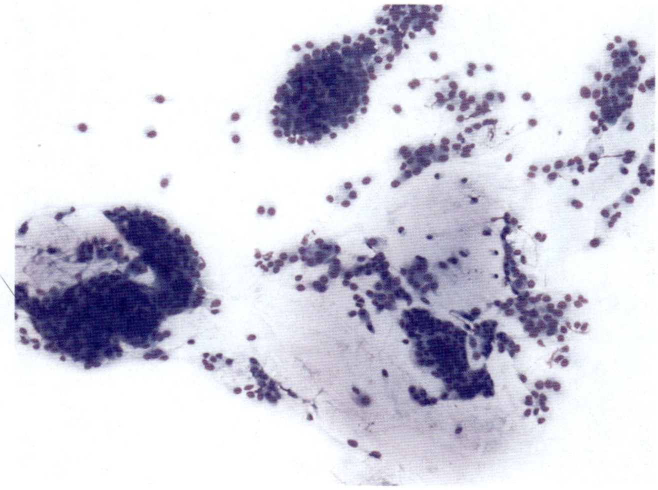

FIGURE 12-1: Mucinous carcinoma. Diff-Quik–stained fine needle aspiration shows islands of cohesive epithelial cells with numerous single cells floating in a lake of pale pink mucin. The cells are fairly bland with round nuclei and smooth nuclear membranes. (Photomicrograph courtesy of Amberly L. Nunez, M.D.)

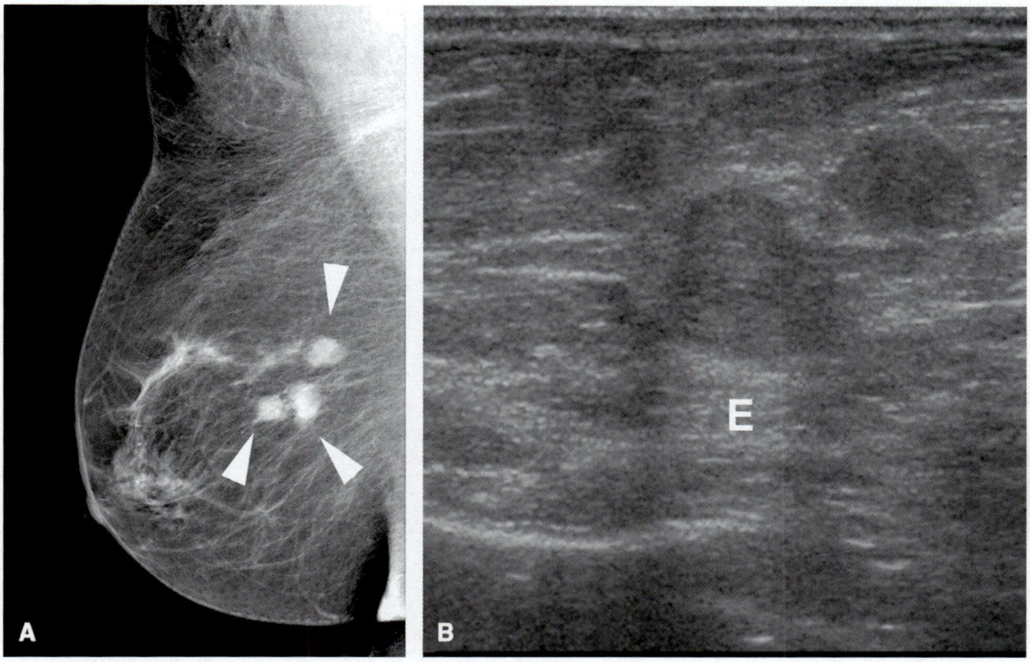

FIGURE 12-2: Imaging features of mucinous carcinoma. A right mediolateral oblique mammographic view reveals three hyperdense round masses with microlobulated margins (*arrowheads*) in the right 9:00 breast (**A**). A gray-scale ultrasound image shows two hypoechoic round masses with indistinct margins and posterior acoustic enhancement (*E*) (**B**).

differentiation is not typical.[4–6] Mucinous carcinoma is often associated with a ductal carcinoma *in situ* (DCIS) component, which may also demonstrate prominent extracellular mucin production. The DCIS may have various patterns, including solid, cribriform, and micropapillary (Figure 12-9).

The diagnosis of a mucinous carcinoma is strictly limited to those comprising greater than 90% of characteristic histology ("pure" mucinous carcinoma),[2] as "mixed" mucinous tumors containing greater than 10% nonmucinous elements (most commonly no special type) are associated with a poorer prognosis than pure mucinous carcinomas.[7–9] Importantly (and as noted above), "mucinous carcinomas" with high-grade nuclei, even if pure, should be regarded as invasive carcinomas with mucinous features as they carry out a worse outcome.

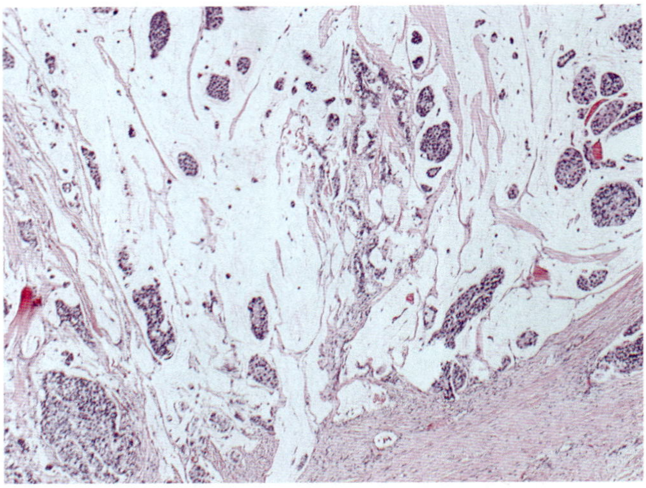

FIGURE 12-3: The presence of abundant extracellular mucin is the hallmark of mucinous carcinoma. The tumor is typically divided into compartments by fibrous septa. The periphery of the lesion is usually circumscribed rather than infiltrative.

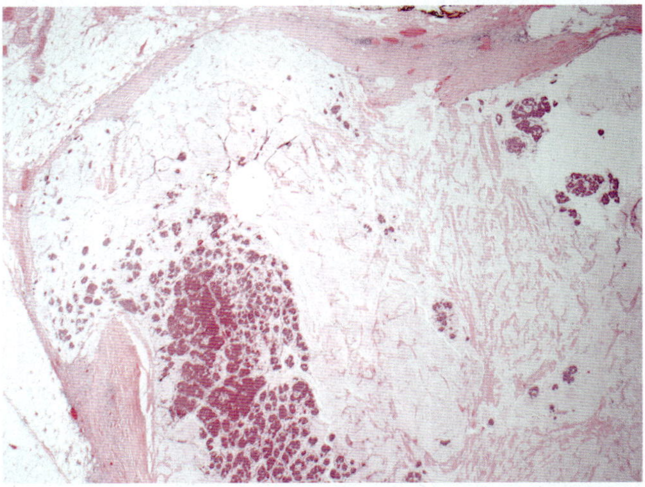

FIGURE 12-4: The cellularity and the extent of stromal mucin vary from region to region in mucinous carcinomas.

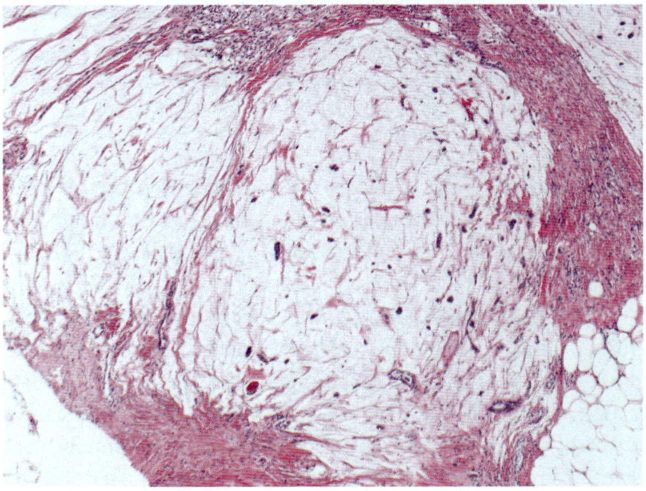

FIGURE 12-5: A mucinous carcinoma with paucicellularity.

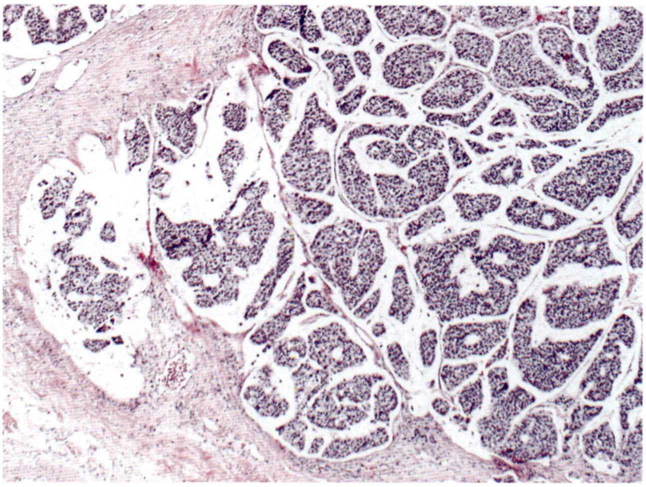

FIGURE 12-6: A "cellular" mucinous carcinoma.

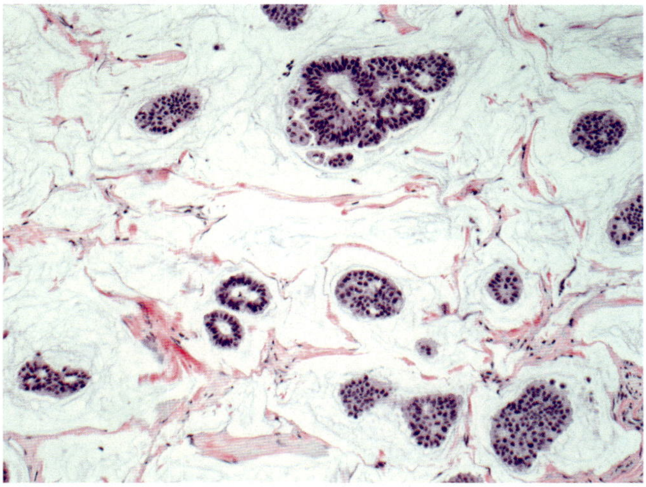

FIGURE 12-7: Mucinous carcinoma with gland formation. Note the low-grade nuclei typical of this tumor.

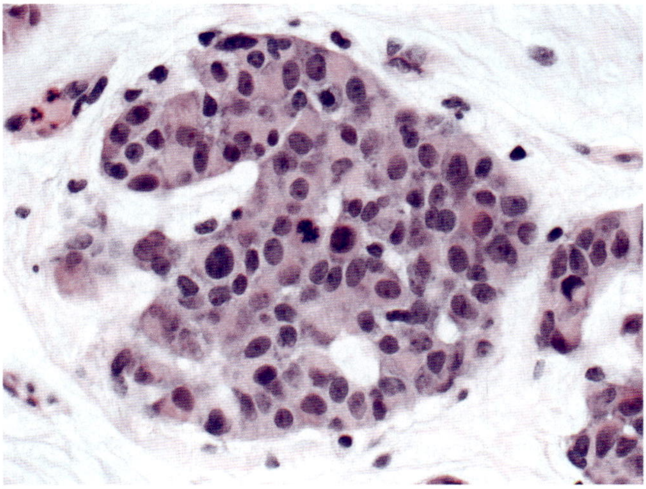

FIGURE 12-8: A "mucinous carcinoma" showing high-grade nuclei and mitotic activity. These lesions should be regarded as invasive carcinoma with mucinous features rather than being classified as conventional mucinous carcinoma.

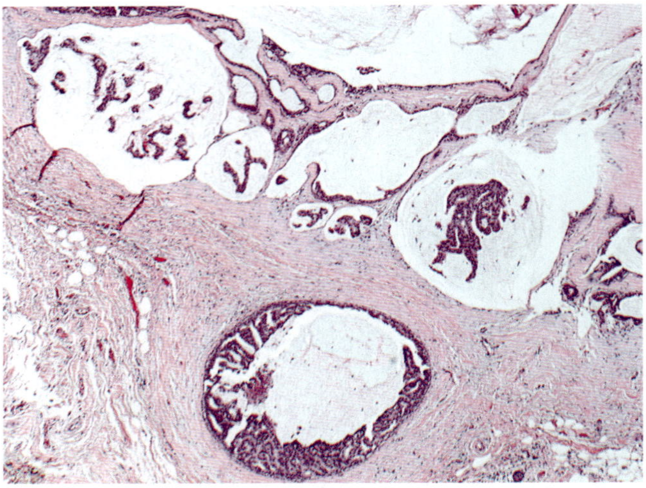

FIGURE 12-9: The coexisting DCIS in mucinous carcinoma commonly produces extracellular mucin.

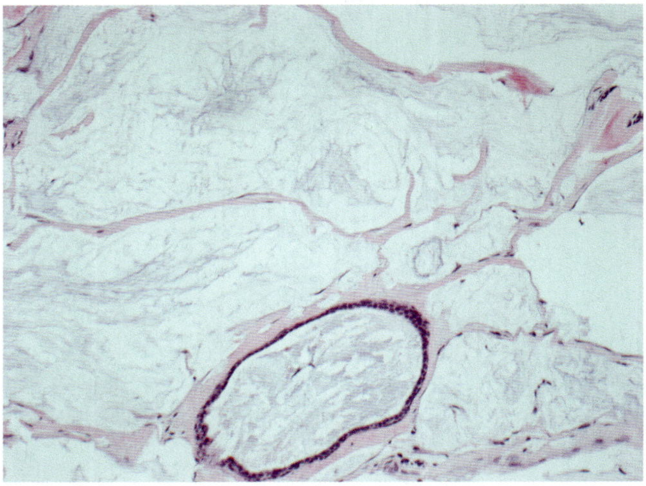

FIGURE 12-10: Mucocele-like lesion showing abundant extravasated stromal mucin. Note the extended, mucin-containing duct lined by attenuated epithelium.

MUCINOUS CARCINOMA, DIFFERENTIAL DIAGNOSIS

The differential diagnosis of mucinous carcinoma includes all mucin-producing lesions of the breast. Among them, mucocele-like lesion may closely resemble mucinous carcinoma and represent a great diagnostic challenge. Mucocele-like lesion is characterized by the presence of cystically dilated, mucin-filled ducts, often associated with abundant extravasated stromal mucin. Features supporting a mucocele-like lesion include the presence of mucin-containing, extended ducts lined by attenuated epithelium (Figure 12-10) or strips/clusters of free floating, cytologically benign epithelium with adherent myoepithelial cells.[10] The diagnostic challenging is amplified by the fact that these lesions may be associated with atypical ductal hyperplasia or DCIS. Occasionally, mucinous carcinoma can be identified in the continuity with mucocele-like lesion.[10] Thus, the distinction between mucocele-like lesion and mucinous carcinoma in core biopsy specimens is difficult and often impossible. In addition, the upstage rate of benign mucoceles on core biopsy to at least atypical ductal hyperplasia on subsequent surgery is up to 17.8% in one series.[11] Therefore, excision is recommended for all mucocele-like lesions diagnosed on biopsy by most authorities.

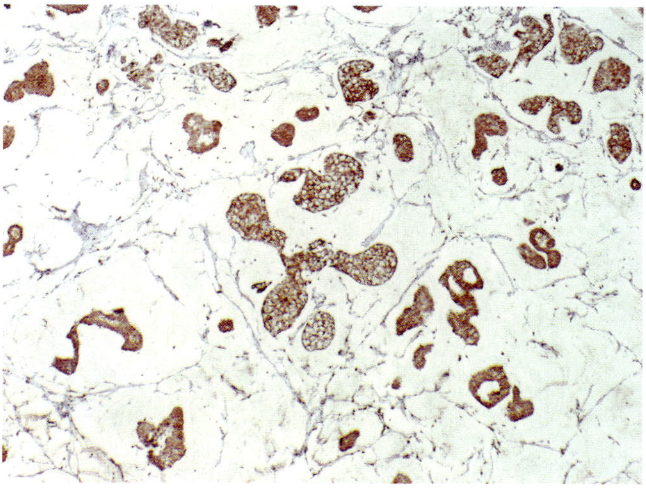

FIGURE 12-11: Mucinous carcinoma with neuroendocrine differentiation as demonstrated by a neuron-specific enolase immunostain.

MUCINOUS CARCINOMA, IMMUNOHISTOCHEMISTRY

Mucinous carcinomas are consistently positive for ER. These tumors mostly show PR expression, ranging from 70% to 84% in different series. HER2 overexpression or gene amplification is extremely rare.[1,6,12,13] Up to 74% of mucinous carcinomas express at least one of the three neuroendocrine markers, including chromogranin, synaptophysin, and neuron-specific enolase (Figure 12-11).[6] The gel-forming secretory-type mucins (MUC2 and MUC6) are highly expressed in mucinous carcinomas.[14,15]

MUCINOUS CARCINOMA, MOLECULAR GENETICS

Gene profiling studies have classified mucinous carcinomas as luminal A molecular subtype.[16] These tumors, along with neuroendocrine carcinomas of the breast, are transcriptionally distinct from grade- and molecular subtype–matched invasive carcinomas of no special type.[17] Further, the hypercellular, so-called mucinous B tumors show a gene expression pattern similar to that of neuroendocrine carcinomas, whereas the paucicellular, mucinous A carcinomas form a discrete subgroup by hierarchical clustering analysis.[17] Furthermore, microarray-based comparative genomic hybridization studies have shown that pure mucinous carcinomas have a relatively low level of genetic instability and rare cytogenetic alterations compared to grade- and ER-matched invasive carcinomas of no special type.[12] Interestingly, both mucinous and nonmucinous components of mixed mucinous tumors are remarkably similar at the molecular level to pure mucinous carcinomas, suggesting that mixed mucinous carcinomas may be best classified as variants of mucinous carcinomas rather than of invasive carcinomas of no special type.[12]

CARCINOMAS WITH SIGNET-RING CELL DIFFERENTIATION

Signet-ring cell is a descriptive term used to designate the light microscopic appearance of cells characterized by a crescent-shaped nucleus displaced to the cell periphery secondarily to the cytoplasmic accumulation of mucin. While breast carcinomas with focal signet-ring cell differentiation are fairly common, those composed of exclusively signet-ring cells are rare. The latter most commonly presents as a variant of invasive lobular carcinoma but can also be seen in nonlobular breast carcinomas.[2] As such, carcinoma with signet-ring cell differentiation is not regarded as a distinct entity by the current WHO classification.[2] These tumors do not produce stromal mucin; thus, it is typically not problematic to distinguish them from mucinous carcinoma.

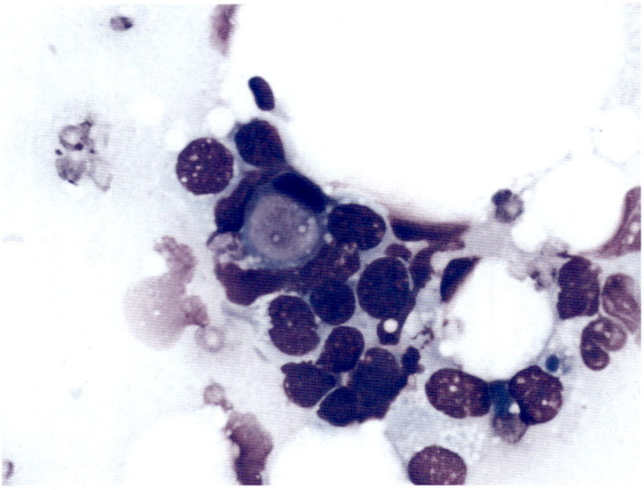

FIGURE 12-12: Carcinoma with signet-ring cell differentiation. Among the group of malignant epithelial cells with enlarged nuclei and irregular nuclear membranes, there is a cell with a large collection of intracytoplasmic mucin that pushes the nucleus to the periphery of the cell, resulting a signet-ring appearance. (Diff-Quik stain; photomicrograph courtesy of Amberly L. Nunez, M.D.)

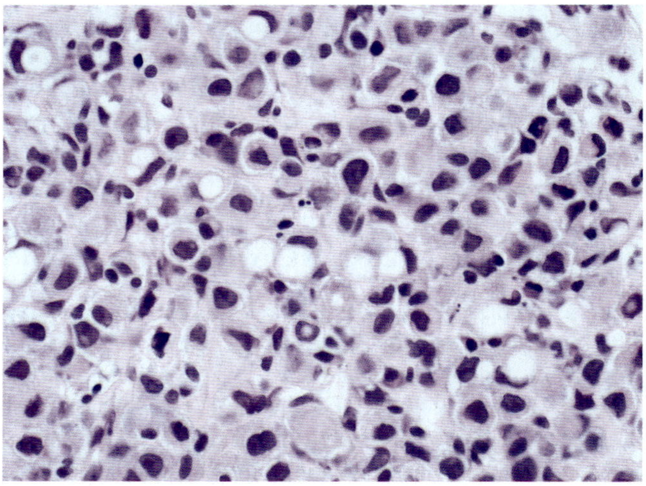

FIGURE 12-13: Histologic appearance of signet-ring cell carcinoma. The cells have clear and vacuolated cytoplasm that indents the nuclei.

CARCINOMAS WITH SIGNET-RING CELL DIFFERENTIATION, CYTOLOGY

Cytologically, the cells with signet-ring cell differentiation typically display a large mucin vacuole in the cytoplasm and an eccentric nucleus and are commonly intermixed with other malignant cells (Figure 12-12).

CARCINOMAS WITH SIGNET-RING CELL DIFFERENTIATION, HISTOLOGY

Similar to their cytologic appearance, carcinoma cells with signet-ring cell differentiation demonstrate abundant intracellular mucin that pushes the nucleus to one side (Figure 12-13). Prominent signet-ring cell differentiation is more commonly seen in invasive lobular carcinoma but may also be seen in invasive carcinoma of no special type and other special types (Figure 12-14).

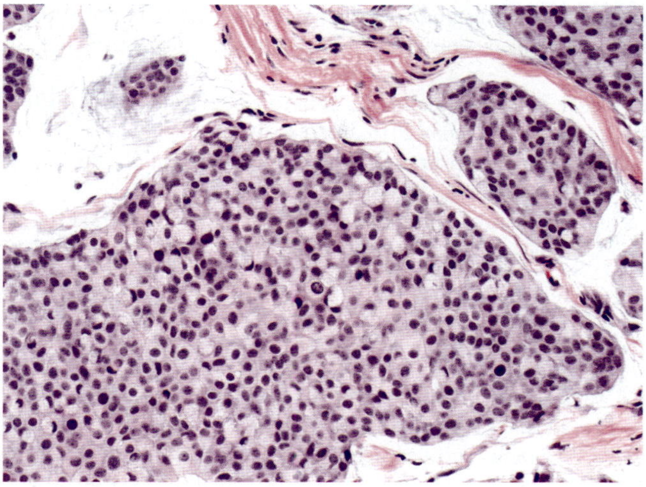

FIGURE 12-14: Mucinous carcinoma with prominent signet-ring cell differentiation.

CARCINOMAS WITH SIGNET-RING CELL DIFFERENTIATION: DIFFERENTIAL DIAGNOSIS

Carcinomas with signet-ring cell differentiation in the breast must be distinguished from metastases to the breast from other sites, of which the most common organ is the stomach.

CARCINOMAS WITH SIGNET-RING CELL DIFFERENTIATION, IMMUNOHISTOCHEMISTRY

Primary mammary carcinomas with signet-ring cell differentiation typically express ER and PR. Thus, lack of hormonal receptor expression strongly suggests a metastasis from another site.

References

1. Barkley CR, Ligibel JA, Wong JS, et al. Mucinous breast carcinoma: a large contemporary series. *Am J Surg* 2008;196:549–551.
2. Bussolati G, Sapino A. Mucinous carcinoma and carcinomas with signet-ring cell differentiation. In: Lakhani SR, Ellis IO, Schnitt SJ, et al., eds. *WHO Classification of Tumours of the Breast*. Lyon, France: IARC Press; 2012:60–61.
3. Liu H, Tan H, Cheng Y, et al. Imaging findings in mucinous breast carcinoma and correlating factors. *Eur J Radiol* 2011;80:706–712.
4. Capella C, Eusebi V, Mann B, et al. Endocrine differentiation in mucoid carcinoma of the breast. *Histopathology* 1980;4:613–630.
5. Rasmussen BB, Rose C, Thorpe SM, et al. Argyrophilic cells in 202 human mucinous breast carcinomas. Relation to histopathologic and clinical factors. *Am J Clin Pathol* 1985;84:737–740.
6. Tse GM, Ma TK, Chu WC, et al. Neuroendocrine differentiation in pure type mammary mucinous carcinoma is associated with favorable histologic and immunohistochemical parameters. *Mod Pathol* 2004;17:568–572.
7. Clayton F. Pure mucinous carcinomas of breast: morphologic features and prognostic correlates. *Hum Pathol* 1986;17:34–38.
8. Andre S, Cunha F, Bernardo M, et al. Mucinous carcinoma of the breast: a pathologic study of 82 cases. *J Surg Oncol* 1995;58:162–167.
9. Komaki K, Sakamoto G, Sugano H, et al. Mucinous carcinoma of the breast in Japan. A prognostic analysis based on morphologic features. *Cancer* 1988;61:989–996.

10. Tan PH, Tse GM, Bay BH. Mucinous breast lesions: diagnostic challenges. *J Clin Pathol* 2008;61:11–19.
11. Jaffer S, Bleiweiss IJ, Nagi CS. Benign mucocele-like lesions of the breast: revisited. *Mod Pathol* 2011;24: 683–687.
12. Lacroix-Triki M, Suarez PH, MacKay A, et al. Mucinous carcinoma of the breast is genomically distinct from invasive ductal carcinomas of no special type. *J Pathol* 2010;222:282–298.
13. Diab SG, Clark GM, Osborne CK, et al. Tumor characteristics and clinical outcome of tubular and mucinous breast carcinomas. *J Clin Oncol* 1999;17:1442–1448.
14. Matsukita S, Nomoto M, Kitajima S, et al. Expression of mucins (MUC1, MUC2, MUC5AC and MUC6) in mucinous carcinoma of the breast: comparison with invasive ductal carcinoma. *Histopathology* 2003;42:26–36.
15. Rakha EA, Boyce RW, Abd El-Rehim D, et al. Expression of mucins (MUC1, MUC2, MUC3, MUC4, MUC5AC and MUC6) and their prognostic significance in human breast cancer. *Mod Pathol* 2005;18: 1295–1304.
16. Weigelt B, Horlings HM, Kreike B, et al. Refinement of breast cancer classification by molecular characterization of histological special types. *J Pathol* 2008;216:141–150.
17. Weigelt B, Geyer FC, Horlings HM, et al. Mucinous and neuroendocrine breast carcinomas are transcriptionally distinct from invasive ductal carcinomas of no special type. *Mod Pathol* 2009;22:1401–1414.

Carcinomas with Neuroendocrine Features

13

Breast carcinomas with variable degrees of neuroendocrine features are not uncommon and can be seen in those of no special type and many of the special types. However, carcinomas exhibiting solely neuroendocrine differentiation are extremely rare, reportedly constituting less than 1% of all breast carcinomas.[1] These tumors are morphologically and immunophenotypically indistinguishable from neuroendocrine tumors of other organ systems such as lung and gastrointestinal tract. In the current WHO classification, the spectrum of carcinomas with neuroendocrine features is divided into three categories, including well-differentiated neuroendocrine tumor, poorly differentiated neuroendocrine carcinoma/small cell carcinoma, and invasive carcinoma with neuroendocrine differentiation.[2]

CARCINOMAS WITH NEUROENDOCRINE FEATURES, CYTOLOGY

Carcinomas with neuroendocrine features often show cohesive sheets and abundant single cells (Figure 13-1), which, on higher magnification, demonstrate scant to inconspicuous pale blue cytoplasm (Figure 13-2). The cells typically show nuclear pleomorphism with irregular nuclear membranes and scattered clumped chromatin.

CARCINOMAS WITH NEUROENDOCRINE FEATURES, GROSS FEATURES

Carcinomas with neuroendocrine features do not have specific characteristics by imaging study or on gross examination (Figure 13-3).

CARCINOMAS WITH NEUROENDOCRINE FEATURES, HISTOLOGY

Well-Differentiated Neuroendocrine Tumor

These tumors are usually densely cellular and form circumscribed solid masses in a background of fibrous stroma (Figure 13-4). The tumor cells are arranged in nests or trabeculae similar to carcinoids/well-differentiated endocrine tumors of other organs (Figure 13-5). The neoplastic cells are round, oval, or spindled; exhibit abundant pale to eosinophilic granular cytoplasm and low- to intermediate-grade nuclei with salt-and-pepper chromatin (Figures 13-6 and 13-7); and show variable expression of neuroendocrine markers (Figure 13-8). Mitotic figures may be seen but not brisk. Because of the presence of a solid growth pattern and uniform small round nuclei, as well as the frequent presence of indistinct cell borders and/or focal areas of single cell infiltration, invasive lobular carcinoma can be a differential diagnostic consideration. The fact that neuroendocrine carcinoma is characterized by intact membranous E-cadherin expression (Figure 13-9) could potentially be utilized in this situation.

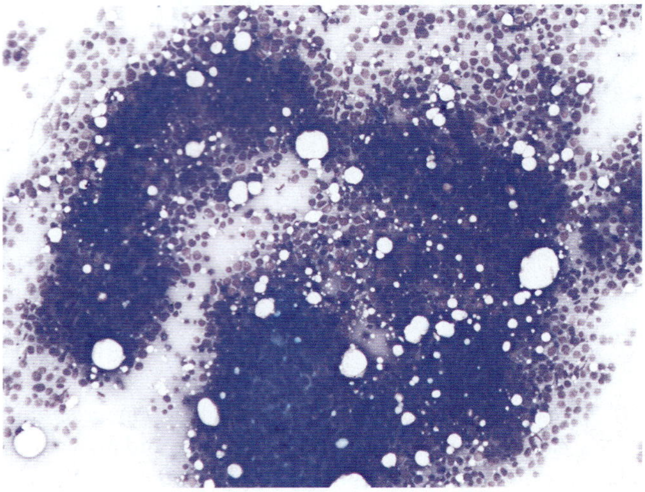

FIGURE 13-1: Carcinoma with neuroendocrine features. Diff-Quik–stained fine needle aspiration shows a highly cellular specimen consisting of an admixture of cohesive sheets and abundant single cells. (Photomicrograph courtesy of Amberly L. Nunez, M.D.)

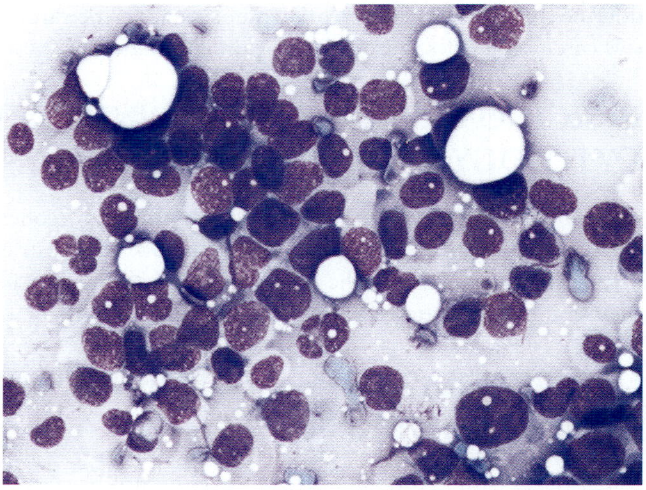

FIGURE 13-2: Carcinoma with neuroendocrine features. The tumor cells show scant to inconspicuous pale blue cytoplasm and pleomorphism nuclei with scattered clumped chromatin and irregular nuclear membranes. (Diff-Quik stain; photomicrograph courtesy of Amberly L. Nunez, M.D.)

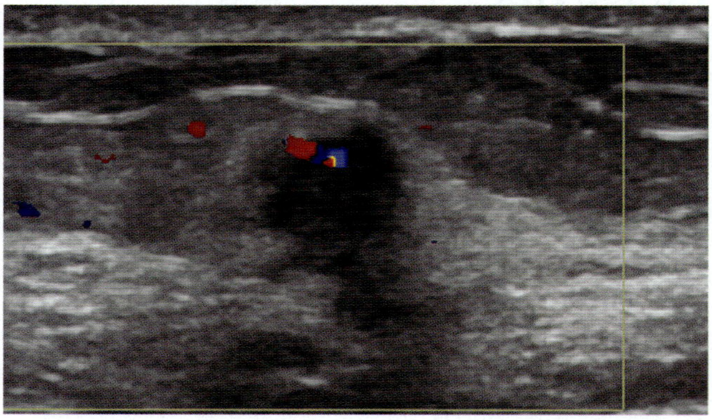

FIGURE 13-3: Color Doppler US image shows a round mass with indistinct margins and increased vascularity.

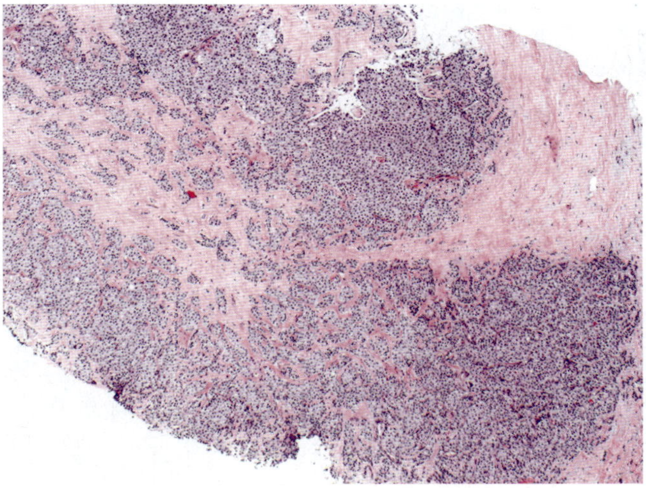

FIGURE 13-4: A low-power view of carcinoma with neuroendocrine features in a core needle biopsy specimen. The tumor is typically hypercellular in a background of densely fibrous stroma, with a somewhat circumscribed periphery.

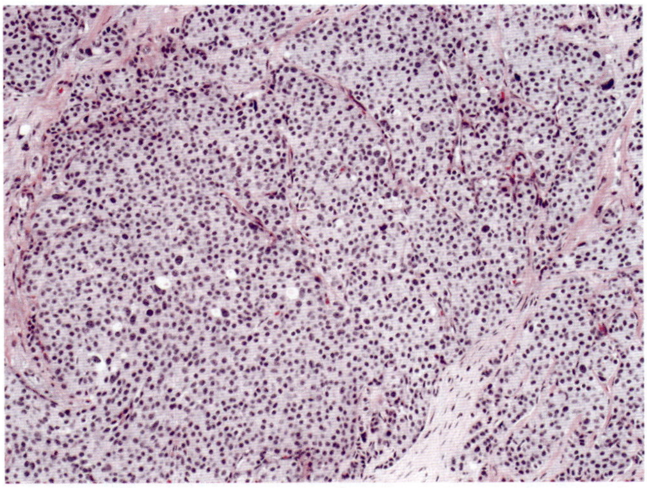

FIGURE 13-5: The cells with neuroendocrine differentiation are typically arranged in solid nests or trabeculae.

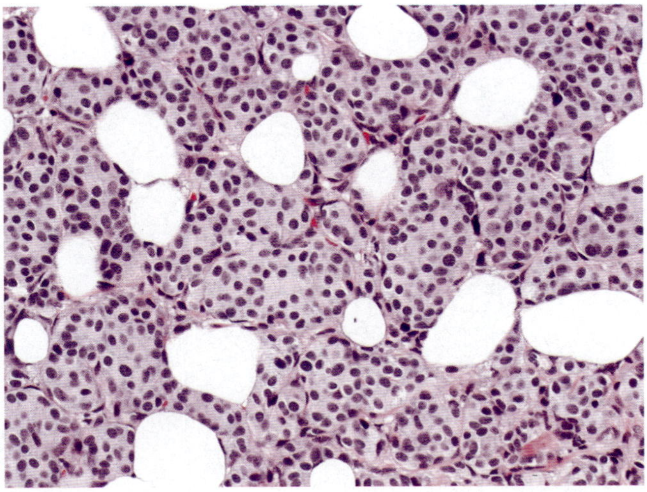

FIGURE 13-6: The nested growth may resemble the appearance of solid DCIS.

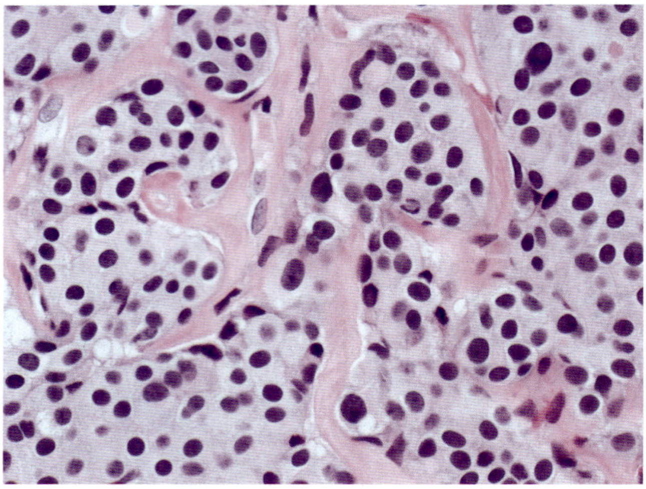

FIGURE 13-7: The neoplastic cells are characteristically round, oval, or short spindled, with abundant pale to eosinophilic granular cytoplasm and low- to intermediate-grade nuclei with salt-and-pepper chromatin. Cell borders may be distinct.

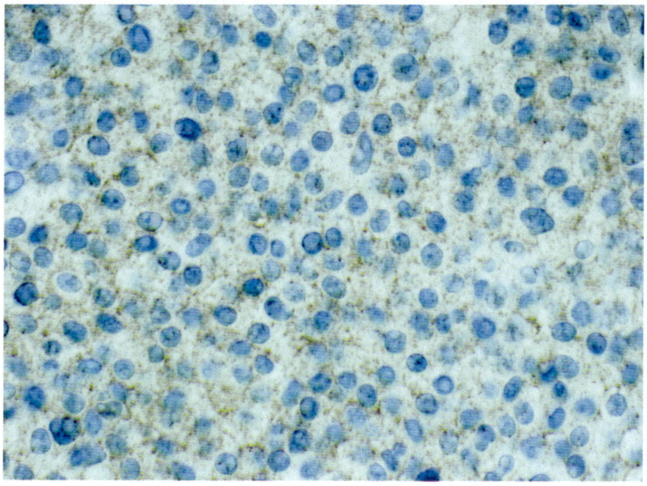

FIGURE 13-8: Given the diverse secretory activity of neuroendocrine tumors, the neoplastic cells typically express one or more neuroendocrine markers with a variable intensity, such as synaptophysin (illustrated in this image), chromogranin, and neuron-specific enolase.

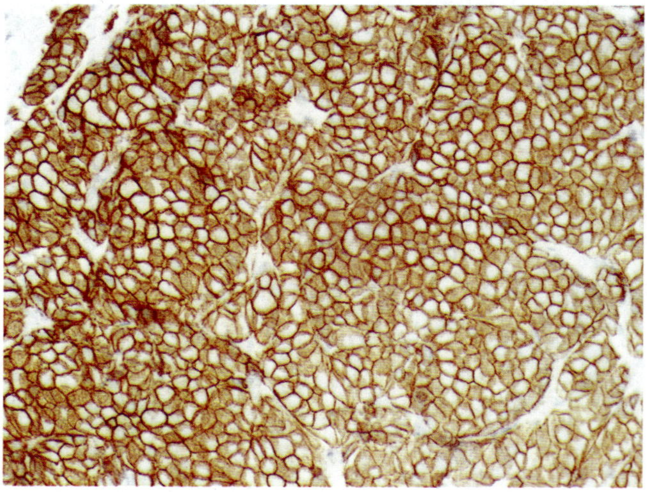

FIGURE 13-9: The combination of uniform small round nuclei and distinct cell borders, along with absence of gland formation in neuroendocrine carcinomas, may cause an erroneous impression of lobular carcinoma. However, intact membranous E-cadherin expression is invariably present, as depicted.

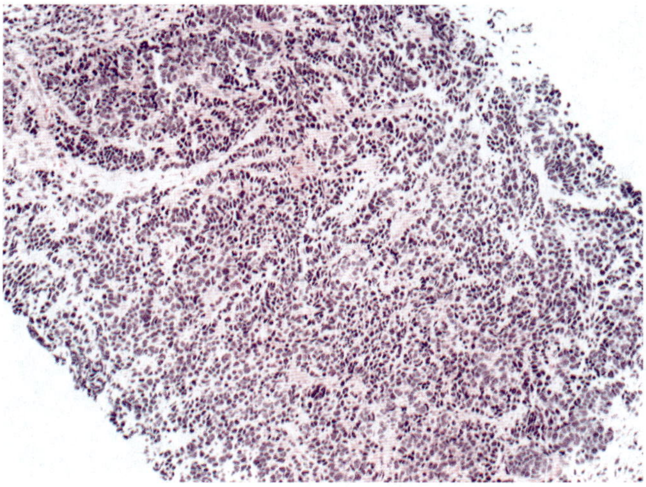

FIGURE 13-10: Mammary small cell carcinoma is histologically indistinguishable from those originating from other organs and is typically composed of highly proliferating malignant cells with hyperchromatic nuclei and scant cytoplasm.

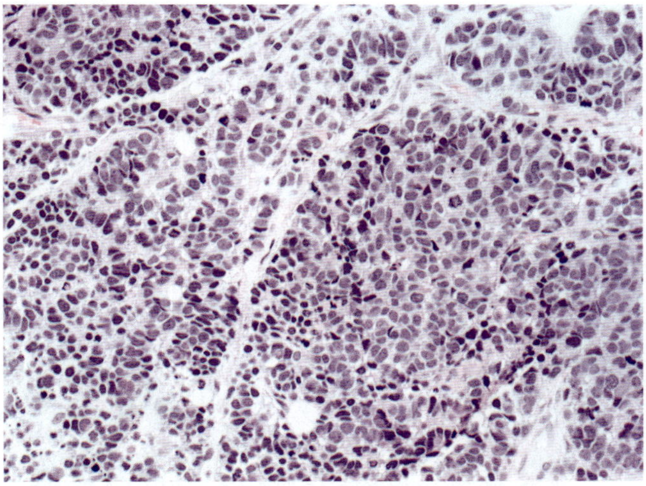

FIGURE 13-11: The constituent cells in mammary small cell carcinomas are typically arranged in nests and trabeculae. The neoplastic cells may vary in size but are generally larger than small lymphocytes.

Poorly Differentiated Neuroendocrine Carcinoma/Small Cell Carcinoma

These tumors are indistinguishable from those in other organs on morphologic grounds or by immunohistochemistry.[3] The tumors are typically composed of closely packed hyperchromatic cells with scant cytoplasm arranged in nests and trabeculae (Figure 13-10). Nuclear molding, mitoses, and tumor necrosis are frequently present (Figures 13-11 and 13-12). Expression of neuroendocrine markers is invariably present (Figure 13-13).

Invasive Carcinoma with Neuroendocrine Features

It is estimated that up to 30% of breast carcinomas demonstrate neuroendocrine differentiation by histochemical or immunohistochemical analysis (Figure 13-14).[2] Neuroendocrine features are most frequently seen in the hypercellular variant of mucinous carcinoma and both *in situ* and invasive components of solid papillary carcinoma (see Chapters 4 and 12).

CARCINOMAS WITH NEUROENDOCRINE FEATURES, DIFFERENTIAL DIAGNOSIS

The chief differential diagnosis is metastasis of neuroendocrine tumor from another site. Thus, clinical workup to exclude an extramammary origin is needed before a definitive diagnosis. In this regard, the presence of associated ductal carcinoma *in situ* (DCIS) (Figure 13-15) can substantiate

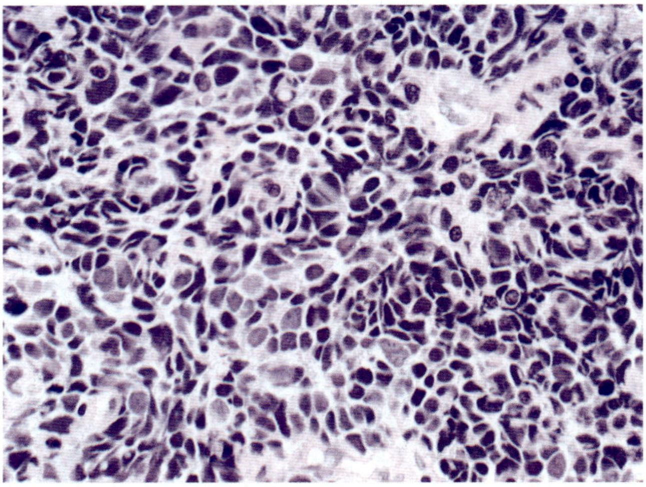

FIGURE 13-12: Nuclear molding, minimal cytoplasm, and stippled chromatin are characteristic of mammary small cell carcinoma. Brisk mitotic activity and tumor necrosis are frequently seen, but prominent nucleoli are typically absent.

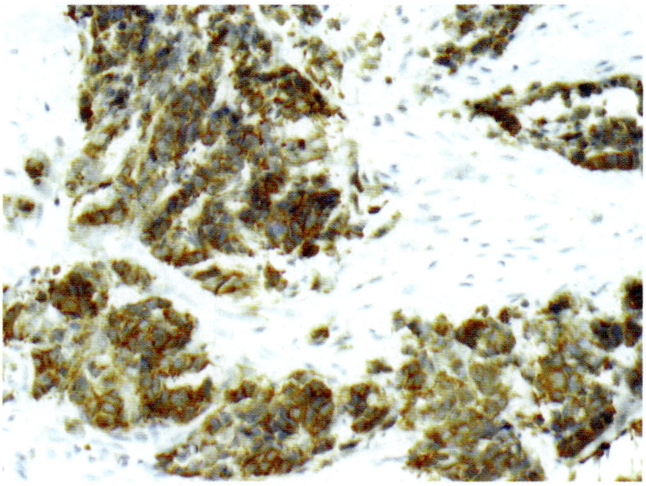

FIGURE 13-13: Synaptophysin expression in mammary small cell carcinoma.

a primary breast neoplasm. As previously discussed, well-differentiated neuroendocrine tumors may mimic invasive lobular carcinomas with a solid or alveolar growth pattern.

CARCINOMAS WITH NEUROENDOCRINE FEATURES, IMMUNOHISTOCHEMISTRY

All these tumors express neuroendocrine markers to a greater or a lesser degree. In addition, thyroid transcription factor-1 (TTF-1) expression in small cell carcinomas of extrapulmonary sites is not uncommon (Figure 13-16), thus reducing its diagnostic utility in this setting. [4,5]

Limited data have shown that ER and PR are expressed in majority of well-differentiated tumors and greater than 50% of poorly differentiated/small cell carcinomas.[2] These tumors typically lack HER2 overexpression or gene amplification.

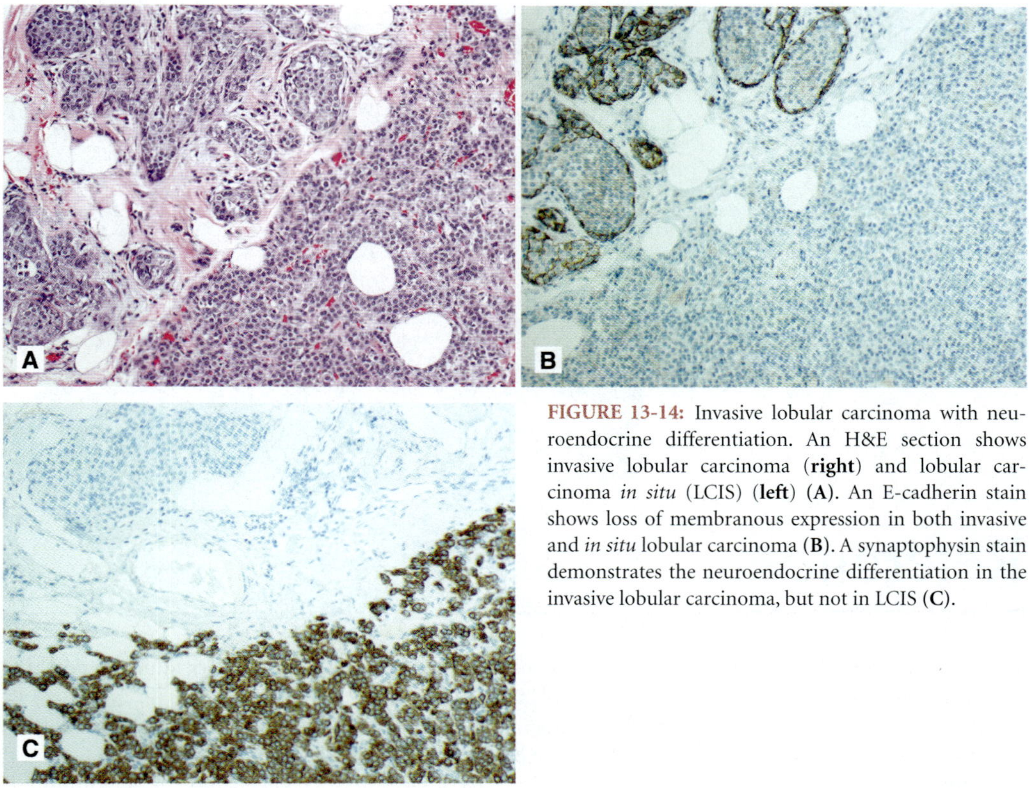

FIGURE 13-14: Invasive lobular carcinoma with neuroendocrine differentiation. An H&E section shows invasive lobular carcinoma (**right**) and lobular carcinoma *in situ* (LCIS) (**left**) (**A**). An E-cadherin stain shows loss of membranous expression in both invasive and *in situ* lobular carcinoma (**B**). A synaptophysin stain demonstrates the neuroendocrine differentiation in the invasive lobular carcinoma, but not in LCIS (**C**).

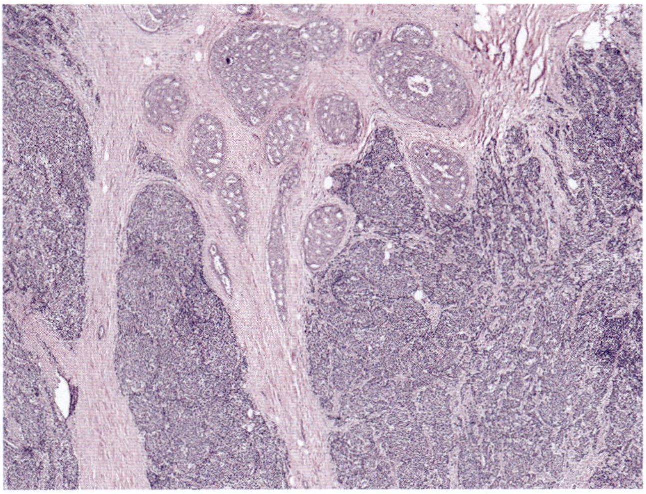

FIGURE 13-15: Mammary small cell carcinoma with associated DCIS.

CARCINOMAS WITH NEUROENDOCRINE FEATURES, HISTOGENESIS

The histogenesis of these tumors is unclear. It is proposed that they may arise from multipotential stem cells capable of divergent differentiation.[6]

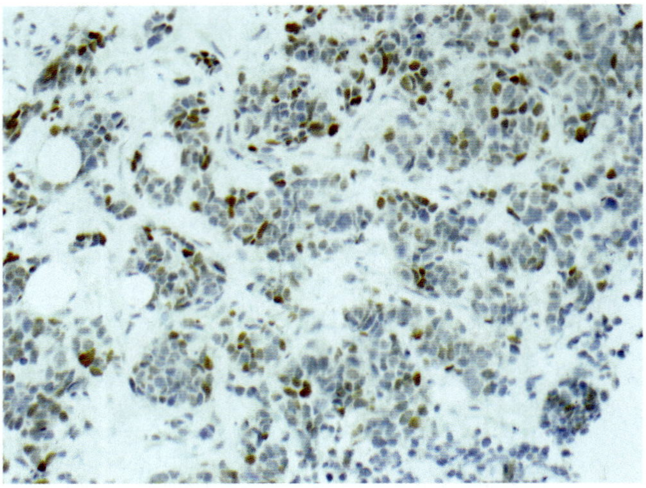

FIGURE 13-16: TTF-1 expression in mammary small cell carcinoma.

References

1. Sapino A, Righi L, Cassoni P, et al. Expression of apocrine differentiation markers in neuroendocrine breast carcinomas of aged women. *Mod Pathol* 2001;14:768–776.
2. Bussolati G, Badve S. Carcinomas with neuroendocrine features. In: Lakhani SR, Ellis IO, Schnitt SJ, et al., eds. *WHO Classification of Tumours of the Breast*. Lyon, France: IARC Press; 2012:62–63.
3. Shin SJ, DeLellis RA, Ying L, et al. Small cell carcinoma of the breast: a clinicopathologic and immunohistochemical study of nine patients. *Am J Surg Pathol* 2000;24:1231–1238.
4. Verset L, Arvanitakis M, Loi P, et al. TTF-1 positive small cell cancers: don't think they're always primary pulmonary! *World J Gastrointest Oncol* 2011;3:144–147.
5. Christie M, Chin-Lenn L, Watts MM, et al. Primary small cell carcinoma of the breast with TTF-1 and neuroendocrine marker expressing carcinoma in situ. *Int J Clin Exp Pathol* 2010;3:629–633.
6. Kinoshita S, Hirano A, Komine K, et al. Primary small-cell neuroendocrine carcinoma of the breast: report of a case. *Surg Today* 2008;38:734–738.

Invasive Micropapillary Carcinoma

14

Invasive micropapillary carcinoma is characterized by small clusters of infiltrating tumor cells surrounded by clear, empty spaces simulating dilated lymphatic channels. The tumor cell clusters lack fibrovascular cores and have a distinct "inside-out" appearance with the apical membrane facing outward. As is the case with micropapillary carcinomas elsewhere, lymph node metastasis is common in this breast neoplasm.

INVASIVE MICROPAPILLARY CARCINOMA, CYTOLOGY

Abundant cell clusters without a fibrovascular core along with other criteria of malignancy are typical cytologic findings in micropapillary carcinomas (Figure 14-1). Occasionally, the characteristic "inside-out" pattern can be appreciated on the fine needle aspiration.

INVASIVE MICROPAPILLARY CARCINOMA, IMAGING AND GROSS FEATURES

Invasive micropapillary carcinoma most frequently presents as a palpable mass. An irregular mammographic asymmetry with microcalcifications is common (Figure 14-2).[1] The gross pathologic findings are typically a solitary mass with poorly defined margins, but these features are nonspecific (Figure 14-3).[2]

INVASIVE MICROPAPILLARY CARCINOMA, HISTOLOGY

The presence of micropapillary features is fairly common in virtually all types of invasive carcinomas, especially no special type. Pure form of invasive micropapillary carcinoma is rare, accounting for up to 2% of all invasive breast carcinomas.[3] The cells in micropapillary carcinoma characteristically form hollow spherules devoid of fibrovascular cores (thus "micropapillary" might be considered a misnomer) or grow as solid aggregates (Figure 14-4). The neoplastic cells display reverse polarity, with the apical aspect of cell membrane facing outward, not to the luminal surface (Figures 14-5 and 14-6). The "inside-out" arrangement of cells can be demonstrated by MUC1[4] or epithelial membrane antigen (EMA) immunostaining, which show a characteristic peripheral staining pattern around the cell clusters (Figure 14-7). The tumoral cells are separated from the surrounding stroma by clear spaces resembling lymphatic channels. While these empty spaces have been argued to represent retraction artifact secondary to poor tissue preservation or fixation, tumor cell clusters from nonmicropapillary carcinomas lack the characteristic reverse polarity seen in micropapillary carcinoma. The tumor cells usually have low- to intermediate-grade nuclei, but can occasionally show significant nuclear pleomorphism. Ductal carcinoma *in situ* (DCIS) is commonly associated with micropapillary carcinomas and is often of micropapillary or cribriform pattern.

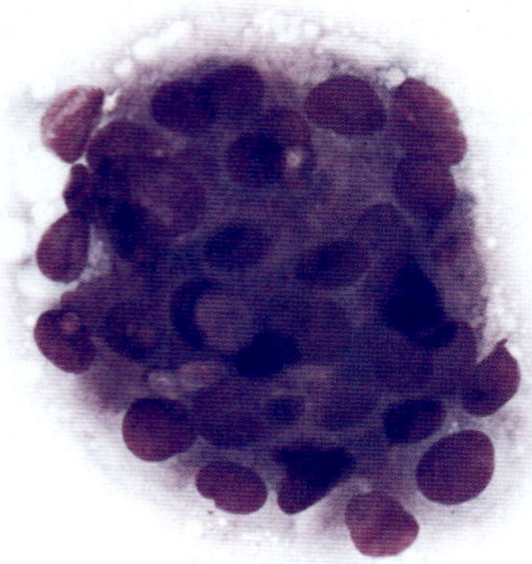

FIGURE 14-1: Invasive micropapillary carcinoma. Diff-Quik–stained fine needle aspiration shows a cohesive ball of atypical ductal cells with round to scalloped outlines. The nuclei are overlapping and enlarged with nuclear membrane irregularities. (Photomicrograph courtesy of Amberly L. Nunez, M.D.)

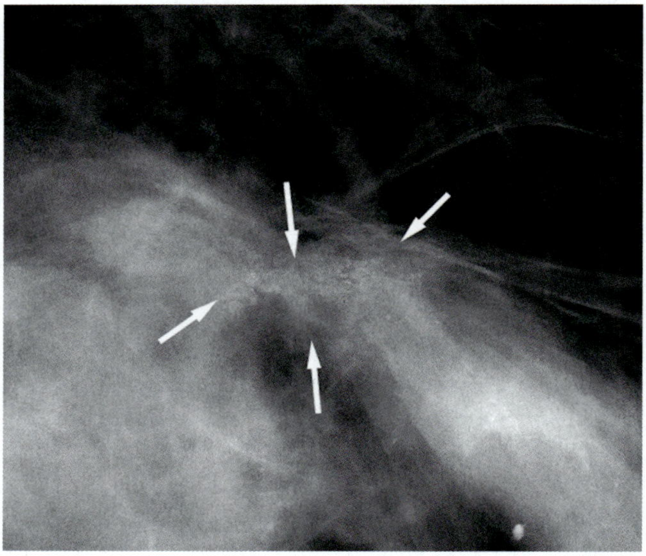

FIGURE 14-2: Invasive micropapillary carcinoma. A magnification craniocaudal mammographic view shows fine pleomorphic calcifications associated with architectural distortion (*arrows*).

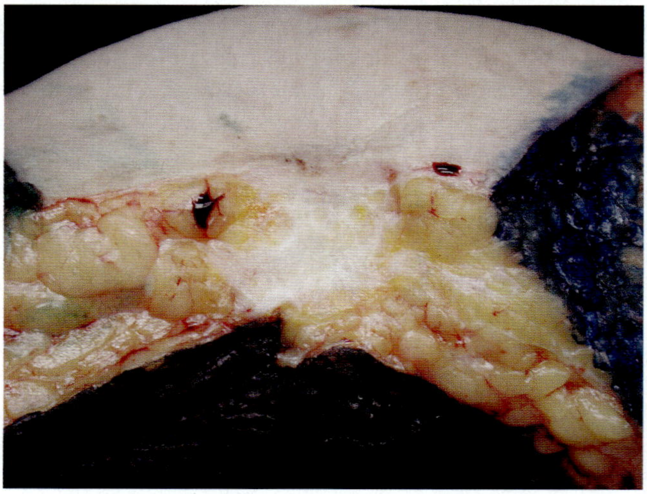

FIGURE 14-3: The gross pathologic features of invasive micropapillary carcinoma. The mass is usually poorly defined with an infiltrative growth pattern (Photograph courtesy of Erik Scott Young, Pennsylvania.)

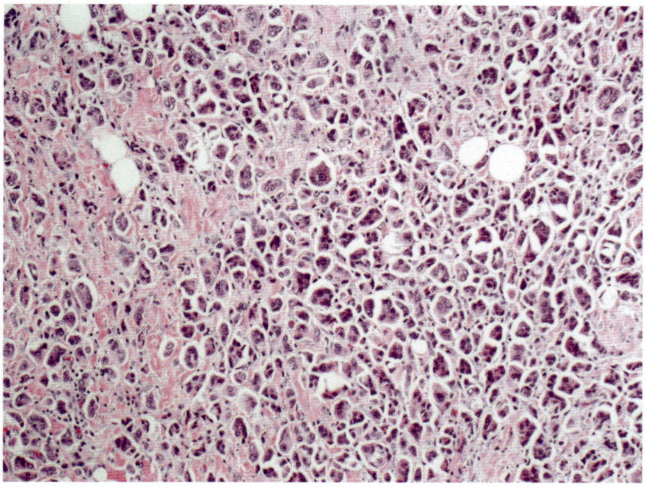

FIGURE 14-4: Micropapillary carcinoma showing avascular hollow spherules and morula-like epithelial clusters within lymphatic-like spaces in a background of fibrotic stroma.

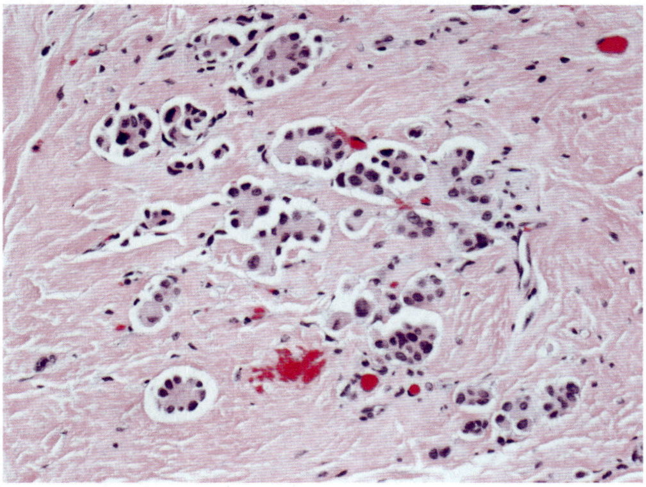

FIGURE 14-5: Characteristic reverse polarity in micropapillary carcinoma, with the apical aspect of cell membrane facing outward.

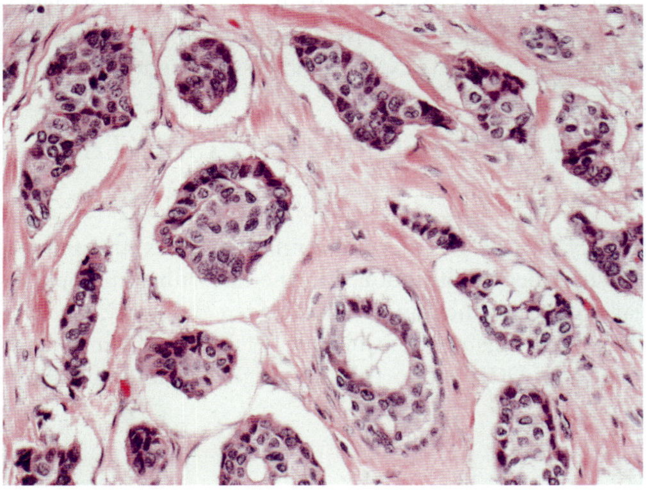

FIGURE 14-6: Micropapillary carcinomas can be of any histologic grade. The cells typically have abundant eosinophilic cytoplasm and vesicular nuclei.

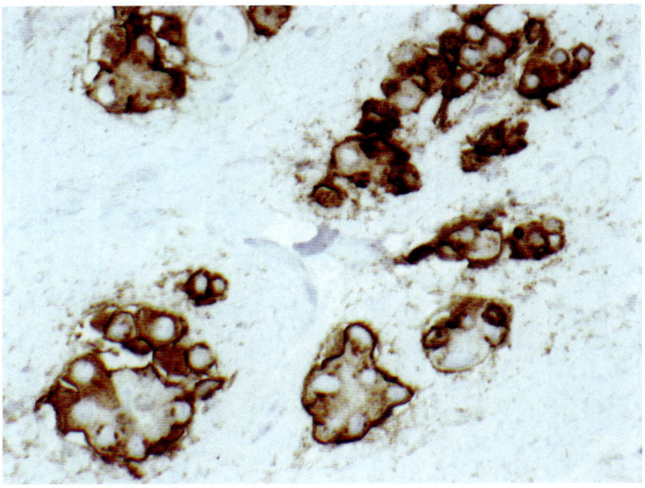

FIGURE 14-7: An EMA stain showing the unique "inside-out" arrangement of cells in micropapillary carcinoma.

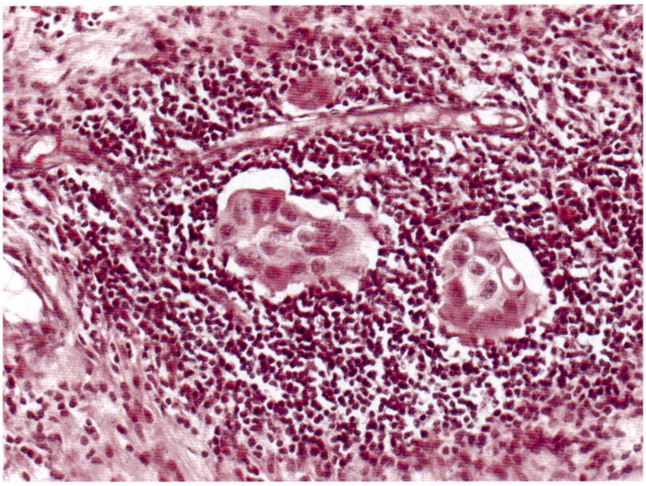

FIGURE 14-8: The micropapillary appearance is typically retained in the lymphatic spaces and nodal metastases.

Lymphovascular invasion and axillary lymph node metastasis are more frequently seen in association with micropapillary carcinomas than other histologic types (Figure 14-8).[5–8] The peculiar micropapillary appearance is usually retained in the lymphatic spaces and nodal metastases. Of note, the diagnosis of lymphovascular invasion is best rendered when present away from main tumor mass and, ideally, in the lymphatics associated with blood vessels (Figure 14-9).

INVASIVE MICROPAPILLARY CARCINOMA, DIFFERENTIAL DIAGNOSIS

Metastatic carcinomas with micropapillary features are chief differential diagnoses encountered in this setting; thus, it is crucial to obtain clinical information. Carcinomas with a micropapillary growth pattern can arise from various organs including lung, bladder, and ovary. Markers that are relatively site specific and helpful in this scenario include TTF-1 (lung), uroplakin (bladder), and PAX8 (ovary). The presence of DCIS supports breast origin of a micropapillary carcinoma.

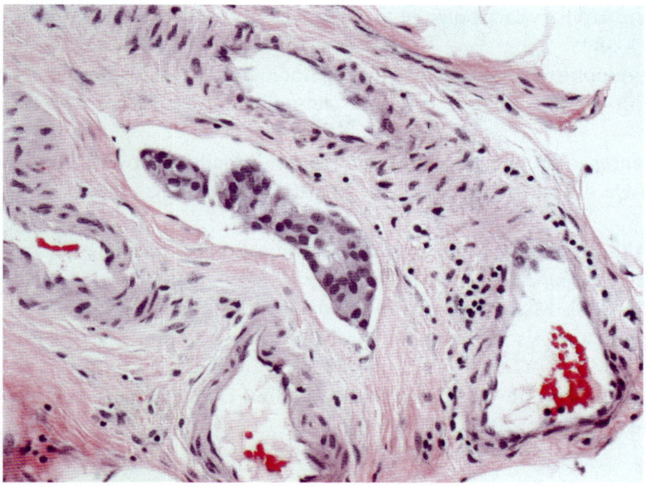

FIGURE 14-9: The diagnosis of lymphatic invasion is best made when present in the lymphatics associated with blood vessels outside of the main tumor mass.

INVASIVE MICROPAPILLARY CARCINOMA, IMMUNOHISTOCHEMISTRY

Micropapillary carcinomas are frequently positive for estrogen (ER) (61% to 100%) and PR (46% to 83%). Published results on HER2 expression are conflicting, ranging from near 100% in early series to about one-third in more recent studies.[2]

INVASIVE MICROPAPILLARY CARCINOMA, MOLECULAR GENETICS

Gene expression profiling studies have classified micropapillary carcinomas as luminal A or B subtypes, consistent with the preponderant high ER expression rate of these tumors.[9] Recurrent gains of chromosome 8q have been demonstrated by array-based comparative genomic hybridization analysis.[10] A significantly high frequency of MYC (8q24) amplification (33%) was found in micropapillary carcinomas when compared to grade- and ER-matched invasive carcinomas of no special type.[11]

References

1. Gunhan-Bilgen I, Zekioglu O, Ustun EE, et al. Invasive micropapillary carcinoma of the breast: clinical, mammographic, and sonographic findings with histopathologic correlation. *AJR Am J Roentgenol* 2002;179:927–931.
2. Reis-Fiho JS, Ellis IO. Invasive micropapillary carcinoma. In: Lakhani SR, Ellis IO, Schnitt SJ, et al., eds. *WHO Classification of Tumours of the Breast*. Lyon, France: IARC Press; 2012:65–66.
3. Paterakos M, Watkin WG, Edgerton SM, et al. Invasive micropapillary carcinoma of the breast: a prognostic study. *Hum Pathol* 1999;30:1459–1463.
4. Li YS, Kaneko M, Sakamoto DG, et al. The reversed apical pattern of MUC1 expression is characteristics of invasive micropapillary carcinoma of the breast. *Breast Cancer* 2006;13:58–63.
5. Nassar H, Wallis T, Andea A, et al. Clinicopathologic analysis of invasive micropapillary differentiation in breast carcinoma. *Mod Pathol* 2001;14:836–841.

6. Walsh MM, Bleiweiss IJ. Invasive micropapillary carcinoma of the breast: eighty cases of an underrecognized entity. *Hum Pathol* 2001;32:583–589.
7. Kim MJ, Gong G, Joo HJ, et al. Immunohistochemical and clinicopathologic characteristics of invasive ductal carcinoma of breast with micropapillary carcinoma component. *Arch Pathol Lab Med* 2005;129:1277–1282.
8. Yu JI, Choi DH, Park W, et al. Differences in prognostic factors and patterns of failure between invasive micropapillary carcinoma and invasive ductal carcinoma of the breast: matched case–control study. *Breast* 2010;19:231–237.
9. Weigelt B, Horlings HM, Kreike B, et al. Refinement of breast cancer classification by molecular characterization of histological special types. *J Pathol* 2008;216:141–150.
10. Marchio C, Iravani M, Natrajan R, et al. Mixed micropapillary-ductal carcinomas of the breast: a genomic and immunohistochemical analysis of morphologically distinct components. *J Pathol* 2009;218:301–315.
11. Marchio C, Iravani M, Natrajan R, et al. Genomic and immunophenotypical characterization of pure micropapillary carcinomas of the breast. *J Pathol* 2008;215:398–410.

Inflammatory Carcinoma

15

Inflammatory carcinoma is not a histologic variant of breast carcinoma, but rather a specific clinical presentation of carcinoma characterized by diffuse skin erythema and edema mimicking an inflammatory process and often resulting in a "peau d'orange" appearance.[1–3] The clinical "inflammatory" symptoms are caused by dermal lymphatic obstruction due to extensive tumor emboli within the lymphovascular spaces. The reported frequency varies between 1% and 10% and is highest among African American women.[4] Inflammatory carcinoma is clinically aggressive regardless of whether histopathologic evidence of dermal lymphatic invasion is present.

INFLAMMATORY CARCINOMA, IMAGING AND GROSS FEATURES

The imaging and gross pathologic features of inflammatory carcinomas are variable. The skin changes include erythema, thickening, tenderness, and induration. The tumor varies from radiographically or grossly indistinct to large masses with associated skin thickening and enhancement on breast MRI (Figure 15-1).[5,6]

INFLAMMATORY CARCINOMA, HISTOLOGY

The characteristic histologic findings in inflammatory carcinomas are the presence of numerous variably sized tumor emboli in dilated dermal lymphatic spaces (Figure 15-2). Significant inflammation is typically absent. However, the emboli may not always be identified in skin biopsies due to limitation of tissue sampling. Conversely, dermal lymphatic invasion is not uncommon in patients without clinical presentation of inflammatory carcinoma. In excisional specimens, extensive tumor emboli are frequently present throughout the breast in addition to skin (Figure 15-3). The tumor is often of high-grade invasive carcinoma of no special type, but less frequently can be other types. Inflammatory carcinoma is classified as T4d for staging purposes.

INFLAMMATORY CARCINOMA, IMMUNOHISTOCHEMISTRY

Inflammatory carcinomas frequently lack ER and PR expression and commonly show HER2 overexpression or gene amplification.[4] High expression of p53 and MUC1 is seen in these tumors.[7–9] Overexpression of E-cadherin is noted paradoxically associated with the aggressive type, probably as a result of altered cadherin function.[10–12]

INFLAMMATORY CARCINOMA, MOLECULAR GENETICS

Inflammatory carcinomas are mostly classified as HER2 and basal-like subtypes.[13] Mutations of p53 are common.[7,9]

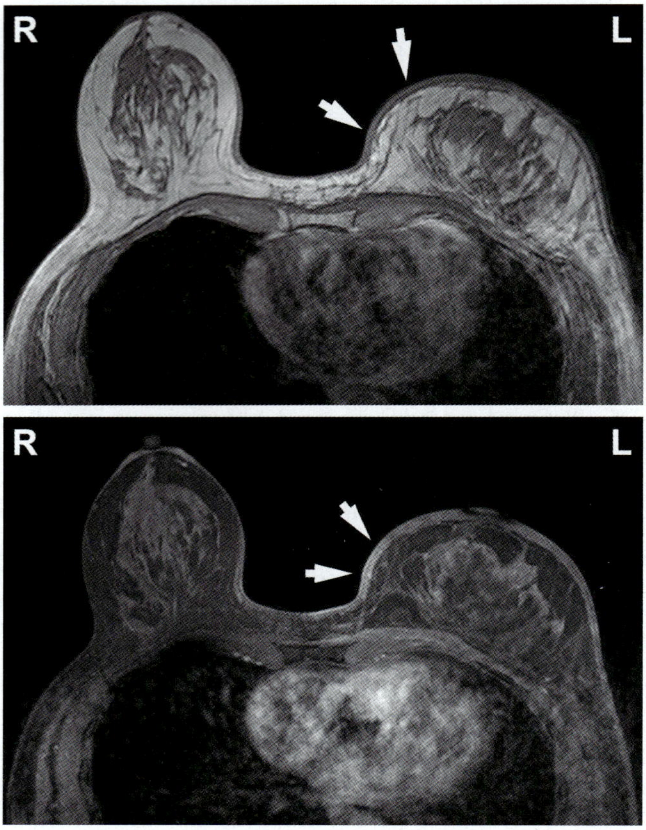

FIGURE 15-1: Imaging features of inflammatory carcinoma. **Upper panel,** axial T1 MR image reveals left medial breast skin thickening (*arrows*). **Lower panel,** axial T1 fat-saturated MR image shows skin thickening with enhancement post–contrast administration consistent with inflammatory carcinoma.

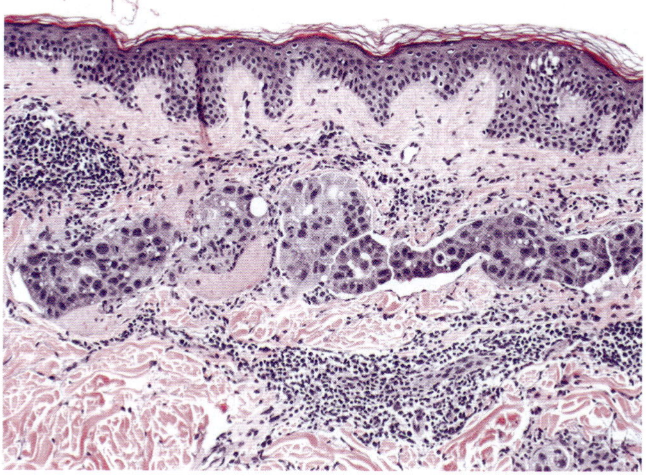

FIGURE 15-2: Inflammatory carcinoma. A punch skin biopsy shows dermal lymphatic invasion.

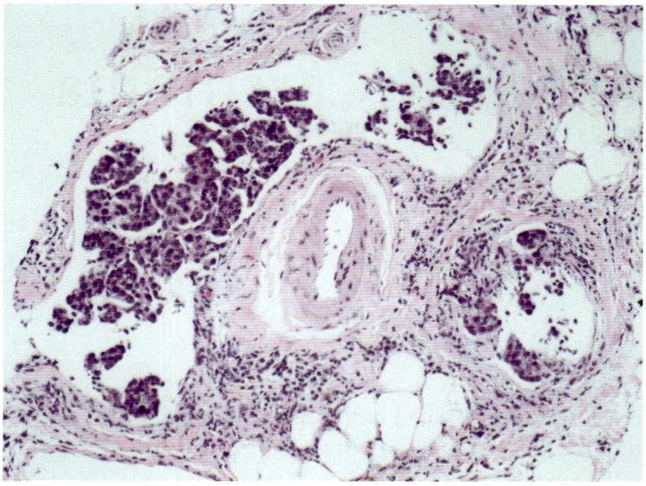

FIGURE 15-3: Numerous tumor emboli with micropapillary features are present in dilated lymphatics. These were adjacent to the invasive tumor in a patient presenting with inflammatory carcinoma.

References

1. Lucas FV, Perez-Mesa C. Inflammatory carcinoma of the breast. *Cancer* 1978;41:1595–1605.
2. Anderson WF, Schairer C, Chen BE, et al. Epidemiology of inflammatory breast cancer (IBC). *Breast Dis* 2005;22:9–23.
3. Hance KW, Anderson WF, Devesa SS, et al. Trends in inflammatory breast carcinoma incidence and survival: the surveillance, epidemiology, and end results program at the National Cancer Institute. *J Natl Cancer Inst* 2005;97:966–975.
4. Charafe-Jauffret E, Tsuda H, Rutgers E. Inflammatory carcinoma. In: Lakhani SR, Ellis IO, Schnitt SJ, et al., eds. *WHO Classification of Tumours of the Breast*. Lyon, France: IARC Press; 2012:67–68.
5. Lee KW, Chung SY, Yang I, et al. Inflammatory breast cancer: imaging findings. *Clin Imaging* 2005;29:22–25.
6. Carbognin G, Calciolari C, Girardi V, et al. Inflammatory breast cancer: MR imaging findings. *Radiol Med* 2010;115:70–82.
7. Faille A, De Cremoux P, Extra JM, et al. p53 mutations and overexpression in locally advanced breast cancers. *Br J Cancer* 1994;69:1145–1150.
8. Van den Eynden GG, Van der Auwera I, Van Laere S, et al. Validation of a tissue microarray to study differential protein expression in inflammatory and non-inflammatory breast cancer. *Breast Cancer Res Treat* 2004;85:13–22.
9. McCarthy NJ, Yang X, Linnoila IR, et al. Microvessel density, expression of estrogen receptor alpha, MIB-1, p53, and c-erbB-2 in inflammatory breast cancer. *Clin Cancer Res* 2002;8:3857–3862.
10. Ye Y, Tellez JD, Durazo M, et al. E-cadherin accumulation within the lymphovascular embolus of inflammatory breast cancer is due to altered trafficking. *Anticancer Res* 2010;30:3903–3910.
11. Kleer CG, van Golen KL, Braun T, et al. Persistent E-cadherin expression in inflammatory breast cancer. *Mod Pathol* 2001;14:458–464.
12. Alpaugh ML, Tomlinson JS, Ye Y, et al. Relationship of sialyl-Lewis(x/a) underexpression and E-cadherin overexpression in the lymphovascular embolus of inflammatory breast carcinoma. *Am J Pathol* 2002;161:619–628.
13. Van Laere S, Van der Auwera I, Van den Eynden GG, et al. Distinct molecular signature of inflammatory breast cancer by cDNA microarray analysis. *Breast Cancer Res Treat* 2005;93:237–246.

16 Secretory Carcinoma

Secretory carcinoma is a rare, translocation-associated carcinoma. It affects both sexes and occurs over a wide age range, but is more commonly seen in children and young adults with a median age of presentation of 25 years; hence, its other designation is "juvenile breast carcinoma." The tumor is associated with a favorable prognosis in young patients.[1–5]

SECRETORY CARCINOMA, IMAGING AND GROSS FEATURES

There are no specific findings for secretory carcinomas on imaging studies. Grossly, they are usually circumscribed masses of variable size.

SECRETORY CARCINOMA, HISTOLOGY

Microscopically, secretory carcinomas are typically well-circumscribed masses with pushing borders, but are rarely infiltrative. The tumors usually have a lobulated growth pattern and can be arranged in microcysts/honeycombs, acini, solid islands or, more commonly, a mixture of these patterns. The striking histologic hallmark is the presence of abundant eosinophilic, PAS-positive, diastase-resistant secretory material within the acini and microcysts simulating thyroid follicles (Figure 16-1). The tumor cells have low-grade nuclei and pale granular or vacuolated cytoplasm and may present as signet-ring cells (Figure 16-2). An *in situ* component may be present and displays similar secretory appearance.[6]

SECRETORY CARCINOMA, DIFFERENTIAL DIAGNOSIS

The main differential diagnoses include cystic hypersecretory carcinoma and lactational changes in normal breast. The vast majority of cystic hypersecretory carcinomas are *in situ* lesions with peripheral myoepithelial lining. The lesional cells typically exhibit pleomorphic nuclei and scant cytoplasm as opposed to the relatively uniform nuclei and abundant cytoplasm seen in secretory carcinomas. When an invasive carcinoma arises, the secretory features usually become inconspicuous. In lactational changes, the underlying normal breast architecture remains.

SECRETORY CARCINOMA, IMMUNOHISTOCHEMISTRY

The majority of secretory carcinomas lack ER and PR expression, HER2 overexpression, and HER2 gene amplification.[6,7] They may express basal cytokeratins (CK5/6, CK14), p63, S100 protein, and smooth muscle actin.[6]

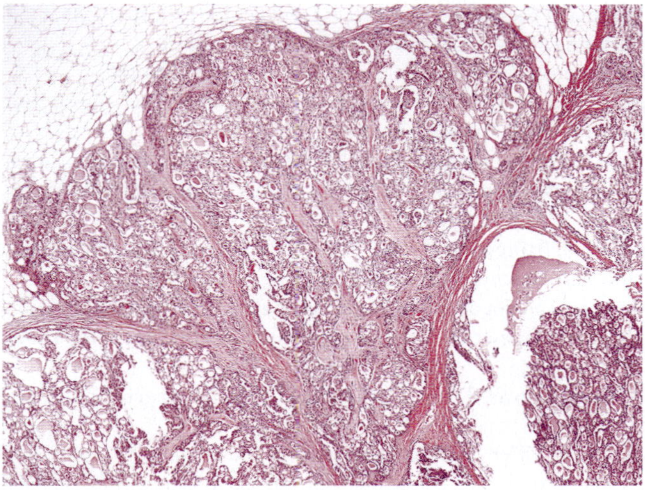

FIGURE 16-1: Secretory carcinoma showing a well-circumscribed mass with pushing borders. The tumor is arranged in acini and cysts separated by fibrous bands with abundant secretory material simulating thyroid follicles.

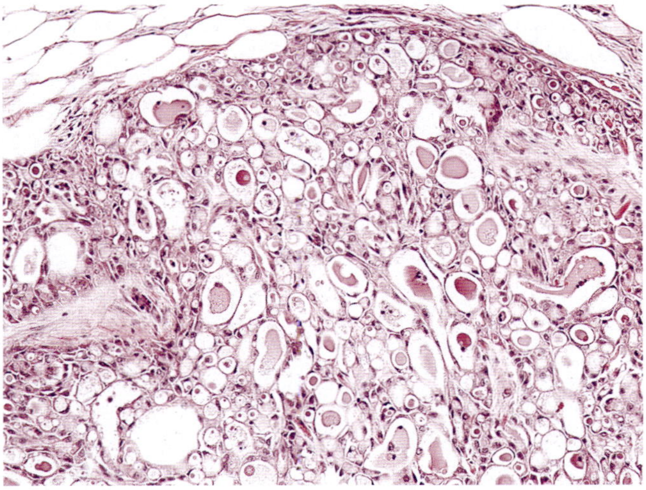

FIGURE 16-2: At higher magnification, the cells of secretory carcinoma have low-grade nuclei and vacuolated clear cytoplasm.

SECRETORY CARCINOMA, MOLECULAR GENETICS

A recurrent balanced translocation, t(12;15)(p13;q25), has been identified as a primary event in secretory carcinomas, which creates a ETV6-NTRK3 gene fusion encoding a chimeric tyrosine kinase.[8] Expression of the fusion gene has been also observed in nearly 100% of secretory carcinomas by other studies and is present in both the invasive and *in situ* components.[6,7] The proposed causal relationship between a single chromosomal translocation and a particular cancer phenotype challenge widely held beliefs concerning breast carcinogenesis. Interestingly, the identical chromosomal rearrangement has also been identified in the histologically similar mammary analog secretory carcinoma that arises in major salivary glands.[9] Further, the same translocation has been known to be oncogenic in a number of nonepithelial malignancies, including congenital fibrosarcoma, mesoblastic nephroma, and acute myeloid leukemia.[10–12]

References

1. McDivitt RW, Stewart FW. Breast carcinoma in children. *JAMA* 1966;195:388–390.
2. Krausz T, Jenkins D, Grontoft O, et al. Secretory carcinoma of the breast in adults: emphasis on late recurrence and metastasis. *Histopathology* 1989;14:25–36.

3. Rosen PP, Cranor ML. Secretory carcinoma of the breast. *Arch Pathol Lab Med* 1991;115:141–144.
4. Tavassoli FA, Norris HJ. Secretory carcinoma of the breast. *Cancer* 1980;45:2404–2413.
5. Oberman HA. Secretory carcinoma of the breast in adults. *Am J Surg Pathol* 1980;4:465–470.
6. Lae M, Freneaux P, Sastre-Garau X, et al. Secretory breast carcinomas with ETV6-NTRK3 fusion gene belong to the basal-like carcinoma spectrum. *Mod Pathol* 2009;22:291–298.
7. Diallo R, Schaefer KL, Bankfalvi A, et al. Secretory carcinoma of the breast: a distinct variant of invasive ductal carcinoma assessed by comparative genomic hybridization and immunohistochemistry. *Hum Pathol* 2003;34:1299–1305.
8. Tognon C, Knezevich SR, Huntsman D, et al. Expression of the ETV6-NTRK3 gene fusion as a primary event in human secretory breast carcinoma. *Cancer Cell* 2002;2:367–376.
9. Skalova A, Vanecek T, Sima R, et al. Mammary analogue secretory carcinoma of salivary glands, containing the ETV6-NTRK3 fusion gene: a hitherto undescribed salivary gland tumor entity. *Am J Surg Pathol* 2010;34:599–608.
10. Knezevich SR, McFadden DE, Tao W, et al. A novel ETV6-NTRK3 gene fusion in congenital fibrosarcoma. *Nat Genet* 1998;18:184–187.
11. Knezevich SR, Garnett MJ, Pysher TJ, et al. ETV6-NTRK3 gene fusions and trisomy 11 establish a histogenetic link between mesoblastic nephroma and congenital fibrosarcoma. *Cancer Res* 1998;58:5046–5048.
12. Eguchi M, Eguchi-Ishimae M, Tojo A, et al. Fusion of ETV6 to neurotrophin-3 receptor TRKC in acute myeloid leukemia with t(12;15)(p13;q25). *Blood* 1999;93:1355–1363.

17 Other Rare Tumors and Variants

There are a number of uncommon tumor types and variants that occur in the breast. These entities are predominantly of skin appendageal (i.e., sebaceous carcinoma) or salivary gland (mucoepidermoid carcinoma, polymorphous carcinoma, oncocytic carcinoma, acinic cell carcinoma) nature. While these tumors are exceptionally rare in the breast, they are still clinically relevant. It is important to note that although most of the salivary gland–type mammary carcinomas (including previously discussed adenoid cystic carcinoma) are "triple negative" and express basal-type markers,[1] these tumors characteristically behave much better than conventional triple-negative breast carcinomas. On the other hand, the rarity of some of the other tumors makes it difficult to accurately determine outcome. Examples of the latter include lipid-rich carcinoma and glycogen-rich carcinoma.

MUCOEPIDERMOID CARCINOMA

Mucoepidermoid carcinoma of the breast is identical to its counterpart in the salivary gland. The clinical features of mucoepidermoid carcinoma are similar to that of invasive carcinomas of no special type. The entity has an estimated incidence of 0.3% of all breast cancers in one series,[2] while there have been only less than 50 cases reported to date in the English language literature. Nipple discharge may be the initial presentation if the tumor is located in the retroareolar region.[3]

Microscopically, mucoepidermoid carcinomas are characterized by the presence of epidermoid (squamoid), mucus-producing cells and intermediate cells, with columnar, clear cell, and oncocytic features (Figures 17-1 to 17-3). A cystic component is frequently present. The proportion of different cell types and architectural pattern varies within and between tumors. The mucocytes are large, with fluffy cytoplasm and peripherally displaced nuclei. These cells contain sialomucin (hence positive for mucicarmine or Alcian blue staining) and may be seen dispersed within the epidermoid or intermediate cells or lining cystic spaces/duct-like structures. Intermediate cells usually predominate. The traditional histologic grading for its salivary gland counterpart includes a numerical grading system using point scoring of five parameters consisting of the proportion of cystic component, neural invasion, necrosis, mitotic index, and anaplasia,[4] although it has been challenged by a recent point-based grading system including the proportion of cystic component, growth pattern, nuclear pleomorphism, lymphovascular and bony invasion, mitotic count, perineural spread, and necrosis.[5] Most of the mucoepidermoid carcinomas of the breast are low grade that tend to be cystic, with abundant mucocytes and minimal atypia or mitotic activity.[6] High-grade tumors are rare and typically consist predominantly of solid sheets of epidermoid cells. Hormonal receptors were negative in the case studies.[7,8]

The differential diagnosis of mucoepidermoid carcinomas essentially includes invasive carcinoma of no special type with squamous differentiation/metaplastic carcinoma. The presence of squamous pearls with true keratinization is supportive of metaplastic carcinoma and argues

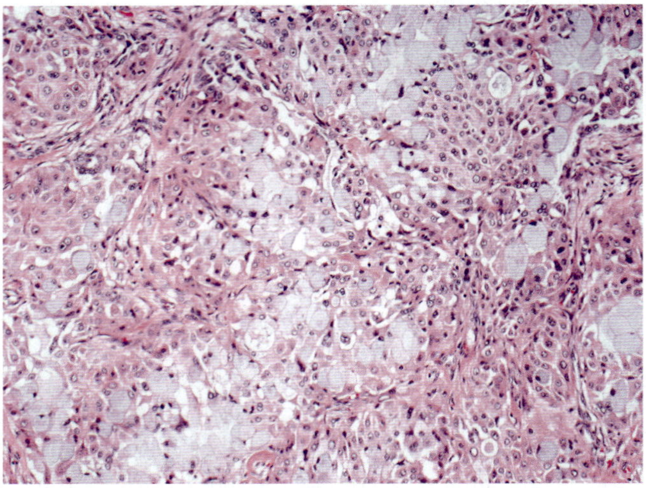

FIGURE 17-1: Mucoepidermoid carcinoma is characterized by the presence of squamoid cells, mucus-producing cells, and cells of intermediate type.

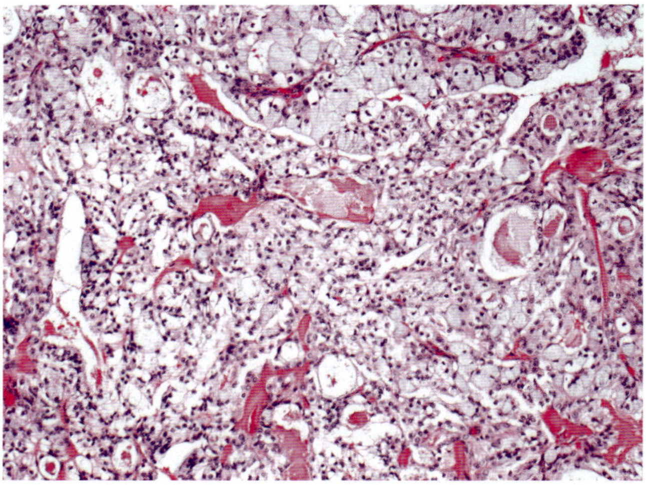

FIGURE 17-2: Mucoepidermoid carcinoma with prominent clear cell features.

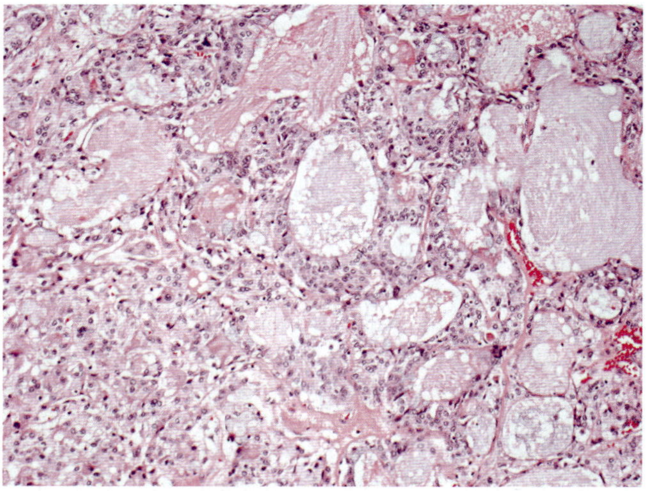

FIGURE 17-3: Mucoepidermoid carcinoma with prominent microcyst formation.

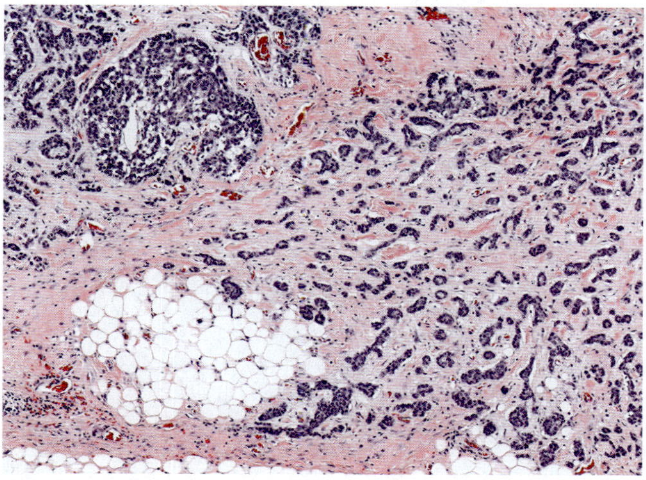

FIGURE 17-4: Polymorphous carcinoma with various growth patterns. (Photomicrograph courtesy of Margaret Brandwein-Gensler, M.D.)

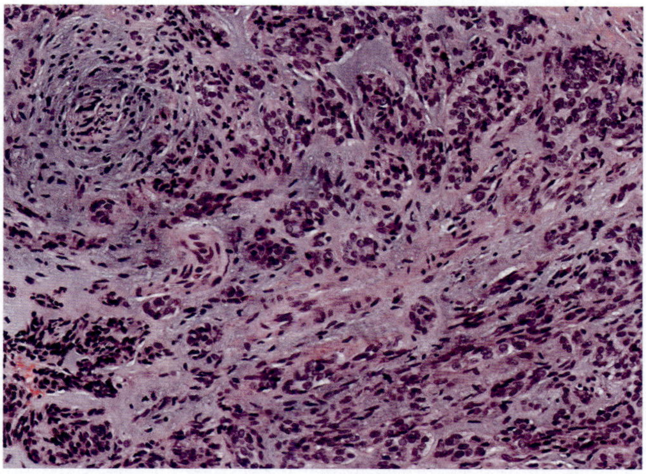

FIGURE 17-5: A higher-power view showing polymorphous carcinoma with low- to intermediate-grade nuclei. Note the targetoid growth pattern in the left upper corner characteristic of lobular carcinoma. (Photomicrograph courtesy of Margaret Brandwein-Gensler, M.D.)

against mucoepidermoid carcinoma.[9] Interestingly, there is at least one case report[6] of a breast mucoepidermoid carcinoma sharing the molecular alteration (partial deletion of 11q21) characteristic of its salivary counterpart.

POLYMORPHOUS CARCINOMA

Polymorphous carcinoma of the breast is histologically similar to its salivary gland counterpart known as polymorphous low-grade carcinoma. Only five cases have been reported to date.[1,10]

Polymorphous carcinoma is characterized by cytologic uniformity, architectural diversity, and an infiltrative growth pattern. The most striking feature is the presence of a wide spectrum of morphologic configurations between tumors and within individual tumors at low magnification (Figure 17-4). The tumor may display solid nests, targetoid, alveolar, cribriform, trabecular, as well as single-file patterns (Figure 17-5). The lesional cells exhibit round to ovoid, low- to intermediate-grade nuclei. Staining for ER, PR, and HER2 was negative.[1]

ACINIC CELL CARCINOMA

Acinic cell carcinoma characteristically consists of acini with serous differentiation and cytoplasmic zymogen-type secretory granules. Acinic cell carcinoma of the breast is very rare, with only scattered case reports described in the literature.[11–15]

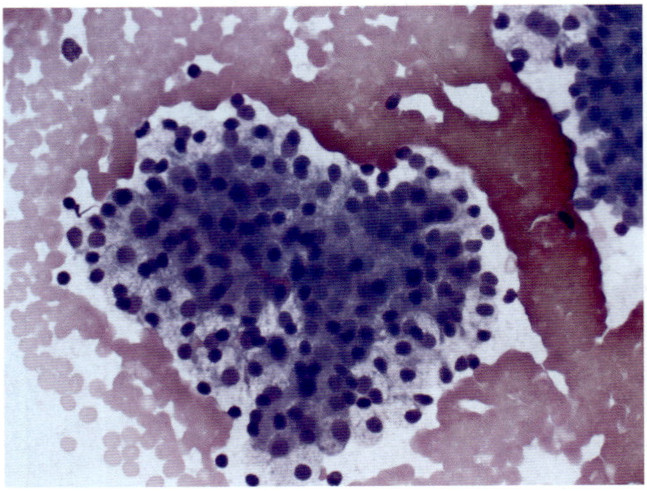

FIGURE 17-6: Cytologic appearance of acinic cell carcinoma. A crowded sheet of acinic cells with round to oval overlapping nuclei and abundant finely granular cytoplasm. (Diff-Quik stain; photomicrograph courtesy of Amberly L. Nunez, M.D.)

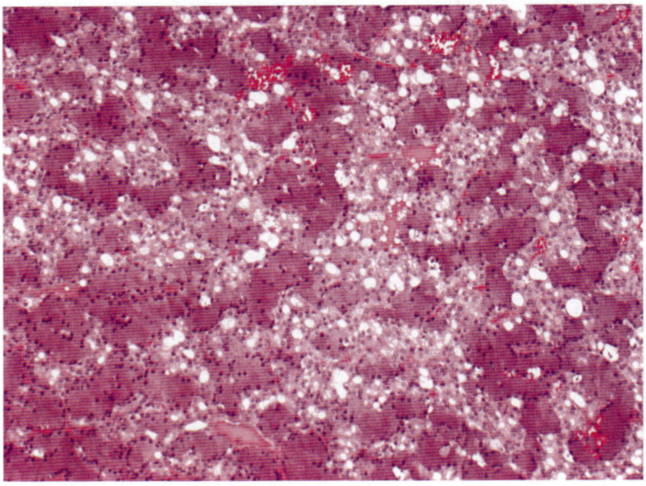

FIGURE 17-7: Acinic cell carcinoma showing sheets of neoplastic cells with abundant pale to eosinophilic granular cytoplasm.

Cytologically, the tumor cells closely resemble normal serous acinic cells of the salivary glands. The lesional cells possess abundant, characteristic coarse zymogen granules that are pinkish in Diff-Quik stain (Figure 17-6). Histologically, the tumor shows a wide variety of morphologic growth patterns ranging from well-formed acini, microcystic, papillary–cystic, follicular, to solid nests. The lesional cells are large and polygonal, with eosinophilic or lightly basophilic cytoplasm and round, eccentric nuclei (Figures 17-7 and 17-8). The cytoplasmic zymogen-like granules are large and course and are periodic acid–Schiff (PAS) positive and resistant to diastase digestion. A clear cell component is frequently seen and may predominate. These cells are similar in size and shape to acinar-type cells but have no cytoplasmic granules.

Acinic cell carcinomas express alpha-1-antichymotrypsin, alpha-1 antitrypsin, amylase, and S100 protein. These tumors are consistently negative for ER, PR, and HER2.[9]

ONCOCYTIC CARCINOMA

An oncocyte (derived from the Greek root onco-, which means mass, bulk) is a cell characterized by an excessive amount of mitochondria that gives rise to voluminous eosinophilic granular cytoplasm. Oncocytic carcinoma of the breast has been defined by the presence of greater than 70% of cells with oncocytic characteristics.[16,17]

Oncocytic carcinoma of the breast typically shows a solid growth pattern with sheets, islands, and nests of large, polygonal cells (Figure 17-9). The oncocytic cells have indistinct cell borders,

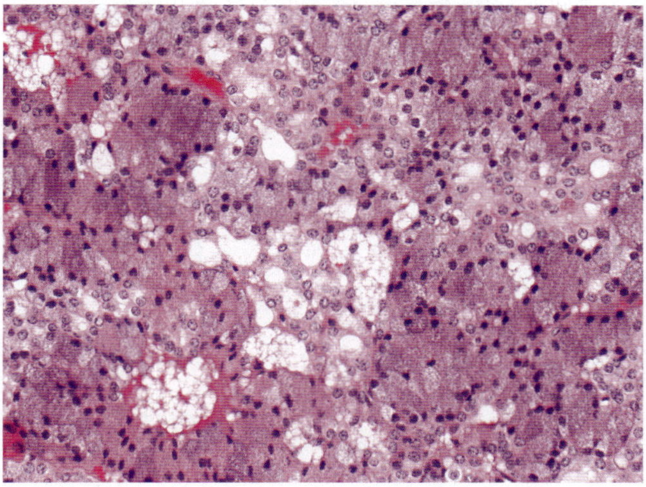

FIGURE 17-8: The constituent cells in acinic cell carcinoma are large and polygonal, with round, eccentric nuclei of low to intermediate grade.

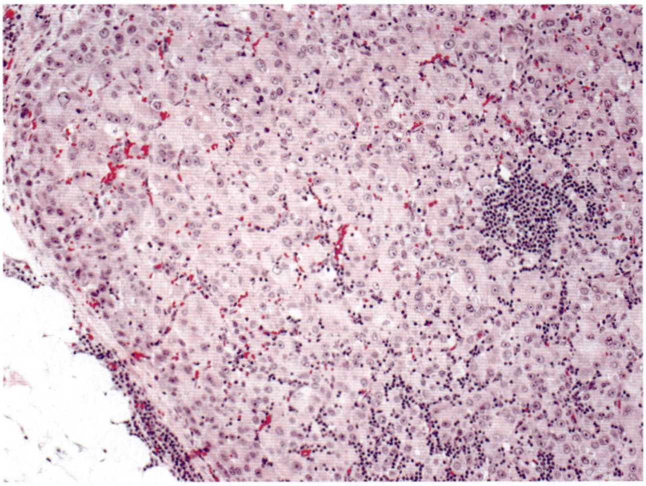

FIGURE 17-9: Oncocytic carcinoma showing a solid growth pattern with sheets of large, polygonal cells.

abundant granular, eosinophilic cytoplasm, and central, round, vesicular nuclei often with prominent nucleoli (Figure 17-10). These cells show strong immunoreactivity for mitochondria. Moreover, a recent series has shown that oncocytic carcinomas of the breast frequently overexpress HER2.[17]

SEBACEOUS CARCINOMA

Primary mammary sebaceous carcinoma is exceedingly rare and is diagnosed when a breast carcinoma demonstrates prominent (>50%) sebaceous differentiation without evidence of origin from cutaneous adnexal sebaceous glands.[18] The sebocytic differentiation is characterized by abundant vesicular and vacuolated clear cytoplasm containing lipid droplets (Figure 17-11). The other cell type in sebaceous carcinoma is that of smaller ovoid to spindle cells with eosinophilic cytoplasm devoid of vacuolization. The tumor cells may be positive for ER and PR. Androgen receptor and HER2 can be expressed.[19–21]

LIPID-RICH CARCINOMA AND GLYCOGEN-RICH CARCINOMA

Lipid-rich carcinoma and glycogen-rich carcinoma are defined by an invasive breast carcinoma with ≥90% of the cells containing abundant cytoplasmic neutral lipid or glycogen, respectively.[18] These lesions typically show a clear cell morphology, although intracytoplasmic glycogen (PAS positive, diastase labile) can also be observed without a significant clear cell appearance in 60% of

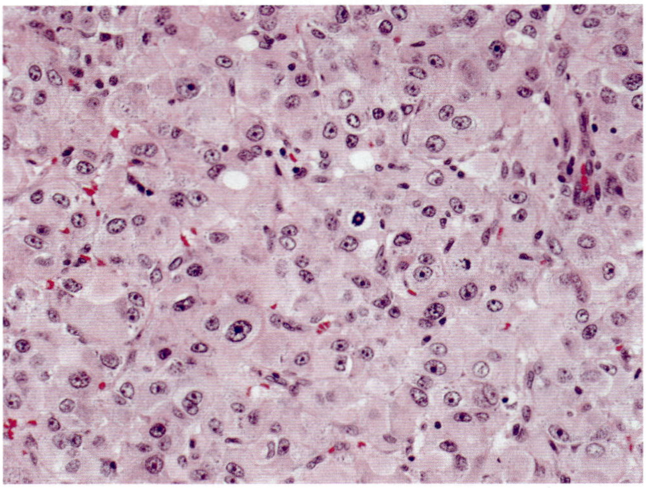

FIGURE 17-10: The cells of oncocytic carcinoma characteristically have indistinct cell borders, abundant granular eosinophilic cytoplasm, and central nuclei with disperse chromatin and prominent nucleoli.

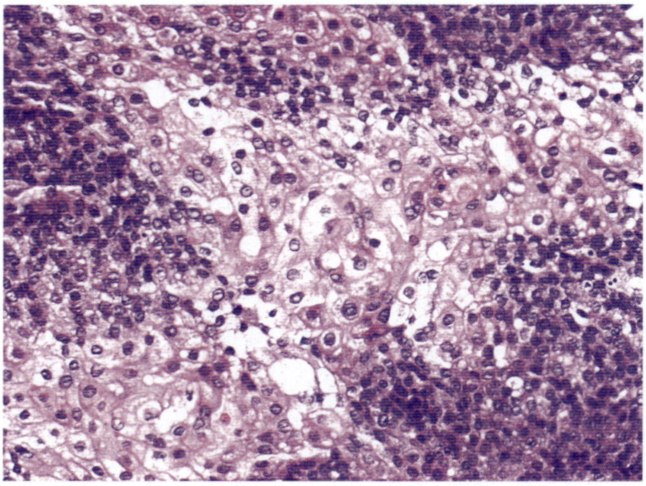

FIGURE 17-11: Sebaceous carcinoma showing vacuolated, lipid-containing clear cytoplasm.

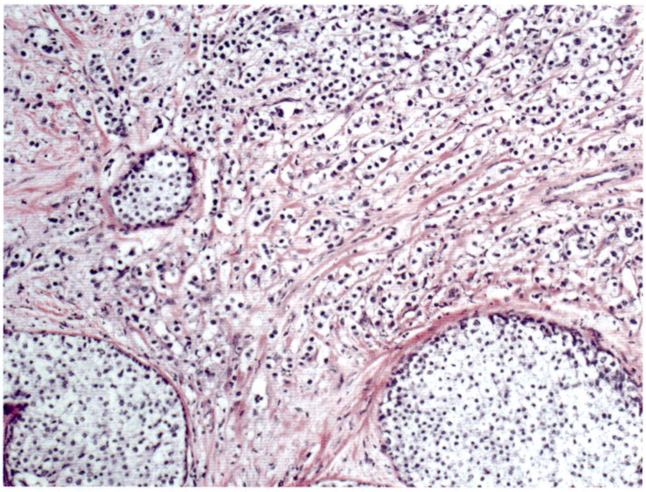

FIGURE 17-12: Lipid-rich carcinoma showing clear cell morphology, which contains cytoplasmic neutral lipid. The coexistence of ductal carcinoma *in situ* supports a mammary origin.

breast carcinomas.[18] It remains controversial if they represent distinct clinicopathologic entities as it has not been proved that these rare histologic variants have a biologic behavior different from that of invasive carcinoma, no special type. The importance of recognizing these variants lies in the fact that they may closely resemble some benign conditions, such as xanthomatous mastitis, or other tumor types with clear cell morphology including metastatic renal cell carcinoma and perivascular epithelioid cell tumor (PEComa). The coexistence of *in situ* carcinoma within the tumor assists with breast primary (Figure 17-12).

References

1. Reyes C, Jorda M, Gomez-Fernandez C. Salivary Gland-like tumors of the breast express basal-type immunohistochemical markers. *Appl Immunohistochem Mol Morphol* 2013;21(4):283–286.
2. Fisher ER, Palekar AS, Gregorio RM, et al. Mucoepidermoid and squamous cell carcinomas of breast with reference to squamous metaplasia and giant cell tumors. *Am J Surg Pathol* 1983;7:15–27.
3. Di Tommaso L, Foschini MP, Ragazzini T, et al. Mucoepidermoid carcinoma of the breast. *Virchows Arch* 2004;444:13–19.
4. Goode RK, Auclair PL, Ellis GL. Mucoepidermoid carcinoma of the major salivary glands: clinical and histopathologic analysis of 234 cases with evaluation of grading criteria. *Cancer* 1998;82:1217–1224.
5. Brandwein MS, Ferlito A, Bradley PJ, et al. Diagnosis and classification of salivary neoplasms: pathologic challenges and relevance to clinical outcomes. *Acta Otolaryngol* 2002;122:758–764.
6. Camelo-Piragua SI, Habib C, Kanumuri P, et al. Mucoepidermoid carcinoma of the breast shares cytogenetic abnormality with mucoepidermoid carcinoma of the salivary gland: a case report with molecular analysis and review of the literature. *Hum Pathol* 2009;40:887–892.
7. Hastrup N, Sehested M. High-grade mucoepidermoid carcinoma of the breast. *Histopathology* 1985;9:887–892.
8. Hornychova H, Ryska A, Betlach J, et al. Mucoepidermoid carcinoma of the breast. *Neoplasma* 2007;54:168–172.
9. Foschini MP, Krausz T. Salivary gland-type tumors of the breast: a spectrum of benign and malignant tumors including "triple negative carcinomas" of low malignant potential. *Semin Diagn Pathol* 2010;27:77–90.
10. Asioli S, Marucci G, Ficarra G, et al. Polymorphous adenocarcinoma of the breast. Report of three cases. *Virchows Arch* 2006;448:29–34.
11. Roncaroli F, Lamovec J, Zidar A, et al. Acinic cell-like carcinoma of the breast. *Virchows Arch* 1996;429:69–74.
12. Schmitt FC, Ribeiro CA, Alvarenga S, et al. Primary acinic cell-like carcinoma of the breast—a variant with good prognosis? *Histopathology* 2000;36:286–289.
13. Winkler N, Morrell G, Factor RE. Invasive carcinoma with acinic cell-like features of the breast. *Breast J* 2013;19:334–335.
14. Damiani S, Pasquinelli G, Lamovec J, et al. Acinic cell carcinoma of the breast: an immunohistochemical and ultrastructural study. *Virchows Arch* 2000;437:74–81.
15. Zhao Y, Li W, Lang R, et al. Primary acinic cell carcinoma of the breast: a case report and review of the literature. *Int J Surg Pathol* 2014;22(2):177–81.
16. Damiani S, Eusebi V, Losi L, et al. Oncocytic carcinoma (malignant oncocytoma) of the breast. *Am J Surg Pathol* 1998;22:221–230.
17. Ragazzi M, de Biase D, Betts CM, et al. Oncocytic carcinoma of the breast: frequency, morphology and follow-up. *Hum Pathol* 2011;42:166–175.
18. Eusebi V, Ichihara S, Vincent-Salomon A, et al. Exceptionally rare types and variants. In: Lakhani SR, Ellis IO, Schnitt SJ, et al., eds. *WHO Classification of Tumours of the Breast*. Lyon, France: IARC Press; 2012:71–76.
19. Murakami A, Kawachi K, Sasaki T, et al. Sebaceous carcinoma of the breast. *Pathol Int* 2009;59:188–192.
20. Hisaoka M, Takamatsu Y, Hirano Y, et al. Sebaceous carcinoma of the breast: case report and review of the literature. *Virchows Arch* 2006;449:484–488.
21. Varga Z, Kolb SA, Flury R, et al. Sebaceous carcinoma of the breast. *Pathol Int* 2000;50:63–66.

18 Pathologic Changes Secondary to Diagnosis or Treatment of Carcinoma

The most common histologic findings associated with diagnostic or surgical procedures include fat necrosis, histiocytic and foreign body giant cell reaction, fibrosis, and hemosiderin deposition. The constellation of these microscopic features commonly referred to as biopsy/surgical site changes is usually not problematic in practice. The diagnostic challenge in this setting is to recognize mechanical displacement of epithelium, whether benign or malignant, into mammary stroma, lymphatics, or lymph node by needling/surgical procedures, as its incorrect categorization can significantly impact subsequent patient management. In light of treatment-associated changes, chemotherapeutic agents may cause variable degrees of morphologic alterations in carcinoma cells as well as benign epithelium, of which the latter may particularly be mistaken for malignancy. Since radiation has become a standardized treatment modality after breast-conserving surgery for invasive and *in situ* carcinoma, radiation-associated atypical vascular lesions (AVLs) and angiosarcoma are increasingly being diagnosed as well.

EPITHELIAL DISPLACEMENT

Iatrogenic displacement of epithelium has long been a well-recognized phenomenon. It typically occurs following a variety of needling procedures including core needle biopsy, fine needle aspiration, anesthetic injection, suture placement, and wire localization. Displaced epithelial cells can be present in the biopsy site, needle tract, lymphovascular spaces, and regional lymph nodes.[1–4] While it may be seen in association with any benign lesion or *in situ* carcinoma, papillary lesions are particularly prone to this artifact owing to the inherent friable nature of lesional tissue; thus, it has been so-called a papillary phenomenon.[5]

Epithelial displacement most commonly occurs in the biopsy tract of mammary stroma.[5] Histologically, it is of particular importance to recognize epithelial displacement as it may produce a pattern that closely simulates invasive carcinoma and thus may result in erroneous diagnosis in patients with benign lesions or *in situ* carcinoma. Displaced epithelium is typically present in the form of isolated, small fragments of epithelium in artificial spaces within the breast stroma. These epithelial aggregates are almost always confined to the traumatized areas that are associated with obvious biopsy site changes such as organizing hemorrhage, acute and chronic inflammation, foreign body giant cell reaction, fat necrosis, hemosiderin deposition, and granulation tissue or scaring, depending on the stage of maturation (Figures 18-1 to 18-4). Rarely, epithelial displacement may reside in breast stroma other than biopsy sites, which can be more problematic. In contrast to true invasive carcinoma, however, the displaced epithelial clusters typically do not elicit a stromal reaction. Thus, in the absence of a prior diagnosis of invasive carcinoma, definitive invasion should be considered only in the context of the simultaneous presence of desmoplastic stromal reaction and in an area away from the previous needling procedure. The absence of

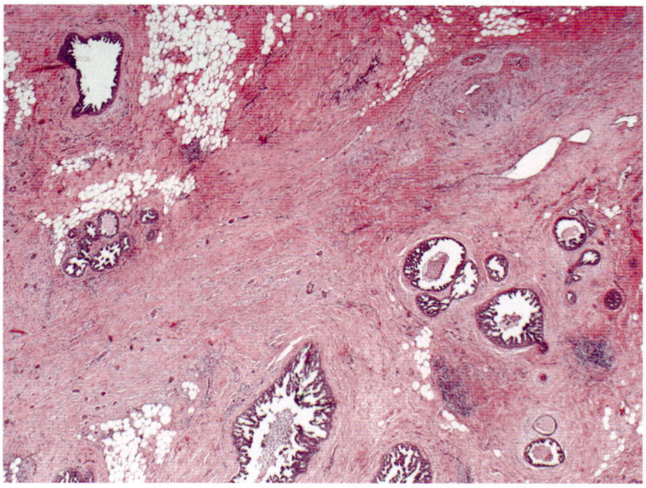

FIGURE 18-1: Displacement of epithelium following needle biopsy of DCIS. A low-power view shows extensive micropapillary DCIS. There is a needle tract in which there are numerous displaced clusters of malignant epithelial cells. Note that the epithelial aggregates are confined to the traumatized area.

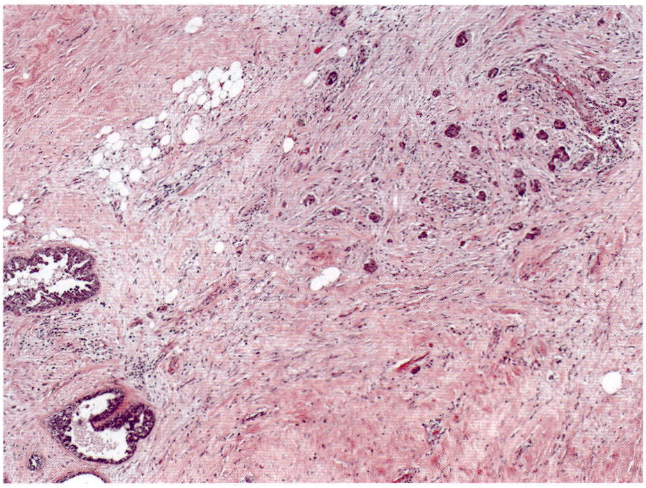

FIGURE 18-2: The stroma surrounding the displaced epithelium shows myofibroblastic proliferation, chronic inflammation, and hemosiderin characteristic of biopsy site changes.

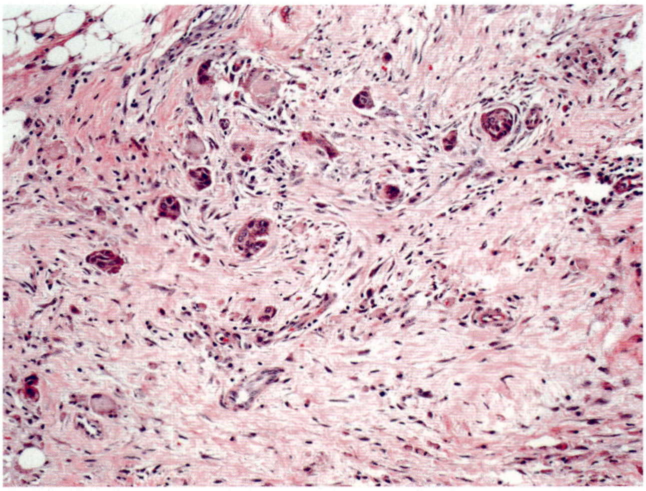

FIGURE 18-3: Foreign body giant cell reaction adjacent to the displaced malignant epithelial cells.

FIGURE 18-4: Displacement of epithelium following needle biopsy of an intraductal papilloma with squamous metaplasia. Note the variably sized clusters of epithelial cells in the neighboring tissue with associated biopsy site changes. The epithelial cells have similar histologic appearance to the cells in the papilloma and also show squamous features.

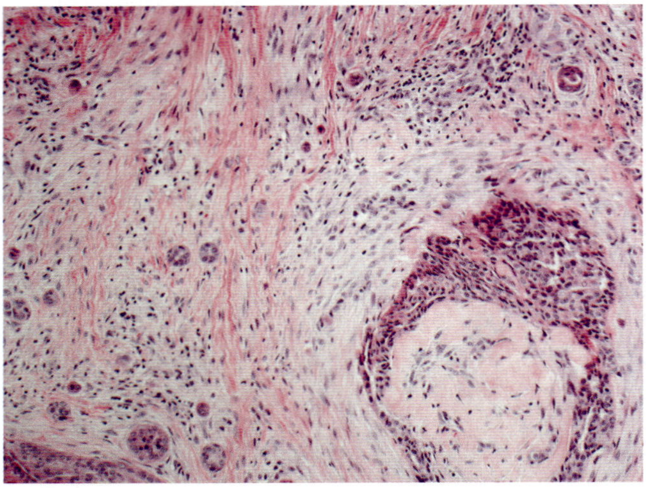

FIGURE 18-5: Displaced malignant epithelial cells in a lymph node. A sentinel lymph node biopsy demonstrates clusters of epithelial cells in the subcapsular sinus from a patient with micropapillary DCIS. Absence of documented invasive carcinoma, cytologic features similar to those in the DCIS, and abundant foamy macrophages surrounding the epithelial clusters point toward the correct interpretation.

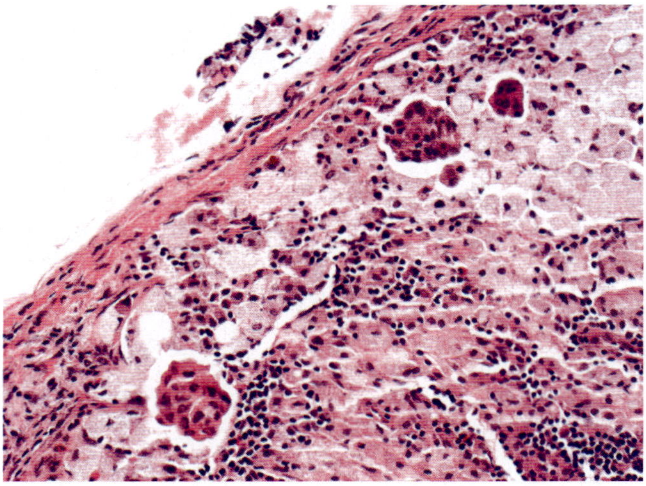

myoepithelial cells in the extralesional epithelial clusters is not, by itself, diagnostic of invasion, particularly in cases of papillary lesions.

Epithelial displacement into lymphatic or vascular spaces can also occur and may be indistinguishable from intrinsic lymphovascular invasion, especially when the displaced epithelia happen to be malignant cells.[5–7] Rarely, this artifact can even be seen in the initial core needle biopsy tissue.[7] Thus, in the absence of bona fide invasive carcinoma, the presence of epithelial clusters in the lymphovascular spaces should be interpreted with extreme caution. When the focus of suspicion is confined to the area of biopsy site, epithelial displacement as a potential manifestation of benign mechanical transport should be considered in the differential diagnosis.

Single or small clusters of epithelial cells in the regional lymph nodes can be even more challenging diagnostically.[4,8] As part of tissue healing process, regional lymph nodes drain traumatized area regardless of its contents (as in the case of silicon lymphadenopathy). In addition, breast massage in women undergoing sentinel lymph node biopsy reportedly may result in epithelial displacement to lymph nodes.[9,10] The features that favor displaced epithelium over true metastasis include degenerative changes such as foamy and/or hemosiderin-laden macrophages, foreign body giant cell reaction, and damaged red blood cells (Figure 18-5). Given that there is no objective method to determine whether an epithelial deposit arrives in a lymph node (or other sites) as a result of metastatic spread or by iatrogenic mechanical transport, it is appropriate to provide an explanatory comment in the pathology report in equivocal cases to emphasize this uncertainty.

The biologic consequence of displaced epithelium in all sites is currently unknown. Whether the displaced malignant cells possess infiltrative or metastatic potential remains a matter of debate. Long-term clinical follow-up is needed to determine the biologic and clinical significance of this unique pathologic phenomenon.

MORPHOLOGIC CHANGES ASSOCIATED WITH NEOADJUVANT THERAPY

Generally, histologic changes associated with neoadjuvant chemotherapy can be seen in both benign breast and tumoral tissues. The most notable histologic alterations in nonneoplastic breast are sclerosis of intralobular stroma, thickening of basement membrane, atrophy of acinar and ductal epithelium, and variable degrees of cytologic atypia. The key to recognize treatment-associated effects is that the altered terminal duct lobular units (TDLUs) in nonneoplastic breast tissue preserve a lobulocentric configuration and lack cellular proliferation on low-power examination (Figure 18-6). The epithelial cells maintain normal nuclear-to-cytoplasmic ratio and cellular polarity. Mitotic activity or necrosis is uncommon, if any. The treatment-associated cytologic atypia in benign epithelial cells typically includes increased cell size with enlarged and hyperchromatic nuclei, small or inconspicuous nucleoli, and eosinophilic, sometimes vacuolated, cytoplasm (Figure 18-7). These effects are more pronounced in TDLUs but are also seen, although less commonly, in larger ducts

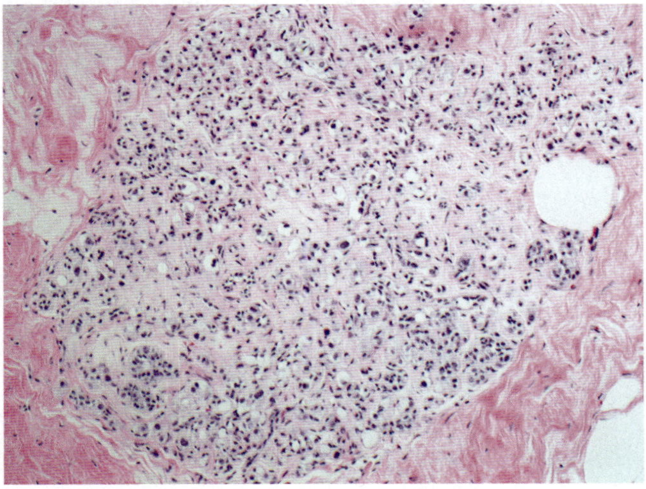

FIGURE 18-6: Therapy-associated changes in a benign breast lobule. Note the well-preserved lobular configuration, absence of epithelial proliferation, fibrosis of intralobular stroma, and thickening of the basement membrane.

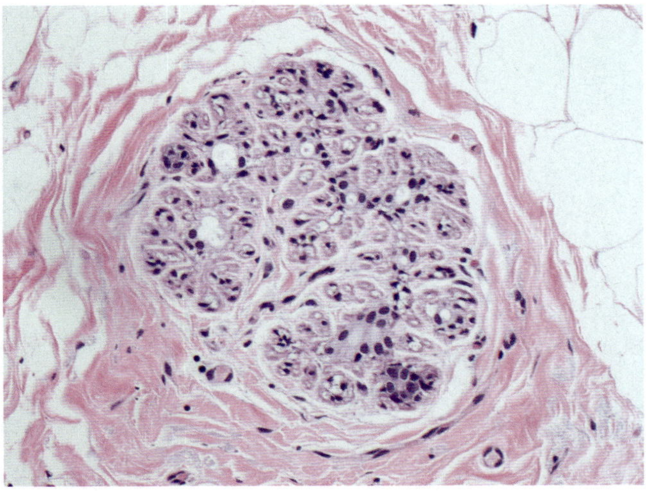

FIGURE 18-7: Another example of atrophic lobule after neoadjuvant therapy showing cytologic atypia including enlarged and hyperchromatic nuclei and vacuolated cytoplasm.

(Figure 18-8). It is important to note that the extent of stromal collagenization is dependent on the interval between therapy and biopsy, and a variable degree of fibrosis is not uncommon in breast tissue without treatment. Thus, stromal fibrosis by itself is not a reliable indicator of therapeutic effects.

Pathologic examination of breast tissue following neoadjuvant chemotherapy is critical in accurately assessing tumor response. In such situation, tumor bed, typically represented as a fibrotic area on gross examination, must be identified and sampled for histologic review. Microscopically, the tumor bed with a complete pathologic response is distinguished by collection of histiocytes, lymphocytes, foreign body giant cells, and hemosiderin deposition in a fibrotic or fibromyxoid stroma without normal glandular elements (Figures 18-9 to 18-11). In cases of partial or no pathologic response, residual carcinoma typically has a haphazard, infiltrative pattern, and the neoplastic cells commonly demonstrate significant nuclear enlargement, multinucleation, vesicular chromatin, and mitotic figures with frequent atypical forms, in addition to hypereosinophilic and/or vacuolated cytoplasm (Figure 18-12). Therapeutic changes in residual ductal carcinoma *in situ* (DCIS) typically demonstrate similar morphologic alterations to invasive carcinoma (Figure 18-13), whereas the cytologic alterations in lobular carcinoma *in situ* (LCIS) may result in an appearance that resembles pleomorphic LCIS or DCIS (Figure 18-14). Histologic features in the lymph nodes previously involved by carcinoma generally resemble those in the mammary stroma (Figures 18-15 and 18-16). The architecture of a lymph node is usually maintained.

FIGURE 18-8: A duct with therapy-related changes, primarily as dense periductal sclerosis.

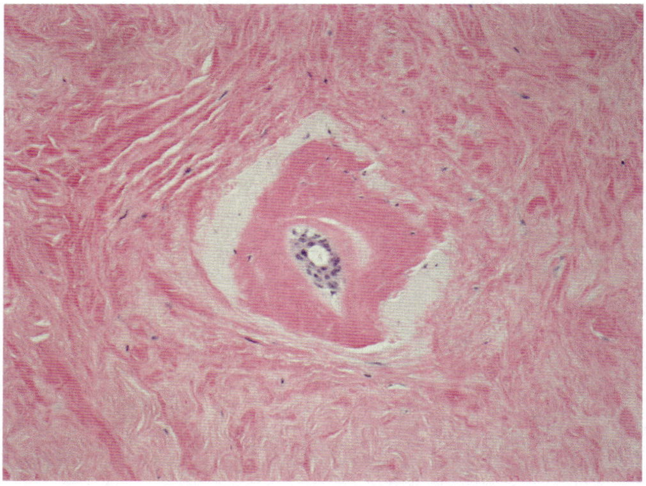

FIGURE 18-9: A low-power view of tumor bed with complete pathologic response. Note the abundant histiocytes, foreign body giant cells, cholesterol clefts, and lymphoid aggregates.

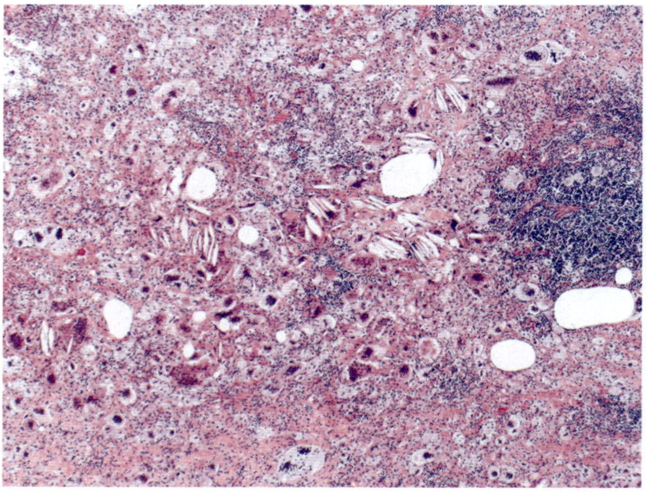

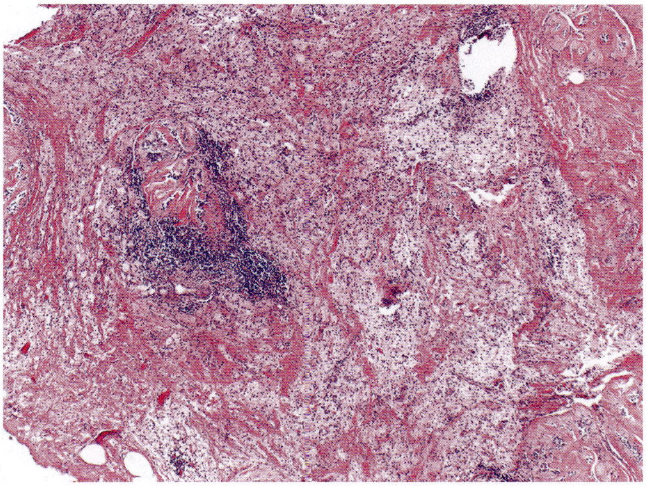

FIGURE 18-10: Another tumor bed showing collection of foamy histiocytes and lymphocytes in the background of collagenized stroma.

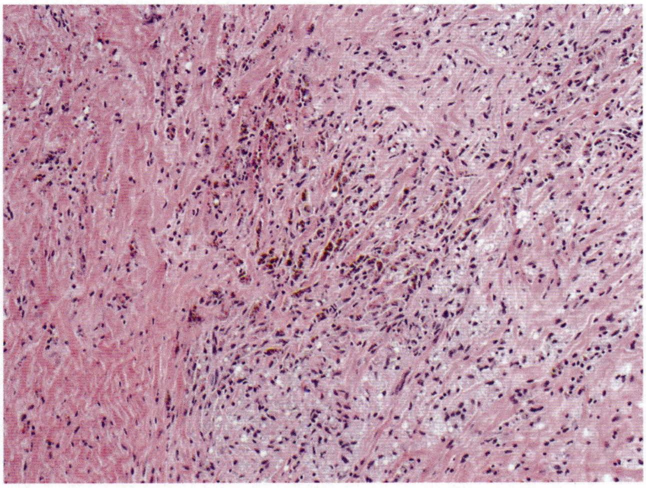

FIGURE 18-11: Hemosiderin deposition is commonly present within the tumor bed following treatment.

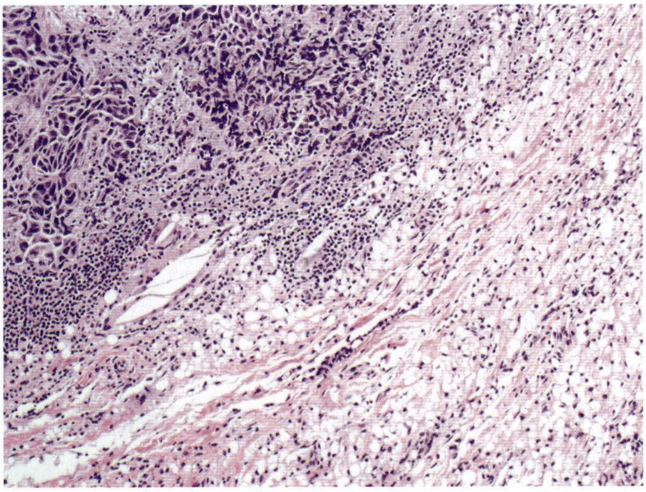

FIGURE 18-12: Partial pathologic response with highly pleomorphic residual carcinoma.

FIGURE 18-13: Therapeutic changes in residual DCIS. Note the highly atypical nuclei yet abundant vacuolated cytoplasm.

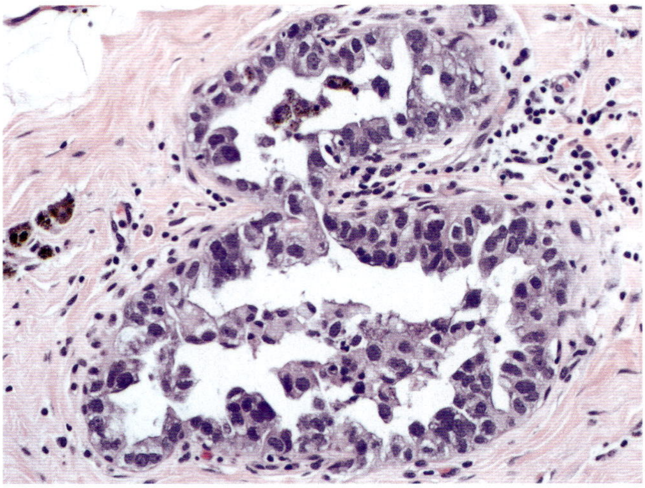

FIGURE 18-14: The cytologic alterations resulting from neoadjuvant therapy in LCIS may mimic pleomorphic LCIS or DCIS.

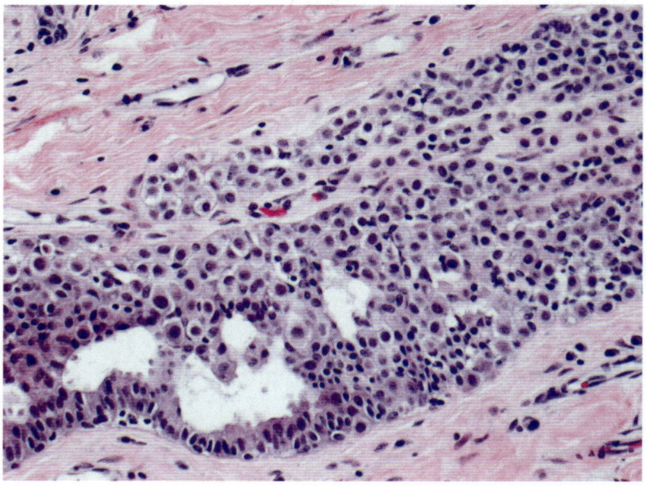

FIGURE 18-15: Complete pathologic response in a previously positive lymph node. The histologic features are generally similar to those in mammary stroma.

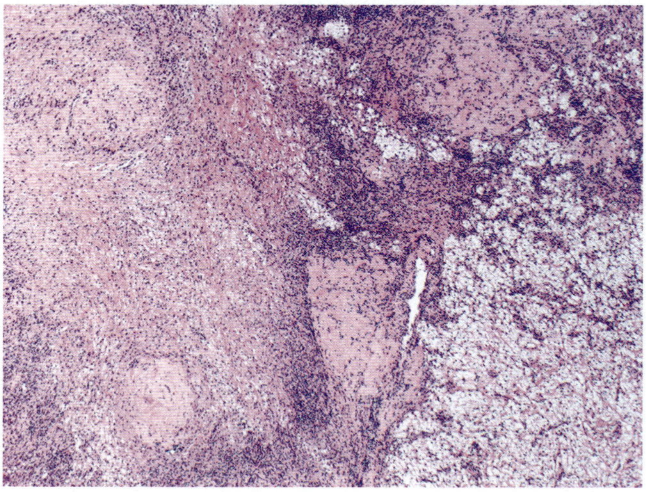

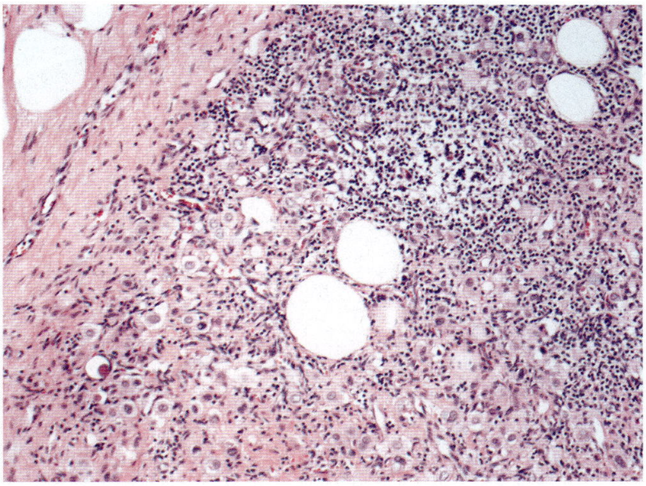

FIGURE 18-16: Partial pathologic response in a lymph node. Note that the subcapsular residual lobular carcinoma cells show significant nuclear atypia and the surrounding stroma is fibrotic.

ATYPICAL VASCULAR LESIONS AND ANGIOSARCOMA

Although the overall incidence is very low, the occurrence of cutaneous vascular lesions has been a well-documented complication of radiation therapy and has been rising in the past decade owing to the increased use of external radiotherapy in the setting of breast-conserving surgery for invasive or *in situ* carcinoma. This group of vascular proliferation has a wide spectrum and overlapping histomorphology, ranging from AVL to high-grade angiosarcoma.

Atypical Vascular Lesions

This group of unusual cutaneous vascular proliferations that develop after external radiation therapy for breast carcinoma was recognized two decades ago.[11] These lesions were thought to have benign clinical behavior and were also termed "benign lymphangiomatous papules," "benign lymphangioendothelioma," "lymphangioma circumscriptum," and "acquired progressive lymphangioma."[12,13]

While AVLs may develop from 1 to 20 years after radiation therapy, the postradiation interval for the occurrence of these lesions is significantly shorter than that of angiosarcoma.[12–15] These lesions typically present clinically as one or more flesh-colored papules, erythematous plaques, or patches in the field of prior radiation. Interestingly, these lesions are closely reminiscent of a variant of hemangioma known as hobnail hemangioma (targetoid hemosiderotic hemangioma).

Histologically, AVLs are generally well circumscribed and consist of ectatic, anastomosing, or irregular-jagged vascular channels lined by a single layer of prominent endothelial cells, often with micropapillary tufts. Nuclear hyperchromasia and hobnailing are frequent findings. Dissection of dermal collagen, a feature often seen in cutaneous angiosarcoma, can also be present. These lesions are typically based in the superficial or middermis and, although may rarely involve the deep dermis, do not extend into subcutaneous tissues (Figures 18-17 to 18-19). In contrast to well-differentiated angiosarcoma, AVLs also lack significant cytologic atypia, multilayering of endothelial cells, mitotic activity, or necrosis.[11–13,16] Nevertheless, there is sufficient morphologic overlap between these entities to make it difficult to reliably classify every radiation-associated vascular lesion. AVLs may also be classified as one of two histologic types. The lymphatic type consists of predominantly thin-walled variably anastomosing lymphatics primarily in superficial dermis, whereas the vascular type comprises primarily small, irregularly dispersed, capillary-type vessels invested by pericytes, often blood filled, in the superficial or deep dermis.[13]

Although the majority of AVLs are associated with a benign clinical outcome,[17] a small proportion of AVLs have been shown to progress to angiosarcoma, supporting the notion that radiation-associated vascular lesions represent a morphologic continuum rather than distinct clinicopathologic

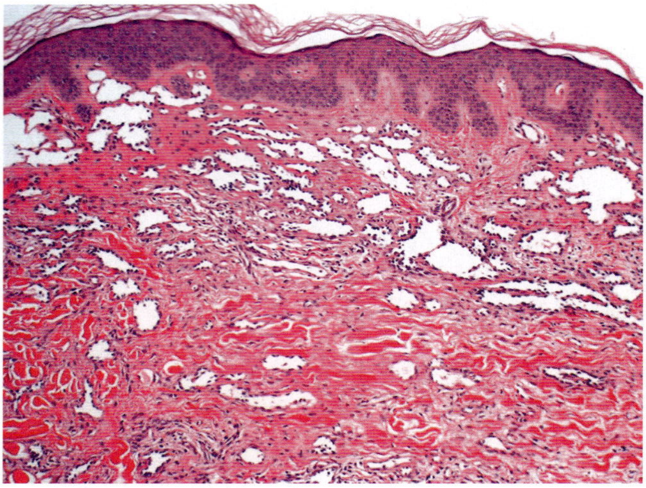

FIGURE 18-17: Atypical vascular lesion. A punch biopsy shows ecstatic and anastomosing vascular channels in the superficial dermis. Dissection of dermal collagen can be appreciated at this power.

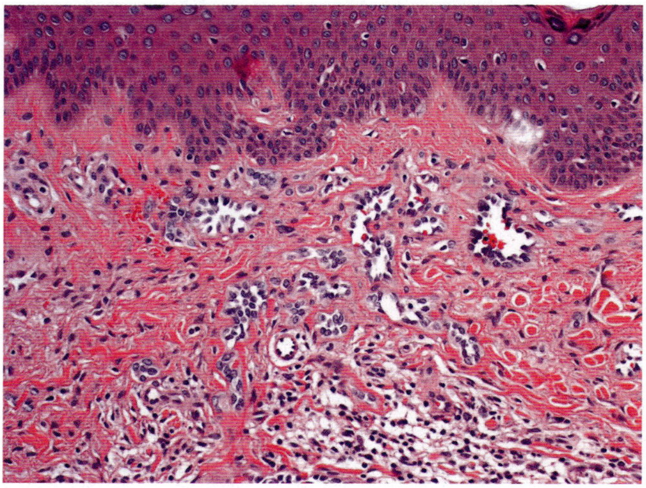

FIGURE 18-18: Atypical vascular lesion. The vascular channels are lined by single layer of prominent endothelial cells with a hobnail-like appearance.

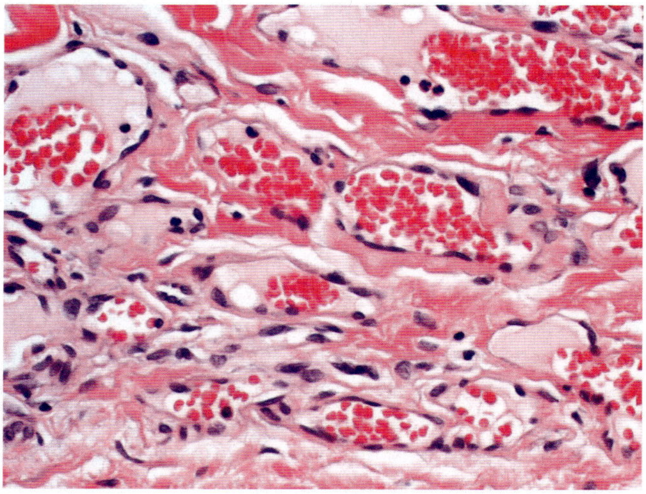

FIGURE 18-19: The endothelial cells in this atypical vascular lesion show enlarged nuclei with hyperchromasia, but significant nuclear pleomorphism or atypical mitosis is absent.

entities.[13,15,18,19] Interestingly, vascular AVLs are more likely to be associated with angiosarcoma.[13] In any case, complete excision with negative margins and close follow-up appear prudent.

Angiosarcoma

Radiotherapy-associated angiosarcoma of the breast typically occurs 2 to 10 years postradiation.[20] While radiation increases the risk for the development of all types of soft tissue sarcomas, the relative risk for angiosarcoma is increased by 9- to10-fold in women treated for breast cancer, although the overall incidence is extremely low (<0.2% of breast malignancies).[12,15,20–22] As in AVLs, the skin of the breast or chest wall within the field of prior radiation is the most frequently affected site, but rarely, mammary parenchyma may also be involved.[12]

Cutaneous angiosarcomas are greatly variable in size, ranging from less than 1 cm to greater than 20 cm. They typically present as one or more erythematous plaques, nodules, or areas of ecchymosis (Figure 18-20). Imaging may reveal skin thickening or an ill-defined mass seen on mammography or US (Figure 18-21).[23] On gross examination, the lesions are commonly ill defined, with spongy and hemorrhagic cut surfaces and soft consistency (Figure 18-22).

Microscopically, freely anastomosing vascular channels that infiltrate the dermis, dissect between collagen fibers, and invade into subcutis are usually appreciated on low magnification (Figure 18-23). The degree of differentiation is variable and ranges from low-grade tumors with minimal cytologic atypia of constituent endothelial cells to overtly malignant cases where the vascular histogenesis cannot be readily determined. Such areas are not infrequently admixed within a single tumor. Multilayering, endothelial tufting, papillary formation, and frequent mitoses are frequently seen and are more pronounced in high-grade tumors (Figures 18-24 to 18-27).

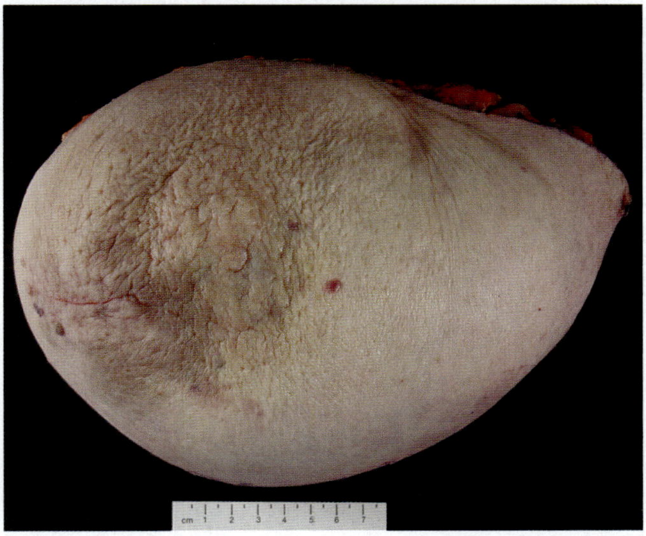

FIGURE 18-20: Radiotherapy-associated cutaneous angiosarcomas typically present as one or more variably sized erythematous plaques, nodules, or areas of ecchymosis (Photograph courtesy of Erik Scott Young, Pennsylvania.)

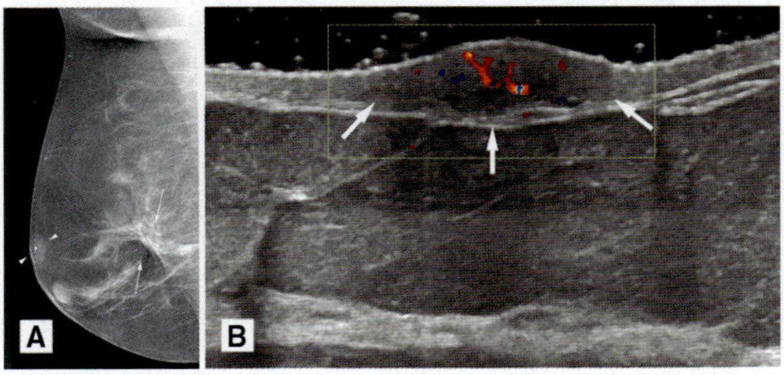

FIGURE 18-21: Imaging features of cutaneous angiosarcoma. A right mediolateral oblique (RMLO) mammographic view demonstrates skin thickening and an ill-defined subcutaneous mass (*arrowheads*) with skin marker denoting area of skin discoloration. Skin retraction and architectural distortion (*arrows*) are noted consistent with patient history of breast-conserving therapy (**A**). A color Doppler US image reveals a hypervascular oval mass in the dermis (**B**).

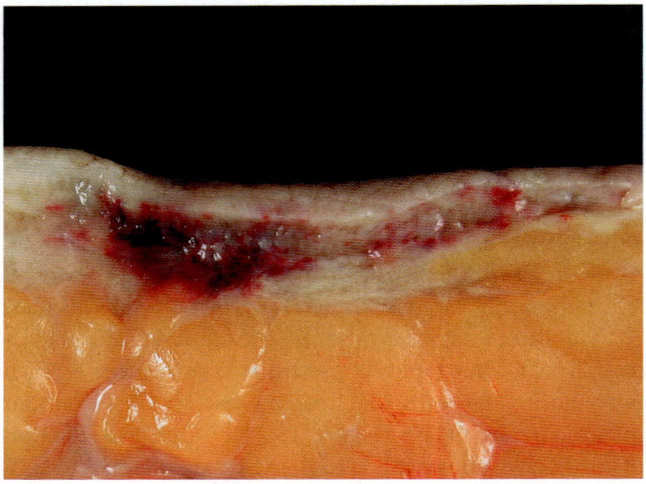

FIGURE 18-22: Cross-section of cutaneous angiosarcoma appearing as a hemorrhagic ill-defined lesion (Photograph courtesy of Erik Scott Young, Pennsylvania.)

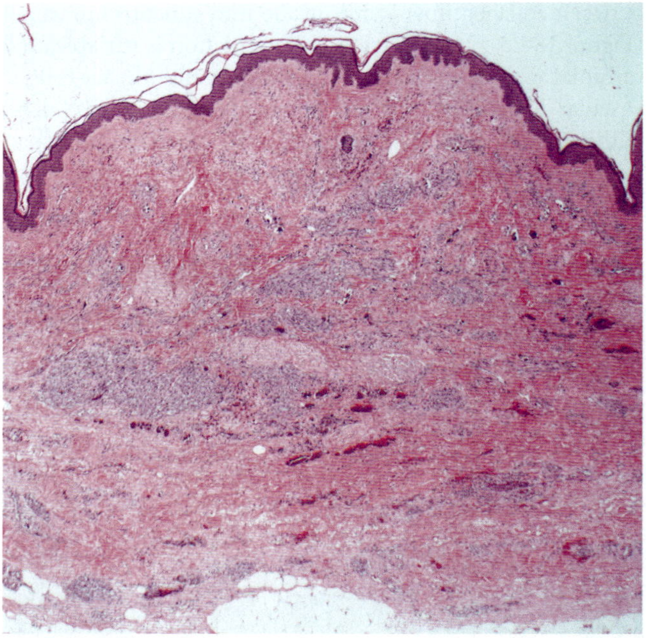

FIGURE 18-23: A low-power view of angiosarcoma. Note that the tumor invades deeply into the subcutis.

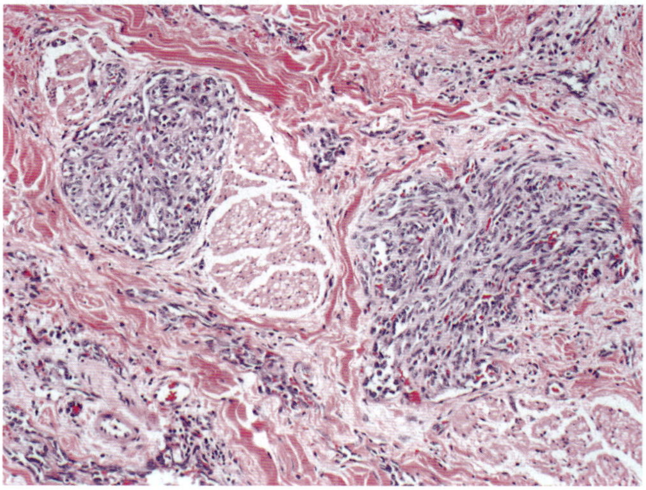

FIGURE 18-24: Dissection of dermal collagen and multilayering are common features in well-differentiated angiosarcomas.

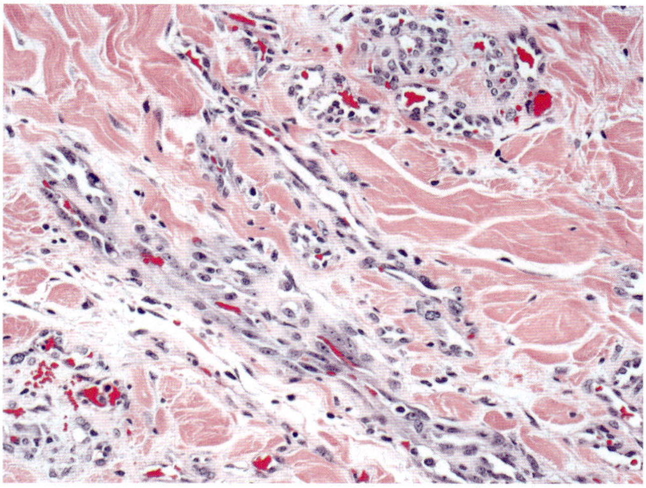

FIGURE 18-25: Readily identified cytologic atypia in well-differentiated angiosarcoma.

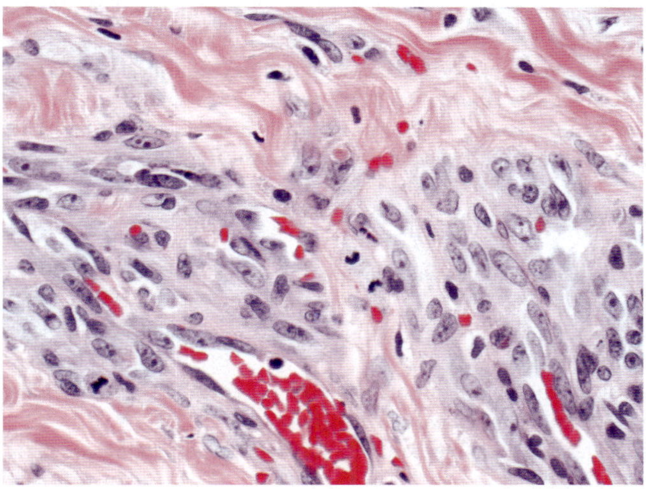

FIGURE 18-26: A high-power view of angiosarcoma showing nuclear pleomorphism and discernible mitotic figures.

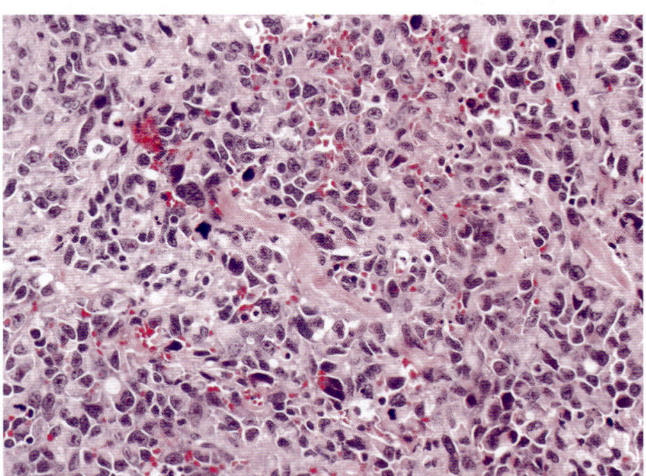

FIGURE 18-27: A high-grade angiosarcoma showing solid growth and epithelioid cytomorphology. The presence of abundant extravasated red blood cells points to its vasoformative nature.

Solid growth of pleomorphic spindled or epithelioid cells and areas of hemorrhage and necrosis (so-called blood lakes) are other characteristics of poorly differentiated tumors.[11,15,24]

While the pathogenesis of postradiation angiosarcoma remains poorly understood, recent studies have shown that these tumors are characterized by MYC gene amplification and protein overexpression, whereas benign breast vascular proliferations, AVLs, and primary skin and soft tissue angiosarcomas that are unrelated to radiotherapy appear to lack such MYC abnormalities.[25–27] This finding suggests a distinct pathogenesis for this unique angiosarcoma subtype and could be utilized for diagnosis and potentially for therapeutic purposes as well. Others, however, have argued against using MYC as a marker for radiation-induced angiosarcoma.[28]

References

1. Youngson BJ, Cranor M, Rosen PP. Epithelial displacement in surgical breast specimens following needling procedures. *Am J Surg Pathol* 1994;18:896–903.
2. Lee KC, Chan JK, Ho LC. Histologic changes in the breast after fine-needle aspiration. *Am J Surg Pathol* 1994;18:1039–1047.
3. Youngson BJ, Liberman L, Rosen PP. Displacement of carcinomatous epithelium in surgical breast specimens following stereotaxic core biopsy. *Am J Clin Pathol* 1995;103:598–602.
4. Bleiweiss IJ, Nagi CS, Jaffer S. Axillary sentinel lymph nodes can be falsely positive due to iatrogenic displacement and transport of benign epithelial cells in patients with breast carcinoma. *J Clin Oncol* 2006;24:2013–2018.
5. Nagi C, Bleiweiss I, Jaffer S. Epithelial displacement in breast lesions: a papillary phenomenon. *Arch Pathol Lab Med* 2005;129:1465–1469.
6. Diaz NM, Mayes JR, Vrcel V. Breast epithelial cells in dermal angiolymphatic spaces: a manifestation of benign mechanical transport. *Hum Pathol* 2005;36:310–313.
7. Koo JS, Jung WH, Kim H. Epithelial displacement into the lymphovascular space can be seen in breast core needle biopsy specimens. *Am J Clin Pathol* 2010;133:781–787.
8. van Deurzen CH, Bult P, de Boer M, et al. Morphometry of isolated tumor cells in breast cancer sentinel lymph nodes: metastases or displacement? *Am J Surg Pathol* 2009;33:106–110.
9. Diaz NM, Vrcel V, Centeno BA, et al. Modes of benign mechanical transport of breast epithelial cells to axillary lymph nodes. *Adv Anat Pathol* 2005;12:7–9.
10. Diaz NM, Cox CE, Ebert M, et al. Benign mechanical transport of breast epithelial cells to sentinel lymph nodes. *Am J Surg Pathol* 2004;28:1641–1645.
11. Fineberg S, Rosen PP. Cutaneous angiosarcoma and atypical vascular lesions of the skin and breast after radiation therapy for breast carcinoma. *Am J Clin Pathol* 1994;102:757–763.
12. Brenn T, Fletcher CD. Postradiation vascular proliferations: an increasing problem. *Histopathology* 2006;48:106–114.
13. Patton KT, Deyrup AT, Weiss SW. Atypical vascular lesions after surgery and radiation of the breast: a clinicopathologic study of 32 cases analyzing histologic heterogeneity and association with angiosarcoma. *Am J Surg Pathol* 2008;32:943–950.
14. Requena L, Kutzner H, Mentzel T, et al. Benign vascular proliferations in irradiated skin. *Am J Surg Pathol* 2002;26:328–337.
15. Brenn T, Fletcher CD. Radiation-associated cutaneous atypical vascular lesions and angiosarcoma: clinicopathologic analysis of 42 cases. *Am J Surg Pathol* 2005;29:983–996.
16. Pan Z, Bland KI, Wei S. Composite cutaneous atypical vascular lesion and Langerhans cell histiocytosis after radiation for breast carcinoma: can radiation induce Langerhans cell histiocytosis? *Dermatol Online J* 2011;17:6.
17. Gengler C, Coindre JM, Leroux A, et al. Vascular proliferations of the skin after radiation therapy for breast cancer: clinicopathologic analysis of a series in favor of a benign process: a study from the French Sarcoma Group. *Cancer* 2007;109:1584–1598.
18. Lucas DR. Angiosarcoma, radiation-associated angiosarcoma, and atypical vascular lesion. *Arch Pathol Lab Med* 2009;133:1804–1809.

19. Weaver J, Billings SD. Postradiation cutaneous vascular tumors of the breast: a review. *Semin Diagn Pathol* 2009;26:141–149.
20. Mery CM, George S, Bertagnolli MM, et al. Secondary sarcomas after radiotherapy for breast cancer: sustained risk and poor survival. *Cancer* 2009;115:4055–4063.
21. Strobbe LJ, Peterse HL, van Tinteren H, et al. Angiosarcoma of the breast after conservation therapy for invasive cancer, the incidence and outcome. An unforseen sequela. *Breast Cancer Res Treat* 1998;47:101–109.
22. Wang XY, Jakowski J, Tawfik OW, et al. Angiosarcoma of the breast: a clinicopathologic analysis of cases from the last 10 years. *Ann Diagn Pathol* 2009;13:147–150.
23. Glazebrook KN, Magut MJ, Reynolds C. Angiosarcoma of the breast. *AJR Am J Roentgenol* 2008;190:533–538.
24. Billings SD, McKenney JK, Folpe AL, et al. Cutaneous angiosarcoma following breast-conserving surgery and radiation: an analysis of 27 cases. *Am J Surg Pathol* 2004;28:781–788.
25. Mentzel T, Schildhaus HU, Palmedo G, et al. Postradiation cutaneous angiosarcoma after treatment of breast carcinoma is characterized by MYC amplification in contrast to atypical vascular lesions after radiotherapy and control cases: clinicopathological, immunohistochemical and molecular analysis of 66 cases. *Mod Pathol* 2012;25:75–85.
26. Fernandez AP, Sun Y, Tubbs RR, et al. FISH for MYC amplification and anti-MYC immunohistochemistry: useful diagnostic tools in the assessment of secondary angiosarcoma and atypical vascular proliferations. *J Cutan Pathol* 2012;39:234–242.
27. Guo T, Zhang L, Chang NE, et al. Consistent MYC and FLT4 gene amplification in radiation-induced angiosarcoma but not in other radiation-associated atypical vascular lesions. *Genes Chromosomes Cancer* 2011;50:25–33.
28. Hadj-Hamou NS, Lae M, Almeida A, et al. A transcriptome signature of endothelial lymphatic cells coexists with the chronic oxidative stress signature in radiation-induced post-radiotherapy breast angiosarcomas. *Carcinogenesis* 2012;33:1399–1405.

SECTION

III

Radiology/Imaging Studies

Breast Cancer Screening

19

INTRODUCTION

As noted in Chapter 1, breast cancer is the second leading cause of cancer mortality in women, and the American Cancer Society (ACS) estimated 232,340 new cases of invasive breast cancer in women in 2013 and 2,240 new cases in men.[1] Since 1990, the mortality rate from breast cancer has decreased more than 30% in the United States,[2] and this is likely related to both the implementation of screening mammography and significant advances in the treatment of breast cancer.[3] Mammography remains the single most effective method for early detection of breast cancer prior to clinical symptoms facilitating treatment of malignancy when it is more likely curable; however, this may also result in a certain amount of overtreatment.[4–7] Additionally, certain women may benefit from additional screening with breast magnetic resonance imaging (MRI)[8]; therefore, a given patient's screening regimen should be optimized after discussion with a health care professional regarding personal risk assessment as well as the benefits and harms of various imaging studies.

SCREENING MAMMOGRAPHY

Several randomized controlled trials and meta-analyses have shown a reduction in breast cancer mortality with general agreement of a 15% to 20% relative risk reduction in breast cancer mortality resulting from invitation to screen.[9–14] While mammography has shown proven benefit, it is not a perfect screening test with documented limitations[15–25] and false-negative rates ranging from 6% to 46%.[26–29] On average, 10% of women undergoing screening mammography will be called back for additional testing, and only 5 of 100 women recalled will have a breast cancer.[30]

The ACS, the National Comprehensive Cancer Network (NCCN), the American Medical Association, the American Congress of Obstetricians and Gynecologists, and the American College of Radiology recommend annual screening mammography for asymptomatic women of average risk starting at 40 years of age.[31–34] Several studies of breast cancer screening with mammography have demonstrated a reduction in breast cancer–associated mortality in women when screening was initiated at age 40[35,36]; however, recommendations for breast cancer screening with mammography for women ages 40 to 49 years have been challenged over the years. In 2009, the U.S. Preventive Services Task Force recommended screening mammography biennially from ages 50 to 74 in women with average risk for breast cancer.[10]

A screening mammogram is a radiographic examination of the breast performed by film or digital technique in women who are asymptomatic. Routine screening mammography includes images of each breast in craniocaudal (CC) and mediolateral oblique projections (Figure 19-1); however, a technologist may perform appropriate views to ensure adequate imaging of breast tissue. Women with breast implants undergo imaging with implants in

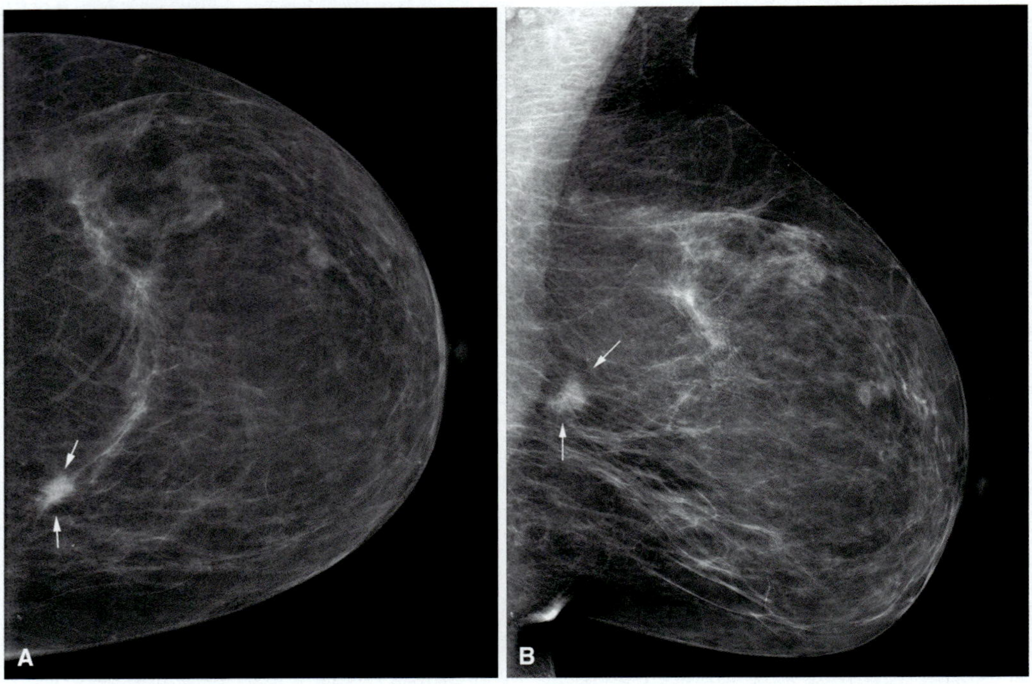

FIGURE 19-1: Left craniocaudal (**A**) and mediolateral oblique (**B**) screening mammogram views demonstrate focal asymmetry (*arrows*) in the left 9:00 breast. Biopsy showed invasive lobular carcinoma.

place and with implants displaced. During a mammogram, the breast tissue is compressed between a compression paddle and a detector plate or film screen (Figure 19-2). Compression is essential for optimal quality with lower radiation. Mean glandular dose per view averaged 2.37 mGy for film mammography and 1.86 mGy for digital mammography in the Digital Mammography Imaging Screening Trial.[37] This trial compared film mammography with digital mammography and revealed that the accuracy rates of the two modalities for the general screening population were very similar.[38] Digital mammography was more accurate than film mammography in pre- or perimenopausal women, women with dense breasts, and women under the age of 50.[39] Digital mammography has largely replaced film mammography for breast cancer screening in the United States and allows for improved acquisition time and ease of storage.

The Mammography Quality Standards Act (MQSA) enacted by Congress in 1992 requires all facilities performing mammography be certified by the U.S. Food and Drug Administration, and this has resulted in improved mammographic technique, lower radiation dose, and better training of personnel.[40] MQSA also requires that mammographic screening reports must be sent to the referring health care provider, and a written report must be sent to the patient in lay language within 30 days of the study.

BREAST IMAGING REPORTING AND DATA SYSTEM

The Breast Imaging Reporting and Data System (BI-RADS) is the standard method for reporting findings originally developed for mammography, and the BI-RADS lexicon is used to describe and categorize findings at mammography, ultrasound (US), or MRI.[41] Mammography reports include an estimate of the fibroglandular composition of breast tissue as compared to adipose tissue (Table 19-1). A patient with findings identified on screening mammography that require additional evaluation will be recalled for those diagnostic imaging studies. The BI-RADS

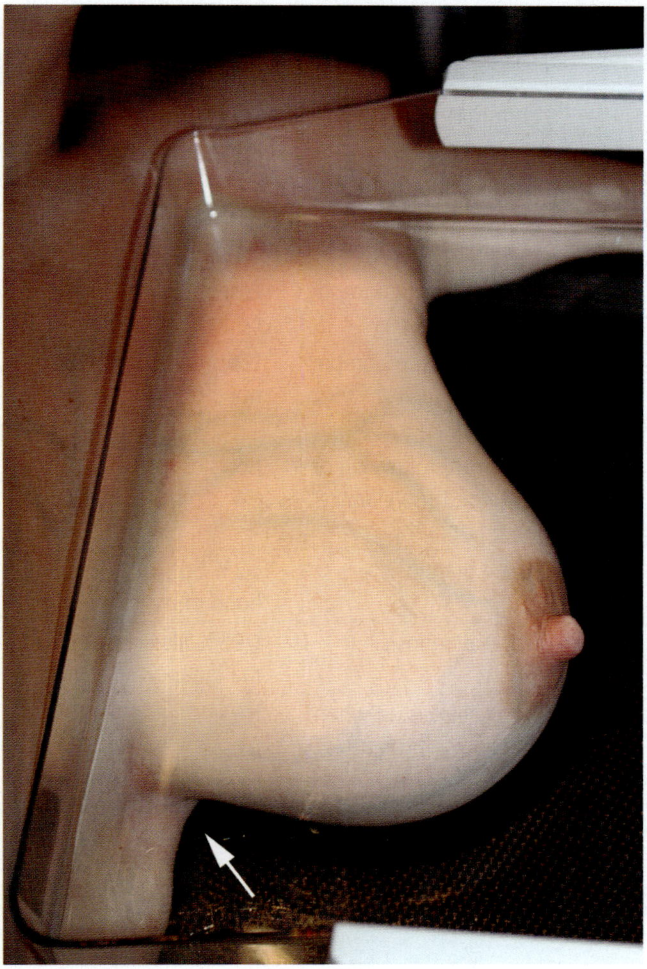

FIGURE 19-2: Positioning for left mediolateral oblique view with compression paddle on medial skin and detector on lateral skin. The nipple is in profile with an open inframammary fold (*arrow*).

lexicon requires a final assessment of one of seven categories (0 to 6) with a recommended follow-up (Table 19-2). For screening mammography, BI-RADS assessment categories 0, 1, and 2 are routinely utilized. Utilizing the BI-RADS assessment categories, a medical audit is performed identifying the number of callbacks, false negatives, false positives, positive predictive values, sensitivity, specificity, and cancer detection rate for a practice as a group and for individual radiologists.

Table 19-1 BI-RADS Breast Composition Categories

	Description
a.	The breasts are almost entirely fatty.
b.	There are scattered areas of fibroglandular density.
c.	The breasts are heterogeneously dense, which may obscure small masses.
d.	The breasts are extremely dense, which lowers the sensitivity of mammography.

American College of Radiology. *Breast Imaging Reporting and Data System* (BI-RADS). 5th ed. Reston, VA: American College of Radiology; 2013. Reprinted with permission of the American College of Radiology (ACR).

Table 19-2 BI-RADS Assessment Categories

Assessment	Assessment	Management	Likelihood of Cancer
Category 0	Need additional imaging evaluation and/or prior mammograms for comparison	Recall for additional imaging and/or comparison with prior examination(s).	N/A
Category 1	Negative	Routine mammography screening	Essentially 0% likelihood of malignancy
Category 2	Benign	Routine mammography screening	Essentially 0% likelihood of malignancy
Category 3	Probably benign	Short-interval (6-month) follow-up or continued surveillance mammography	>0% but ≤2% likelihood of malignancy
Category 4	Suspicious	Tissue diagnosis	>2% but <95% likelihood of malignancy
Category 5	Highly suggestive of malignancy	Tissue diagnosis	≥95% likelihood of malignancy
Category 6	Known biopsy-proven malignancy	Surgical excision when clinically appropriate	N/A

American College of Radiology. *Breast Imaging Reporting and Data System* (BI-RADS). 5th ed. Reston, VA: American College of Radiology; 2013. Reprinted with permission of the American College of Radiology (ACR).

SCREENING WOMEN AT INCREASED RISK FOR BREAST CANCER

The ACS recommends annual breast MRI as an adjunct to mammography for women with BRCA mutations or a first-degree relative of a mutation carrier, women with a lifetime risk of 20% to 25% or greater based on family history risk assessment models, women with a history of chest radiation between the ages of 10 and 30, and women with Li-Fraumeni syndrome or Cowden/Bannayan-Riley-Ruvalcaba syndromes and their first-degree relatives.[8] The NCCN defines six increased risk categories: (a) women with a personal history of breast cancer, (b) women ≥35 years of age with a 5-year risk of developing breast cancer of ≥1.7%, (c) women with prior history of lobular carcinoma *in situ*, (d) women with lifetime risk of greater than 20% as defined by risk assessment models largely based on family history, (e) women with prior chest radiation therapy between the ages of 10 and 30, and (f) women with a known BRCA mutation or untested first-degree relatives of mutation carriers.[32] Women with a personal history of breast cancer are screened annually following a period of 6-month follow-up mammography after diagnosis that varies according to practice. The NCCN recommends that women ≥35 years of age with a 5-year risk of developing breast cancer of ≥1.7% and women with a prior history of lobular carcinomas *in situ* should undergo annual screening mammography.[32] On the other hand, women in the latter three categories are recommended to undergo annual mammogram, annual breast MRI, and clinical breast exam every 6 to 12 months starting at age 30.[8,32]

BREAST CANCER SCREENING WITH MRI

Using magnetic fields and a dedicated breast coil, MRI obtains cross-sectional imaging of the breasts. Breast MRI performed for the detection of breast cancer requires administration of an

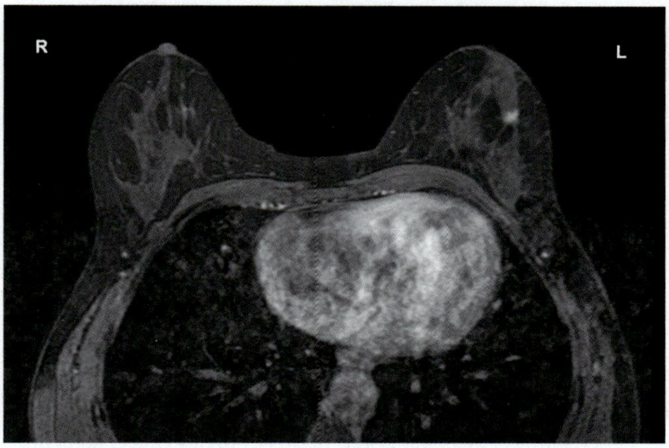

FIGURE 19-3: Screening MRI. Axial T1 postcontrast image reveals an enhancing round 5-mm mass with spiculated margins in the left 3:00 breast. This proved to be an invasive carcinoma.

intravenous gadolinium contrast agent. Breast MRI is usually performed on a magnet of 1.5-T field strength or greater to obtain a slice thickness of 3 mm or less with in plane resolution of 1 mm or less. T1- and T2-weighted sequences are obtained, and chemical fat suppression and subtraction techniques are employed to optimize lesion detection. Kinetic curves to assess lesion enhancement are generated by calculating lesion enhancement prior to and throughout the dynamic postcontrast sequences. High spatial and temporal resolution allow for the detection of small lesions.

Retrospective and prospective studies have shown screening breast MRI is valuable for early detection in women at increased risk for breast cancer (Figure 19-3).[42–49] Breast MRI has been shown to have a higher sensitivity for detecting breast cancer (71% to 93.8%) when compared to mammography (19% to 58.8%).[43,46–50]

OTHER MODALITIES

Ultrasound is primarily used with diagnostic mammography for lesion characterization and to guide lesion biopsy. Since US uses high-frequency sound waves to produce an image without radiation, ultrasound was thought to have a promising role in screening women with dense breast tissue at increased risk for breast cancer. A large prospective study evaluated the diagnostic yield of screening ultrasound in addition to mammography in high-risk women with at least heterogeneously dense breasts to reveal increased cancer detection that was accompanied by increased false positives over mammography alone.[51] The median time to complete a high-quality bilateral screening US was 19 minutes during this study.[51] Given the time of exam and increased false positives, the role of US in breast cancer screening is evolving.

References

1. Siegel R, Niashadham MA, Jemal A. Cancer statistics. *CA Cancer J Clin* 2013;63:11–30.
2. Howlader N, Noone AM, Krapcho M, et al. SEER Cancer Statistics Review, 1975-2011, National Cancer Institute. Bethesda, MD, http://seer.cancer.gov/csr/1975_2011, based on November 2013 SEER data submission, posted to the SEER web site April 2014. Accessed January 25, 2014.
3. Berry DA, Cronin KA, Plevritis SK, et al. Effect of screening and adjuvant therapy on mortality from breast cancer. *N Engl J Med* 2005;353:1784–1972.
4. Duffy SW, Tabar L, Olsen AH, et al. Absolute numbers of lives saved and overdiagnosis in breast cancer screening, from a randomized trial and from the Breast Screening Programme in England. *J Med Screen* 2010;17:25–30.
5. Yen MF, Tabar L, Vitak B, et al. Quantifying the potential problem of overdiagnosis of ductal carcinoma in situ in breast cancer screening. *Eur J Cancer* 2003;29:1746–1754.

6. Welch HG, Black WC. Overdiagnosis in cancer. *J Natl Cancer Inst* 2010;102:605–613.
7. Zahl PH, Strand SH, Maehlen J. Incidence of breast cancer in Norway and Sweden during introduction of nationwide screening; prospective cohort study. *BMJ* 328;2004:921–924.
8. Saslow D, Boetes C, Burke W, et al. American Cancer Society guidelines for breast screening with MRI as an adjunct to mammography. *CA Cancer J Clin* 2007;55:75–89.
9. Tabar L, Fagerberg CJ, Gad A, et al. Reduction in mortality from breast cancer after mass screening with mammography. Randomized trial from the Breast Cancer Screening Working Group of the Swedish National Board of Health and Welfare. *Lancet* 1985;1:829–832.
10. Nystrom L, Andersson I, Bjurstam N, et al. Long-term effects of mammography screening; updated overview of the Swedish randomized trials. *Lancet* 2002;359:909–919.
11. Gotzche PC, Nielson M. Screening for breast cancer with mammography. *Cochrane Database Syst Rev* 2011;1:CD001877.
12. Nelson HD, Tyne K, Naik A, et al. Screening for breast cancer: an update for the U.S. Preventive Services Task Force. *Ann Intern Med* 2009;151:727–37, W237–W242.
13. Independent UK Panel on Breast Cancer Screening. The benefits and harms of breast cancer screening: an independent review, *Lancet* 2012;3,80:1778–1786.
14. Tabar L, Vitak B, Chen TH, et al. Swedish two-country trial; impact of mammographic screening on breast cancer mortality during 3 decades. *Radiology* 2011;260:658–663.
15. Bird RE, Wallace TW, Yankaskas BC. Analysis of cancers missed at screening mammography. *Radiology* 1992;184:613–617.
16. Kalisher L. Factors influencing false negative rates in xeromammography. *Radiology* 1979;133:297–301.
17. Goergen SK, Evans J, Cohen GP, et al. Characteristics of breast carcinomas missed by screening radiologists. *Radiology* 1997;204:131–135.
18. Holland R, Hendricks JH, Mravunac M. Mammographically occult breast cancer: a pathologic and radiologic study. *Cancer* 1983;52:1810–1819.
19. Boyd NF, Martin LJ, Bronskill M, et al. Breast tissue composition and susceptibility to breast cancer. *J Natl Cancer Inst* 2010;102:1224–1237.
20. Harvey JA, Fajardo LL, Innis CA. Previous mammograms in patients with impalpable breast carcinoma: retrospective vs. blinded interpretations. *AJR Am J Roentgenol* 1993;161:1167–1172.
21. Feig SA, Shaber GS, Patchefsky A, et al. Analysis of clinically occult and mammographic occult breast tumors. *AJR Am J Roentgenol* 1977;128:403–408.
22. Wallis MG, Walsh MT, Lee JR. Review of false negative mammography in a symptomatic population. *Clin Radiol* 1991;44:13–15.
23. Martin JE, Moskowitiz M, Milbrath JR, et al. Breast cancer missed by mammography. *AJR Am J Roentgenol* 1979;132:737–739.
24. Cahill CJ, Boulter PS, Gibbs NM, et al. Features of mammographically negative breast tumors. *Br J Surg* 1981;68:883–884.
25. Mann BD, Giuliano AE, Bassett LW, et al. Delayed diagnosis of breast cancer as a result of normal mammograms. *Arch Surg* 1983;118:23–24.
26. Warren Burhenne LJ, Wood SA, D'Orsi CJ, et al. Potential contribution of computer-aided detection to the sensitivity of screening mammography. *Radiology* 2000;215:554–562.
27. Rosenberg RD, Hunt WC, Williamson MR, et al. Effects of age, breast density, ethnicity, and estrogen replacement therapy on screening mammographic sensitivity and cancer stage at diagnosis: review of 183,134 screening mammograms in Albuquerque, New Mexico. *Radiology* 1998;209;511–518.
28. Kerlikowske K, Grady D, Barclay J, et al. Likelihood ratios for modern screening mammography. Risk of breast cancer based on age and mammographic interpretation. *JAMA* 1996;276:39–43.
29. Porter PL, El-Bastawissi AY, Mandelson MT, et al. Breast tumor characteristics as predictors of mammographic detection: comparison of interval-and screen–detected cancers. *J Natl Cancer Inst* 91;1999:2020–2028.
30. Rosenberg RD, Yankaskas BC, Abraham LA, et al. Performance benchmarks for screening mammography. *Radiology* 2006;241:55–66.
31. Smith RA, Cokkinides V, Brooks D, et al. Cancer screening in the United States 2010 a review of current American Cancer Society guidelines and issues in cancer screening. *CA Cancer J Clin* 2010;60:99–119.
32. National Comprehensive Cancer Network. Breast cancer screening and diagnosis. Version 2, 2013.
33. American College of Obstetricians-Gynecologists. Practice bulletin no. 122: breast cancer screening. *Obstet Gynecol* 2011;118:372–382.

34. American College of Radiology. Breast imaging and interventions guidelines. http://www.acr.org/Quality-Safety/Standards-Guidelines/Practice-Guidelines-by-Modality/Breast-Imaging. Accessed June 2, 2013.
35. Hellquist BN, Duffy SW, Abdsaleh S, et al. Effective of population-based service screening with mammography for women ages 40 to 49 years; evaluation of the Swedish Mammography Screening in Young Women (SCRY) cohort. *Cancer* 2011;117:714–722.
36. Tabar L, Yen MF, Vitak B, et al. Mammography service screening and mortality in breast cancer patients; 20-year follow-up before and after introduction of screening. *Lancet* 2003;361:1405–1410.
37. Hendrick RE, Pisano ED, Averbukh A, et al. Comparison of acquisition parameters and breast dose in digital mammography and screen-film mammography in the American College of Radiology Imaging Network Digital Mammographic Imaging Screening Trial. *AJR Am J Roentgenol* 2010;194:362–369.
38. Pisano ED, Gatsonis C, Hendrick E, et al. Digital Mammographic Imaging Screening Trail (DMIST) Investigators Group. Diagnostic performance of digital versus film mammography for breast-cancer screening. *N Engl J Med* 2005;353:1773–1783.
39. Pisano ED, Hendrick RE, Yaffe MJ, et al. DMIST Investigators Group Diagnostic accuracy of digital versus film mammography; exploratory analysis of selected population subgroups in DMIST. *Radiology* 2008;246:376–383.
40. Monsees BS. The Mammography Quality Standards Act. An overview of the regulations and guidance. *Radiol Clin North Am* 2000;28:759–772.
41. American College of Radiology (ACR). *Breast Imaging Reporting and Data System Atlas (BI-RADS Atlas)*. Reston, VA: American College of Radiology; 2013.
42. Morris EA, Liberman L, Ballon DJ, et al. MRI of occult breast carcinomas in high-risk population. *AJR Am J Roentgenol* 2003;181:619–626.
43. Warner E, Plewes DB, Hill KA, et al. Surveillance of BRCA1 and BRCA2 mutation carriers with magnetic resonance imaging, ultrasound, mammography, and clinical breast examination. *JAMA* 2004;292:1317–1325.
44. Warner E, Plewes DB, Hill KA, et al.; Magnetic Resonance Imaging Screening Study Group. Efficacy of MRI and mammography for breast-cancer screening in women with a familial or genetic predisposition. *N Engl J Med* 2004;29;351:427–437.
45. Lehman CD, Isaacs C, Schnall MD, et al. Cancer yield of mammography, MR, and US in high-risk women: prospective multi-institution breast cancer screening study. *Radiology* 2007;244:381–388.
46. Leach MO, Boggis CR, Dixon AK, et al. Screening with magnetic resonance imaging and mammography of a UK population at high familial risk of breast cancer: a prospective multicenter cohort study (MARIBS). *Lancet* 2005;365:1769–1778.
47. Passaperuma K, Warner E, Causer PA, et al. Long-term results of screening with magnetic resonance imaging in women with BRCA mutations. *Br J Cancer* 2012;107:24–30.
48. Kreige M, Brekelmans CT, Boetes C, et al. Efficacy of MRI and mammography for breast cancer screening in women with a familial or genetic predisposition. *N Engl J Med* 2004;351:427–437.
49. Sardenelli F, Podo F, D'Agnolo G, et al. Multicenter comparative multimodality surveillance of women at genetic-familial high risk for breast cancer (HIBCRIT study): interim results. *Radiology* 2007;242:698–715.
50. Weinstein SP, Localio AR, Conant EF, et al. Multimodality screening of high-risk women: a prospective cohort study. *J Clin Oncol* 2009;27:6124–6128.
51. Berg WA, Blume JD, Cormack JB, et al. Combined screening with ultrasound and mammography vs mammography alone in women with elevated risk of breast cancer. *JAMA* 2008;299:2151–2163.

20 Diagnostic Breast Imaging

INTRODUCTION

Diagnostic breast imaging plays an essential role in the diagnosis, staging, and treatment planning of patients with breast cancer. While screening mammography is crucial for breast cancer detection, diagnostic mammography, ultrasound (US), breast MRI, and other imaging modalities play a pivotal role in the diagnosis and evaluation of patients with breast cancer. Breast cancer often presents as a mass and/or suspicious calcifications identified at screening mammography and may also present clinically as a palpable abnormality. A mass with malignant features is usually indicative of invasive breast cancer, whereas malignant calcifications often represent ductal carcinoma *in situ* (DCIS). When a patient is diagnosed with breast cancer, an imaging evaluation for extent of disease and staging is performed and tailored for each patient based on clinical findings. It is important to determine extent of disease within the ipsilateral breast since multicentric disease, malignancy involving more than one-quadrant of a breast, is not amenable to breast-conserving therapy.

Diagnostic Mammography

Diagnostic mammography utilizes mammographic views in addition to the routine screening views to localize a lesion, to further characterize a lesion, or to confirm or exclude the presence of a lesion. The location of a lesion is described in a clock face manner as if the observer is standing in front of the patient or localized to a quadrant of the breast (Figure 20-1). Exaggerated lateral or medial views increase visualization of axillary tail (Figure 20-2) or medial lesions, respectively. Spot compression views maximally compress and immobilize an area of interest, reducing superimposition distinguishing between true lesions (Figure 20-3) or summation artifact.[1,2] Magnification views are obtained by generating an air gap between the breast and the image receptor to increase object-to-image distance, thereby increasing the magnification factor. Magnification views are utilized to evaluate masses,[1,2] calcifications (Figure 20-4), architectural distortion,[1,2] and specimen imaging.

Invasive carcinomas are typically characterized by masses, asymmetries, architectural distortions, and calcifications on mammography. A mass is a space-occupying lesion identified in two separate planes. Masses are further characterized by shape, margins, and density.[3] Irregular shape and spiculated margins are more often associated with malignant lesions (Figure 20-5).[4] A focal asymmetry is identified in two planes but lacks the borders and conspicuity of a mass and could also represent an island of normal glandular tissue; alternatively, an asymmetry is only seen in one mammographic plane.[5] Additional mammographic evaluation of asymmetries may identify an underlying mass or architectural distortion. Architectural distortion can be seen with or without an associated mass and describes radiating spiculations and focal retraction seen mammographically (Figure 20-6). Indeterminant or suspicious calcifications are further assessed with magnification mammographic views. Calcifications of intermediate suspicion for malignancy are coarse

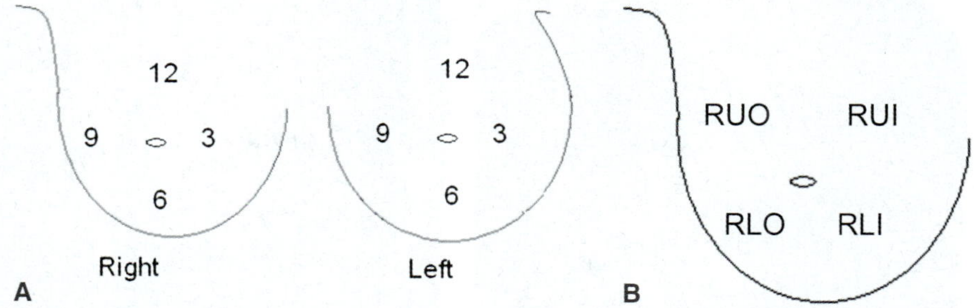

FIGURE 20-1: Breast lesion localization. Breast lesions are localized by clock face as if facing the patient. A 3:00 lesion is in the lateral left breast and medial right breast **(A)**. Breast lesions can also be localized by quadrants. Right upper outer (RUO), right upper inner (RUI), right lower outer (RLO), and right lower inner (RLI) **(B)**.

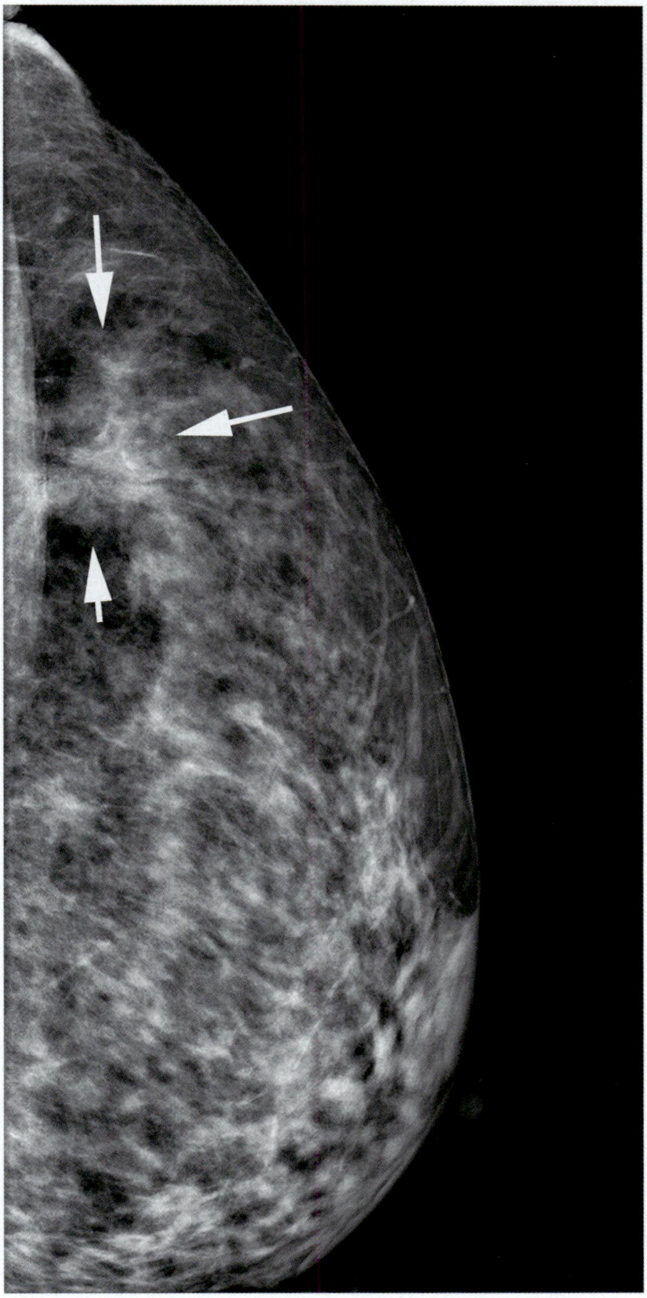

FIGURE 20-2: Left exaggerated craniocaudal view allows for visualization of spiculated mass (*arrows*) in the axillary tail, IDC.

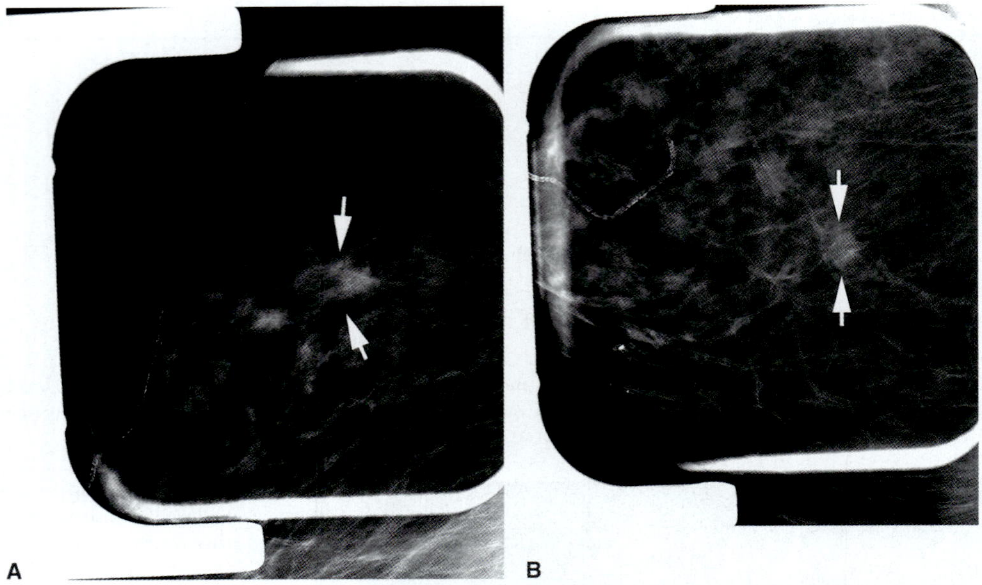

FIGURE 20-3: Right mediolateral (ML) (**A**) and craniocaudal (CC) (**B**) spot compression views confirm suspicious right 12:00 focal asymmetry, (*arrows*). Biopsy revealed invasive lobular carcinoma.

FIGURE 20-4: Right medial lateral magnification (RMML) view characterizes pleomorphic and fine-linear branching calcifications in a segmental distribution. Biopsy revealed ductal carcinoma *in situ*.

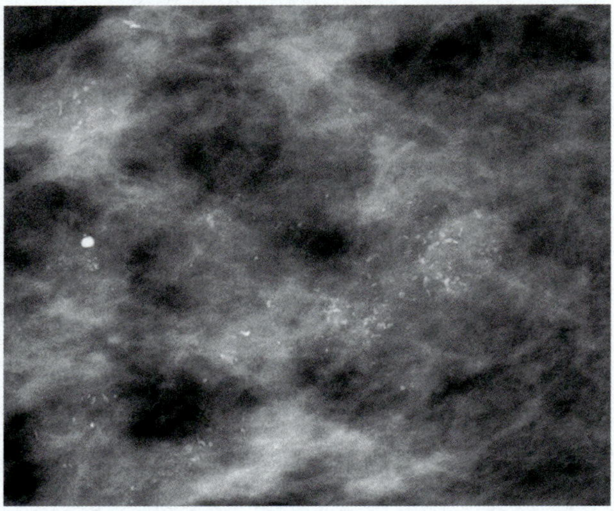

FIGURE 20-5: Left magnification craniocaudal (LMCC) view demonstrates an irregular hyperdense mass with spiculated margins. Biopsy revealed invasive lobular carcinoma.

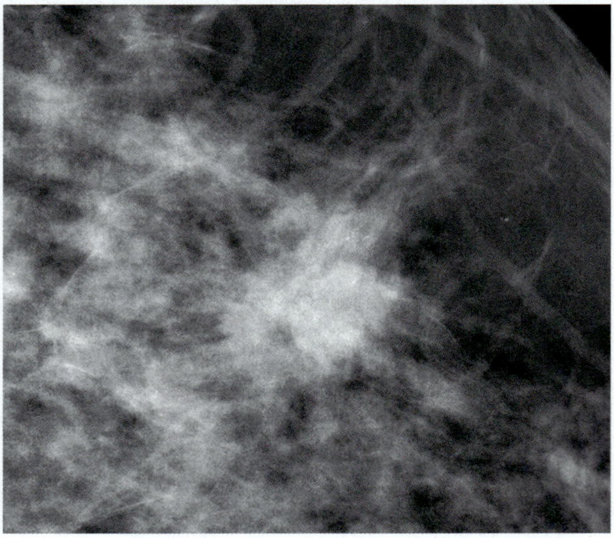

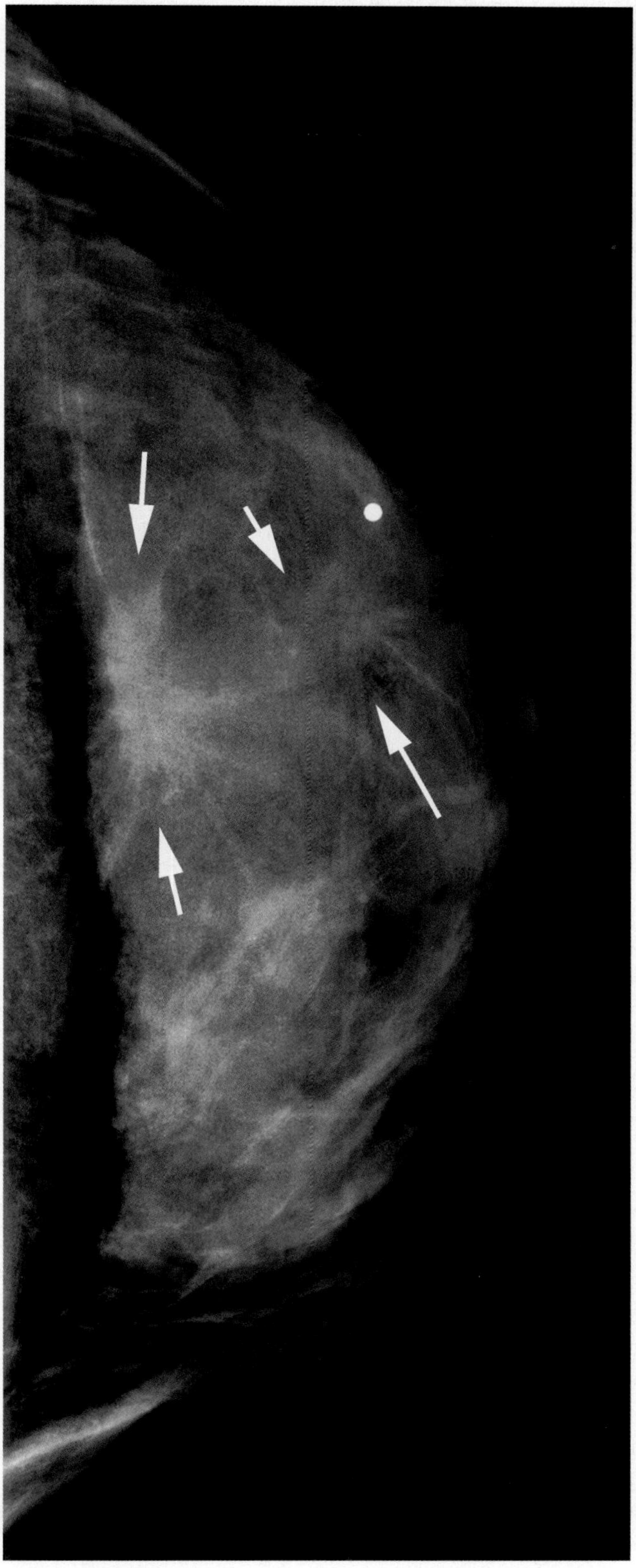

FIGURE 20-6: Left craniocaudal view shows two areas of architectural distortion (*arrows*) in the left 12:00 breast. Note the spiculations associated with this multifocal invasive ductal carcinoma.

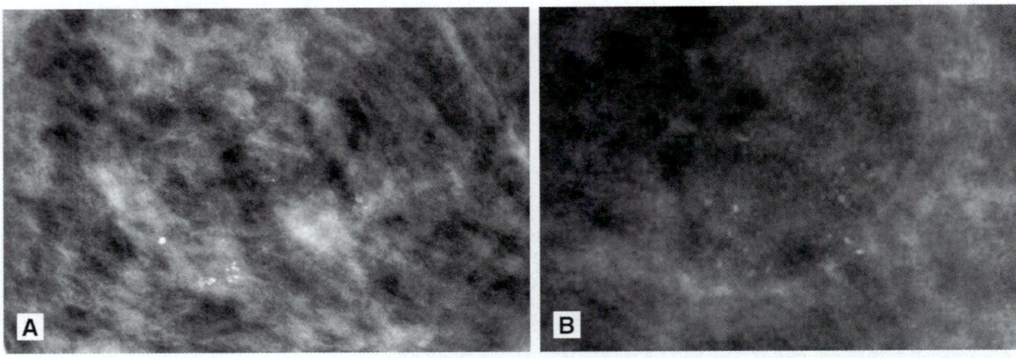

FIGURE 20-7: Coarse heterogeneous calcifications in a grouped distribution (**A**). Amorphous calcifications in a segmental distribution (**B**). Biopsy of both lesions revealed ductal carcinoma *in situ*.

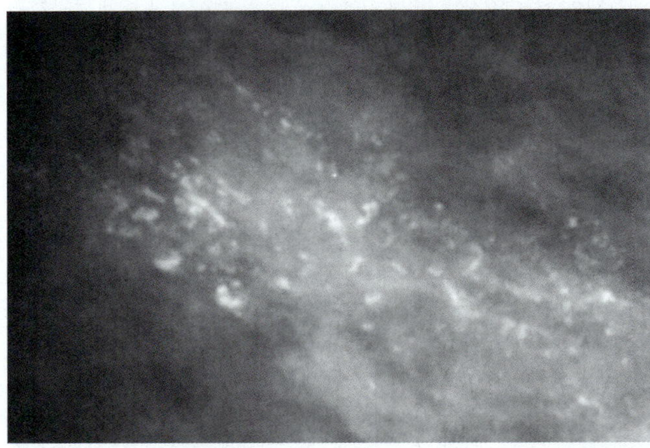

FIGURE 20-8: Fine pleomorphic and fine-linear branching calcifications in a segmental distribution. Biopsy revealed ductal carcinoma *in situ*.

FIGURE 20-9: Punctate and amorphous calcifications in a linear distribution denoted by *asterisk*. Biopsy showed ductal carcinoma *in situ*.

heterogeneous (Figure 20-7A) or amorphous (Figure 20-7B).[6,7] Fine pleomorphic and fine-linear branching calcifications have a higher probability of malignancy (Figure 20-8).[7] Malignant calcifications are more likely to be in a linear (Figure 20-9), segmental, or grouped distribution.[7] Malignant calcifications may or may not be associated with a mass (Figure 20-10).

Ultrasound Imaging

US imaging uses high-frequency sound waves to generate images without ionizing radiation. Breast US is performed for the evaluation of palpable abnormalities, breast pain, suspected

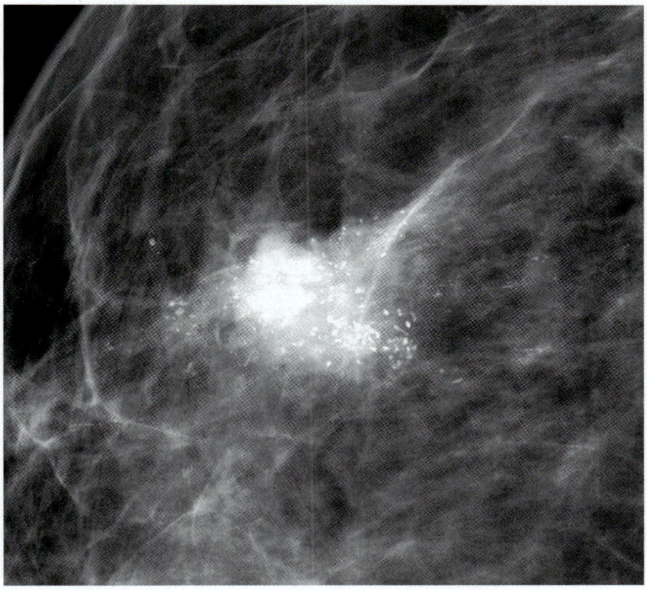

FIGURE 20-10: Round hyperdense mass with spiculated margins with associated fine pleomorphic and fine-linear branching calcifications. Biopsy revealed invasive mixed with *in situ* ductal.

abnormalities on mammography or MRI, suspected abnormalities of breast implants, and suspected or palpable axillary adenopathy. US is the initial imaging study for palpable breast abnormalities in women under 30 or women who are pregnant or lactating. Real-time imaging can be performed with US, making it optimal for image-guided procedures. Breast US imaging should be performed with the highest frequency linear transducer that provides appropriate tissue penetration. US is valuable in determining whether a mammographic mass is cystic or solid.

Lesions identified at US are further characterized by shape, margin, size, lesion orientation relative to the skin surface, lesion boundary, posterior acoustic features, and vascularity.[3] The echogenicity of a mass is reported as compared with a normal fat lobule and described as hypoechoic, isoechoic, hyperechoic, or mixed echogenicity. US is a valuable tool to further evaluate suspected breast cancer identified at mammography.[8–10] Sonographic findings of malignancy include spiculated margins, nonparallel orientation (taller than wide), angular margins, shadowing, branch pattern, hypoechogenicity, calcifications, duct extension, and microlobulation in decreasing order of positive predictive value for malignancy[11] (Figure 20-11). When a breast

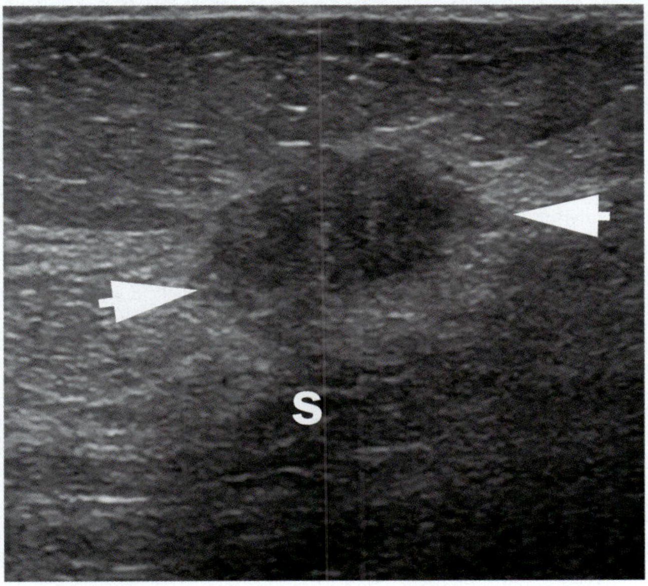

FIGURE 20-11: Grayscale US image reveals a hypoechoic oval mass with spiculated and angular margins (*arrows*) with posterior acoustic shadowing (s). Biopsy revealed invasive ductal carcinoma.

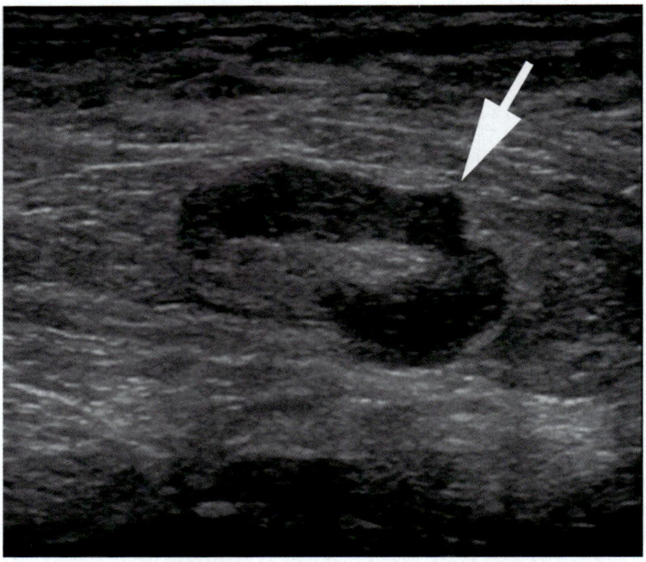

FIGURE 20-12: Grayscale US image of the ipsilateral axilla shows a lymph node with a thickened cortex and a focal cortical prominence (*arrow*), positive for malignant involvement by FNA.

cancer is suspected, US evaluation of the ipsilateral breast and axillary region can be useful for staging[12–14] (Figure 20-12).

Magnetic Resonance Imaging

Breast MRI is a valuable tool for the diagnosis and management of breast cancer. Current indications for breast MRI include high-risk screening (as discussed in Chapter 19), silicone implant evaluation, extent of disease assessment in patients newly diagnosed with breast cancer (Figure 20-13), evaluation of response to neoadjuvant therapy (Figure 20-14), and identification of an unknown primary in patients with metastatic axillary disease and negative mammogram and

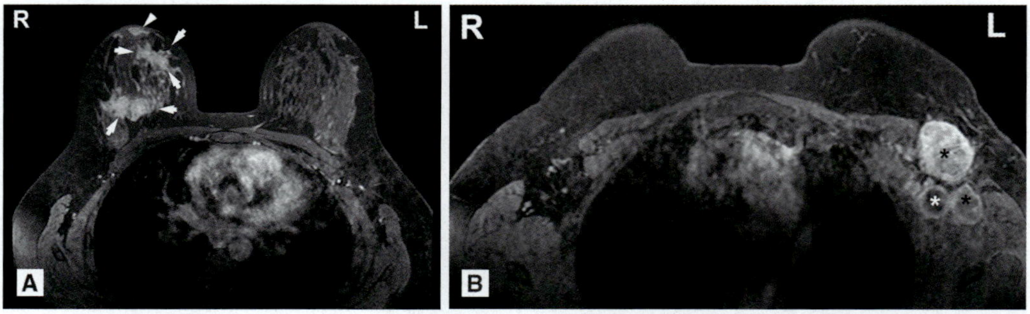

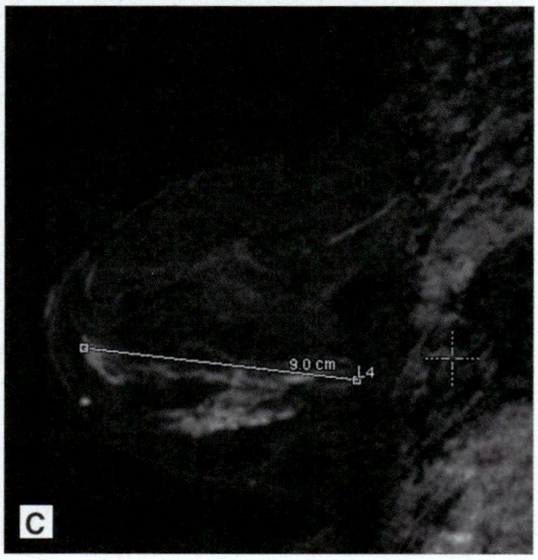

FIGURE 20-13: MRI for extent of disease. Delayed axial T1 fat-saturated image reveals right multicentric malignancy. Irregular enhancing masses with spiculated margins are noted in the right upper outer posterior and right upper inner anterior breast (*arrows*). Also, note the superficial irregular mass in the anterior breast extending to the skin surface (*arrowhead*) (**A**). Delayed axial postcontrast T1 fat-saturated image reveals multiple enlarged left axillary lymph nodes (*black asterisk*) in this patient with left breast invasive ductal carcinoma; one lymph node shows central necrosis (*white asterisk*) (**B**). Sagittal subtraction image reveals clumped linear non–mass enhancement spanning 9.0 cm in maximal AP dimension in the left 6:00 breast and extending close to the skin surface. Malignant calcifications representing biopsy-proven ductal carcinoma *in situ* only spanned an area of 4.5 cm on mammography (**C**).

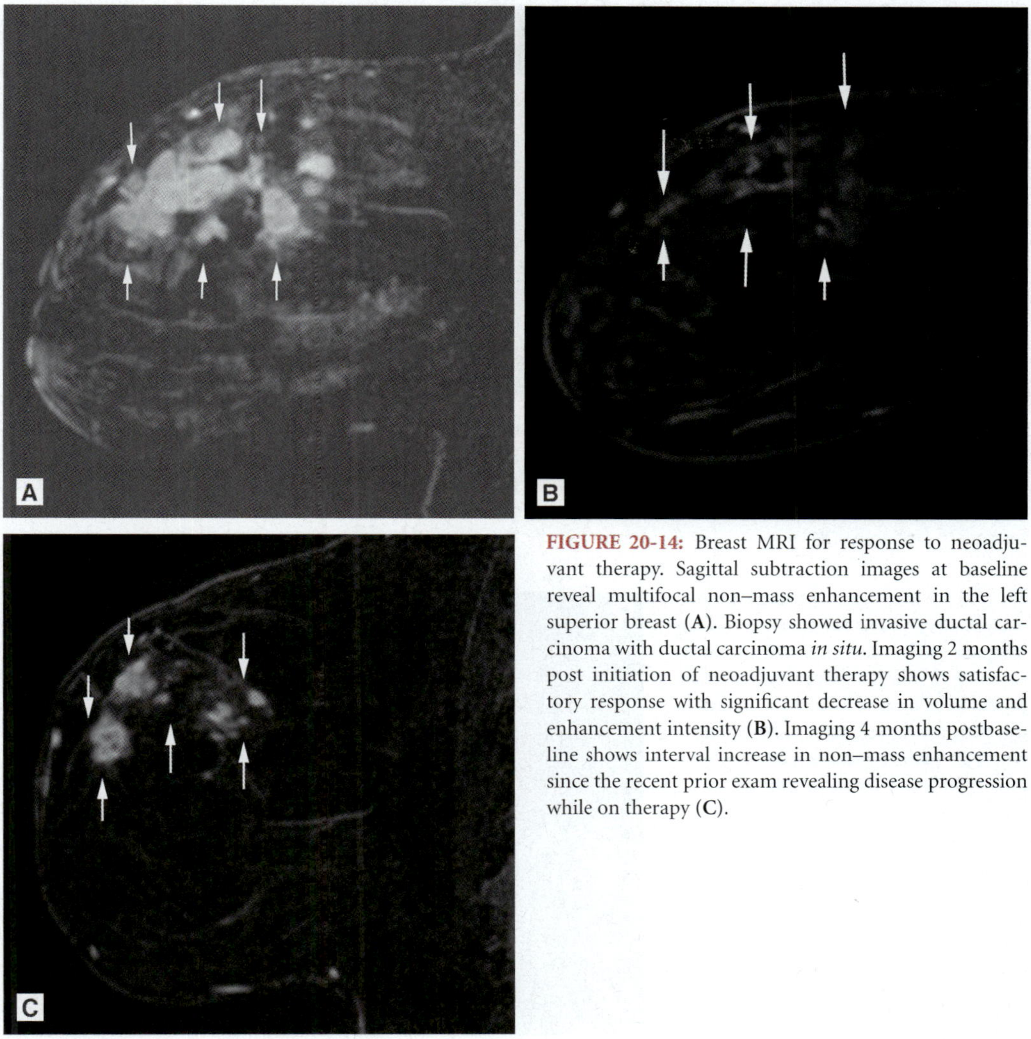

FIGURE 20-14: Breast MRI for response to neoadjuvant therapy. Sagittal subtraction images at baseline reveal multifocal non–mass enhancement in the left superior breast (**A**). Biopsy showed invasive ductal carcinoma with ductal carcinoma *in situ*. Imaging 2 months post initiation of neoadjuvant therapy shows satisfactory response with significant decrease in volume and enhancement intensity (**B**). Imaging 4 months postbaseline shows interval increase in non–mass enhancement since the recent prior exam revealing disease progression while on therapy (**C**).

US (Figure 20-15) and less often for resolving inconclusive findings on clinical examination, mammography, and/or US. Breast MRI has been shown to identify additional malignancy in the ipsilateral breast in patients with newly diagnosed breast cancer[15] (Figure 20-13A) as well as unsuspected contralateral malignancy in 3% to 5% of patients (Figure 20-16).[16–18] The routine use of breast MRI for extent of disease is controversial as there are little data related to improvements in recurrence rates, mortality, or reexcision rates.[18–23] False-positive findings at MRI may lead to additional imaging or biopsies that delay treatment.[18,19] Breast MRI has been shown to be valuable in predicting response to neoadjuvant therapy by changes in volumetric measurements early in treatment.[24]

Breast MR findings are classified as a mass, a focus, or non–mass enhancement.[3] Masses are further characterized by shape, margins, internal enhancement, and kinetics.[3] Malignant masses are more likely to have an irregular shape, spiculated margins, heterogeneous internal enhancement, and rapid rise and wash-out kinetics (Figure 20-17).[3] A focus is a dot of enhancement measuring less than 5 mm.[3] Non–mass enhancement is further characterized by internal enhancement, distribution, and enhancement kinetics. Distributions for non–mass enhancement include focal, linear (Figure 20-18), segmental, regional, multiple regions or diffuse.[3] Internal enhancement patterns can include homogenous, heterogeneous, clumped, or clustered ring.[3,25] Non–mass enhancement can represent DCIS (Figure 20-19). DCIS most commonly presents as

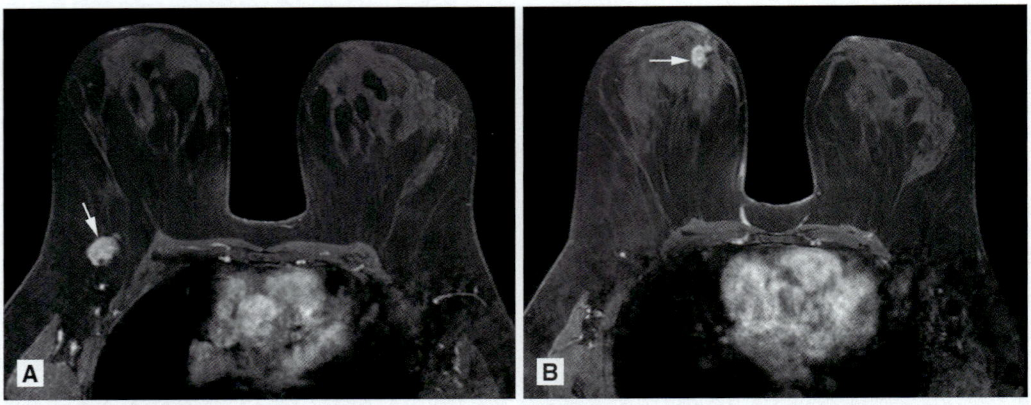

FIGURE 20-15: Axial T1 fat-saturated delayed postcontrast image reveals an enlarged right axillary lymph node (*arrow*) biopsy-proven metastatic adenocarcinoma consistent with breast primary with negative right mammogram and ultrasound (**A**). Axial T1 fat-saturated delayed postcontrast image identifies the enhancing right 3:00 subareolar oval breast mass with irregular margins and heterogeneous internal enhancement with rapid rise and wash-out kinetics, invasive mammary carcinoma (**B**).

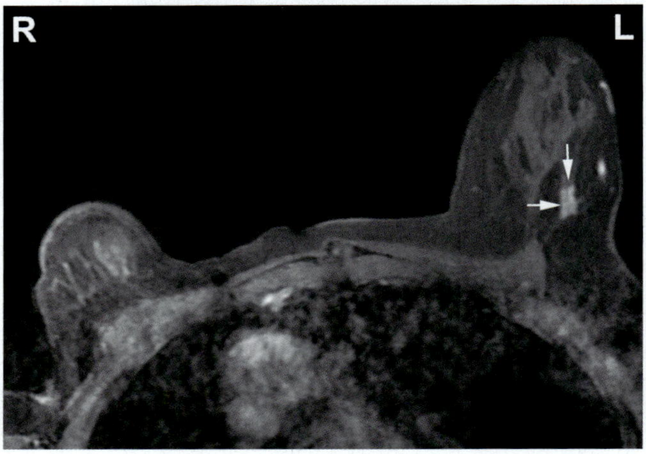

FIGURE 20-16: Axial T1 fat-saturated delayed postcontrast MR image reveals an irregular area of non–mass enhancement (*arrows*) in the left upper outer breast, proved to be invasive lobular carcinoma, in this patient with recently diagnosed recurrent right invasive ductal carcinoma 4 years post–right breast–conserving therapy.

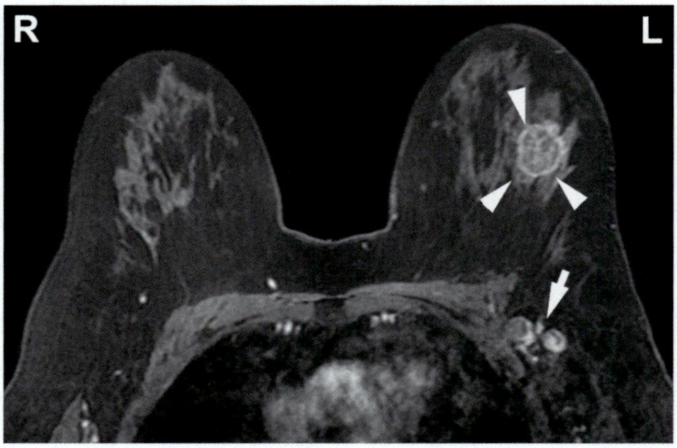

FIGURE 20-17: Axial T1 fat-saturated delayed postcontrast MR image demonstrates an oval mass (*arrowheads*) with irregular margins, heterogeneous internal enhancement with peripheral rim enhancement, which proved to be triple-negative invasive ductal carcinoma. Mass has rapid rise and wash-out kinetics. Note ipsilateral axillary nodal involvement (*arrow*).

clumped non–mass enhancement in a segmental distribution.[25] Dynamic MRI allows for assessment of enhancement kinetics within a lesion. Initial uptake of contrast within a lesion usually within the first 2 minutes is described as rapid, medium, or slow, and delayed enhancement kinetics are characterized as persistent (gradually increasing), plateau (stable over time), or wash-out

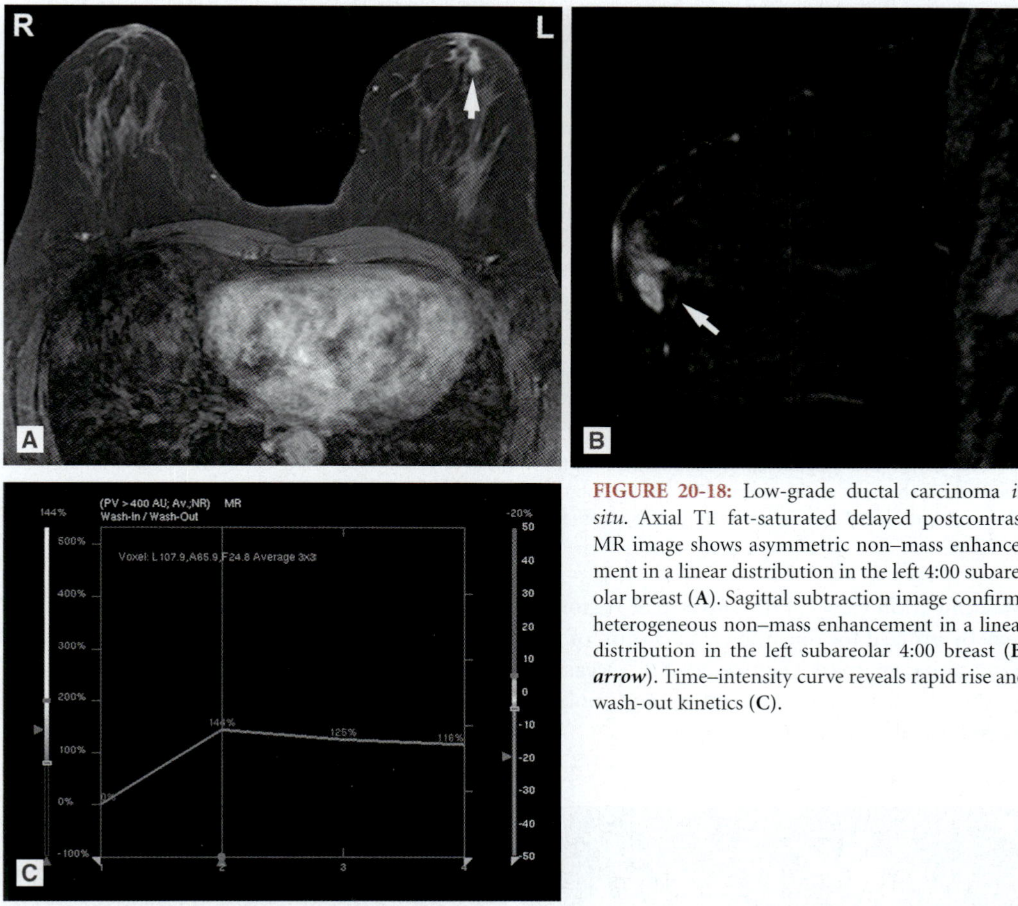

FIGURE 20-18: Low-grade ductal carcinoma *in situ*. Axial T1 fat-saturated delayed postcontrast MR image shows asymmetric non–mass enhancement in a linear distribution in the left 4:00 subareolar breast (**A**). Sagittal subtraction image confirms heterogeneous non–mass enhancement in a linear distribution in the left subareolar 4:00 breast (**B,** ***arrow***). Time–intensity curve reveals rapid rise and wash-out kinetics (**C**).

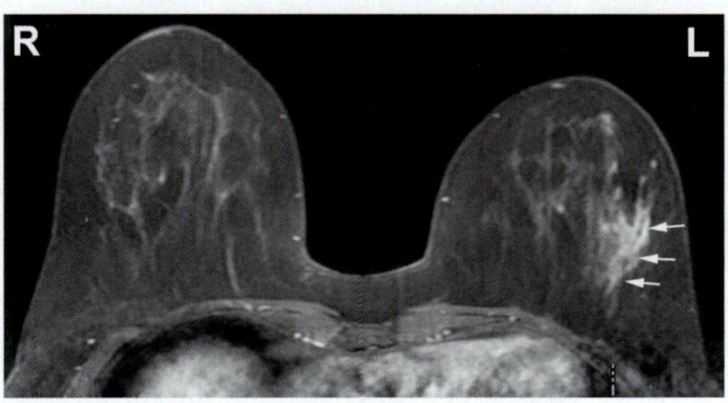

FIGURE 20-19: Ductal carcinoma *in situ*. Axial T1 fat-saturated delayed postcontrast MR image shows asymmetric non–mass clumped linear enhancement in the left lower outer breast (*arrows*).

(decreasing over time). There is overlap of kinetic patterns within malignant lesions with the most common pattern being rapid rise with wash-out kinetics.

DUCTOGRAPHY

Ductography can identify pathology in patients with unilateral single duct spontaneous nipple discharge. Physical exam is performed to elicit the discharge and assist in guiding the placement of a 30- or 32-gauge blunt-tipped cannula. The cannula is inserted into the discharging duct and approximately 0.2 to 0.3 mL of undiluted iodinated, water-soluble contrast is injected.

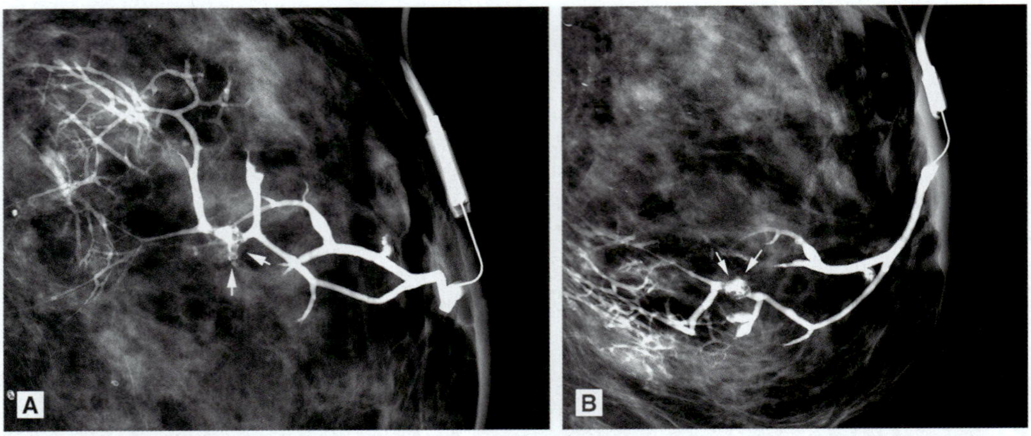

FIGURE 20-20: Left magnification craniocaudal (LMCC) image reveals an oval filling defect consistent with an intraductal mass (*arrows*) in the retroareolar breast, solid papillary carcinoma (**A**). Orthogonal magnification lateral view places the intraductal mass (*arrows*) in the left 6:00 breast, solid papillary carcinoma (**B**).

Magnification views of the subareolar region are obtained in orthogonal planes. Additional views may be utilized for optimal visualization of the ducts. Filling defects may represent ductal debris, hematoma, or mass (Figure 20-20). Occasionally, air bubbles may present and can be distinguished by sharp circumscription and mobility. Ductography may be useful in localizing intraductal papillary lesions for surgery.

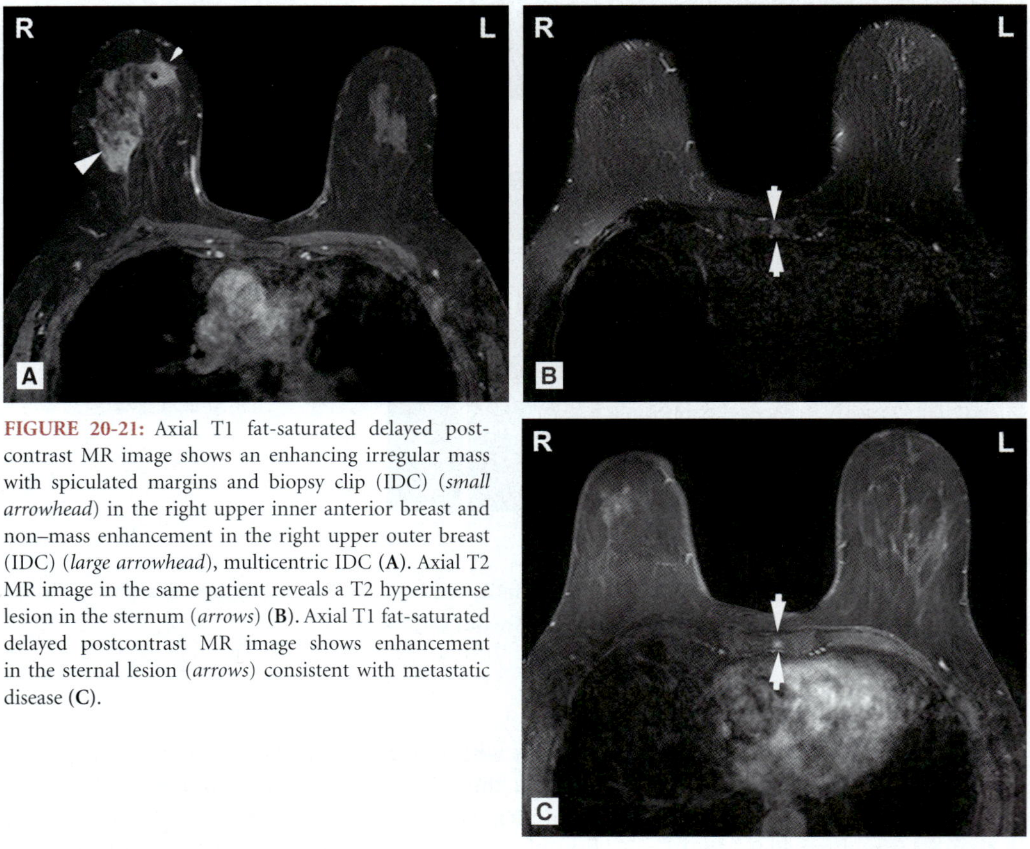

FIGURE 20-21: Axial T1 fat-saturated delayed postcontrast MR image shows an enhancing irregular mass with spiculated margins and biopsy clip (IDC) (*small arrowhead*) in the right upper inner anterior breast and non–mass enhancement in the right upper outer breast (IDC) (*large arrowhead*), multicentric IDC (**A**). Axial T2 MR image in the same patient reveals a T2 hyperintense lesion in the sternum (*arrows*) (**B**). Axial T1 fat-saturated delayed postcontrast MR image shows enhancement in the sternal lesion (*arrows*) consistent with metastatic disease (**C**).

STAGING

Imaging studies are used to stage patients with newly diagnosed breast cancer and help determine subsequent therapy. The disease within the breasts is evaluated with bilateral mammography and US and, if indicated, breast MRI. Multicentric disease is defined as malignancy identified in more than one quadrant of the breast and is not amenable to breast-conserving therapy (Figure 20-21). Multifocal disease is defined as more than one site of malignancy within the same quadrant of the breast (Figure 20-14). Patients suspected or diagnosed with breast cancer undergo US evaluation of the ipsilateral axillary region and, if indicated, internal mammary chain and supraclavicular lymph nodes as well. Additional imaging evaluation can be performed as directed by clinical signs or symptoms or by tumor characteristics; these include chest, abdomen, and pelvis computed tomography (CT), bone scan, or positron emission tomography with computed tomography (PET-CT) (Figure 20-22).[26,27]

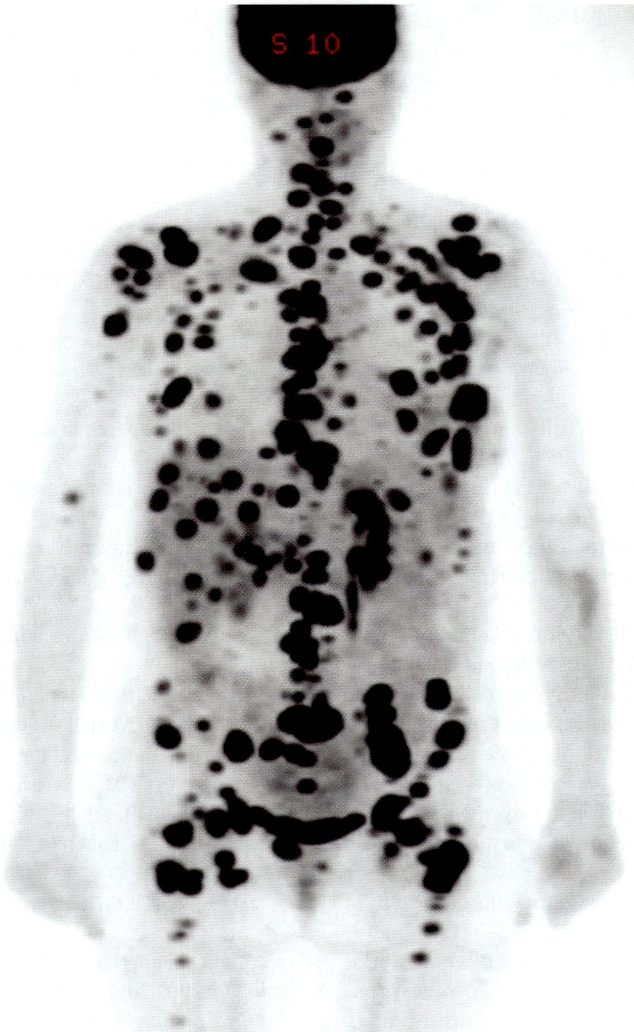

FIGURE 20-22: Whole body PET-CT image for staging in a patient with breast cancer reveals numerous FDG-avid osseous and hepatic lesions consistent with diffuse metastases.

References

1. Berkowitz JE, Gatewood OMB, Gayler BW. Equivocal mammographic findings: evaluation with spot compression. *Radiology* 1989;171:369–371.
2. Sickles EA. Practical solutions to common mammographic problems: tailoring the examination *AJR Am J Roentgenol* 1988;151:31–39.
3. American College of Radiology (ACR). *Breast Imaging Reporting and Data System Atlas (BI-RADS).* 5th ed. Reston, VA: American College of Radiology; 2013.
4. Newstead GM, Baute PB, Toth HK. Invasive lobular and ductal carcinoma: mammographic findings and stage of diagnosis. *Radiology* 1992;184:623–627.
5. Sickles EA. The spectrum of breast asymmetries: imaging features, work-up, management. *Radiol Clin North Am* 2007;45:765–771.
6. Berg WA, Arnoldus CL, Teferra E, et al. Biopsy of amorphous breast calcifications: pathologic outcome and yield at stereotactic biopsy. *Radiology* 2001;221:495–503.
7. Burnside ES, Ochsner JE, Fowler KJ, et al. Use of microcalcification descriptors in BI-RADS 4th edition to stratify risk of malignancy. *Radiology* 2007;242:388–395.
8. Jacob D, Brombart JC, Muller C, et al. Analysis of the results of 137 subclinical breast lesions excisions. Value of ultrasonography in the early diagnosis of breast cancer. *J Gynecol Obstet Biol Reprod* 1997;26:27–31.
9. Jackson VP, Reynolds HE, Hawes DR. Sonography of the breast. *Semin Ultrasound CT MR* 1996;17:460–475.
10. Lamb PM, Perry NM, Vinnicombe SJ, et al. Mammographic findings and histologic grade in patients with invasive ductal carcinoma of the breast. *Clin Radiol* 2000;55:40–44.
11. Stavros AT, Thickman D, Rapp CL, et al. Solid breast nodules: use of sonography to distinguish between benign and malignant lesions. *Radiology* 1995;196:123–134.
12. Pamilo M, Soiva M, Lavast EM. Real- time ultrasound, axillary mammography and clinical examination in the detection of axillary lymph node metastases in breast cancer patients. *J Ultrasound Med* 1989;8:115–120.
13. Bruneton JN, Caramella E, Hery M, et al. Axillary node metastases in breast cancer: preoperative detection with ultrasound. *Radiology* 1986;158:325–326.
14. Vassallo P, Wernecke K, Roos N, et al. Differentiation of benign from malignant superficial lymphadenopathy: the role of high resolution US. *Radiology* 1992;183:215–220.
15. Girardi V, Carbognin G, Baglio I, et al. Multifocal, multicentric and contralateral breast cancers: breast MR imaging in the preoperative evaluation of patients with newly diagnosed breast cancer. *Radiol Med* 2011;116(8):1226–1238.
16. Liberman L, Morris EA, Kim CM, et al. MR imaging findings in the contralateral breast of women with recently diagnosed breast cancer. *AJR Am J Roentgenol* 2003;180:333–341.
17. Lehman CD, Gastonic C, Kuhl CK, et al; ACRIN Trial 6667 Investigators Group. MRI evaluation of the contralateral breast in women with recently diagnosed breast cancer. *N Engl J Med* 2007;356(13):1295–1303.
18. Brennan ME, Houssami N, Lord S, et al. Magnetic resonance imaging screening of the contralateral breast in women with newly diagnosed breast cancer: systematic review and meta-analysis of incremental cancer detection and impact on surgical management. *J Clin Oncol* 2009;27:5640–5649.
19. Morrow M. Magnetic resonance imaging in breast cancer: one step forward, two steps back? *JAMA* 2004;292:2779–2780.
20. Turnbill L, Brown S, Harvey I, et al. Comparative effectiveness of MRI in breast cancer (COMICE) trial: a randomized controlled trial. *Lancet* 2010;375:563–571.
21. Bleicher RJ, Ciocca RM, Egleston BL, et al. Association of routine pre-treatment magnetic resonance imaging with time to surgery, mastectomy rate, and margin status. *J Am Coll Surg* 2009;209:180–187.
22. Hwang N, Schiller DE, Crystal P, et al. Magnetic resonance imaging in the planning of initial lumpectomy for invasive breast carcinoma: its effect on ipsilateral breast tumor recurrence after breast-conservation therapy. *Ann Surg Oncol* 2009;16:3000–3009.

23. Pengel KE, Loo CE, Teertstra HJ, et al. The impact of preoperative MRI on breast-conserving surgery of invasive cancer: a comparative cohort study. *Breast Cancer Res Treat* 2009;116:161–169.
24. Hylton NM, Blume JD, Bernreuter WK, et al. Locally advanced breast cancer: MR imaging for prediction of response to neoadjuvant chemotherapy—results from ACRIN 6657/I-SPY trial. *Radiology* 2012;263:663–672.
25. Rosen EL, Smith-Foley SA, De Martini WB, et al. BI-RADS MRI enhancement characteristics of ductal carcinoma in situ. *Breast J* 2007;13(6):545–550.
26. Rosen EL, Eubank WB, Mankoff MD. FDG PET, PET/CT, and breast cancer imaging. *Radiographics* 2007;33(4):S215–S229.
27. Groheux D, Espie M, Giacchetti S, et al. Performance of FDG PET/CT in the clinical management of breast cancer. *Radiology* 2013;266(2):388–405.

21 Image-Guided Procedures and Radiologic–Pathologic Correlation

Advances in breast imaging and increased utilization have resulted in greater detection of clinically occult suspicious breast lesions. The implementation of image-guided biopsy methods to obtain histologic diagnoses has also increased since the early 1990s due to technologic advancements for both surgical and percutaneous image-guided breast biopsies. The use of image guidance for breast needle biopsy has emphasized the importance of radiologic–pathologic correlation to ensure accurate diagnosis, and this clinical goal is best achieved with collaboration between breast radiologists, surgeons, and pathologists.

In 2004, over 144,000 breast biopsy procedures were performed, and 86% were performed with image guidance.[1] Initially, fine needle aspiration (FNA) was utilized to percutaneously biopsy breast masses until the 1990s when the use of core needle biopsy (CNB) increased. CNB can be performed with various needle gauges, vacuum assistance, and by various modalities of image guidance including mammography (stereotactic), ultrasound (US), and magnetic resonance imaging (MRI). Image-guided CNB has become the preferred biopsy method for suspicious breast lesions.

Needle-localized excisional biopsy has a high accuracy rate; however, the differences in sensitivity and specificity between needle-localized excisional biopsy and image-guided percutaneous biopsy have decreased with improved technology. Image-guided percutaneous biopsy is minimally invasive without significant scarring or breast deformation[2,3] and is associated with minimal patient discomfort. Since the majority of breast lesions referred for biopsy are benign, an image-guided biopsy revealing a concordant benign histologic diagnosis may eliminate the need for a surgical procedure.[4] Patients diagnosed with breast cancer by image-guided breast biopsy generally undergo fewer operative procedures.[4–7] The diagnosis of suspicious mammographic lesions by image-guided biopsy can decrease the overall cost of diagnosis and treatment by up to 56%.[4,8–14] To obtain the most accurate histologic diagnosis and ultimately the best outcomes for patients, the most appropriate procedure for tissue diagnosis should be determined for each patient.

BIOPSY TECHNIQUES

Fine Needle Aspiration

Fine needle aspiration (FNA) was first reported as a method to sample suspicious palpable lesions in the 1930s[15,16] followed by the development of image-guided techniques.[17–20] The technique for obtaining a cytologic specimen includes use of a small gauge needle (18 to 27 gauge) attached to a 10-mL syringe. After the entry site is appropriately cleansed and anesthetized, the tip of the needle is advanced into the lesion, agitating the needle by varying the angle of insertion and passing the needle within the lesion to dislodge cells. The aspirate is smeared onto a glass slide or placed in a preservation solution and submitted for cytologic evaluation. In some centers where rapid cytopathology interpretation is available, FNA allows for immediate preliminary diagnosis. FNA can diagnose breast lesions with high accuracy rates.[19–21] False-positive results are less common than false-negative results, and discordant results require additional tissue sampling. Image-guided FNA biopsy may decrease the number of inadequate samples obtained and may improve accuracy with minimal additional costs.[22,23]

Since FNA is limited to cytologic diagnosis and cannot distinguish between *in situ* or invasive carcinomas or consistently provide hormone receptor status, it is rarely recommended as the sole biopsy technique for a suspicious breast lesion. However, it remains a valuable technique for the evaluation of axillary lymph nodes (Figure 21-1)[24,25] or lesions near the chest wall or breast implants.

Core Needle Biopsy

Spring-Loaded Automatic Needle

CNB was first described in 1975[26] and samples intact pieces of tissue for histologic evaluation revealing important structural information and has been widely implemented in practice since successful reports in the 1990s.[27,28] After skin cleansing and administration of local anesthesia, a small skin incision is made for insertion of the CNB device, usually an 18- to 14-gauge spring-loaded automated needle. The needle is positioned adjacent to the targeted lesion, and the CNB device is deployed. A small core of the tissue is collected from the lesion. Several passes are made through the lesion to obtain adequate sampling. Masses usually require fewer samples than microcalcifications or architectural distortion.[29–31] Appropriate patient positioning and needle orientation parallel to the chest wall decrease the probability of injury to muscle, intrathoracic, or pericardial structures (Figure 21-2). After an adequate number of samples are obtained, a radiopaque biopsy marker may be placed and local pressure is applied to the site of biopsy for hemostasis. Although CNB retrieves a larger sample than with FNA, underestimation of disease is a limitation.

Vacuum-Assisted Biopsy

CNB can be performed with vacuum-assisted biopsy (VAB) devices to obtain larger specimen samples and decrease the rate of sampling error especially when targeting suspicious microcalcifications. Specimen radiography is useful to confirm sampling of the targeted lesion (Figure 21-3). The technique of VAB is similar to CNB with a spring-loaded device. After skin cleansing and local anesthesia administration, a small nick is made in the skin, and an 8- to 11-gauge VAB device is inserted into the breast under image guidance and positioned either

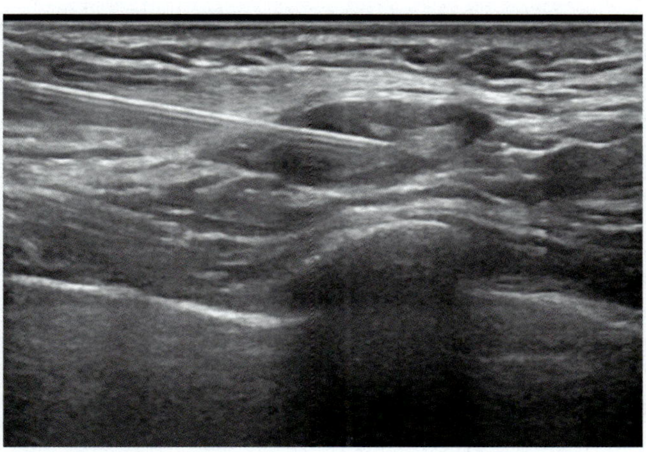

FIGURE 21-1: Ultrasound-guided FNA of an axillary lymph node with increased cortical thickening; aspirate revealed metastatic disease. Note orientation of the needle parallel to the chest wall.

FIGURE 21-2: Ultrasound-guided core needle biopsy of a round mass with indistinct margins. Note the needle tip (*arrow*) through the superficial aspect of the mass that was found to be an example of invasive ductal carcinoma. Needle is parallel to chest wall to avoid chest wall injury.

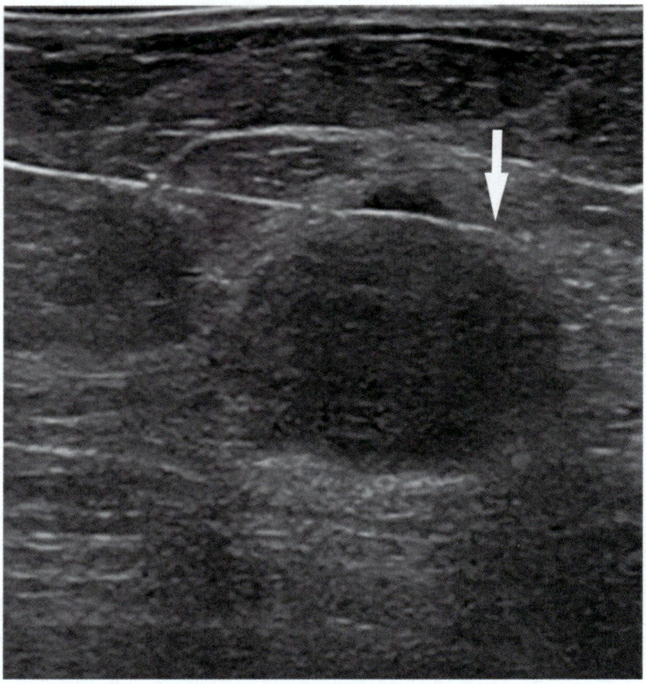

FIGURE 21-3: Specimen radiograph of 11-gauge samples obtained during stereotactic biopsy reveals successful sampling of pleomorphic calcifications in the cores obtained. These revealed intermediate-grade ductal carcinoma *in situ*.

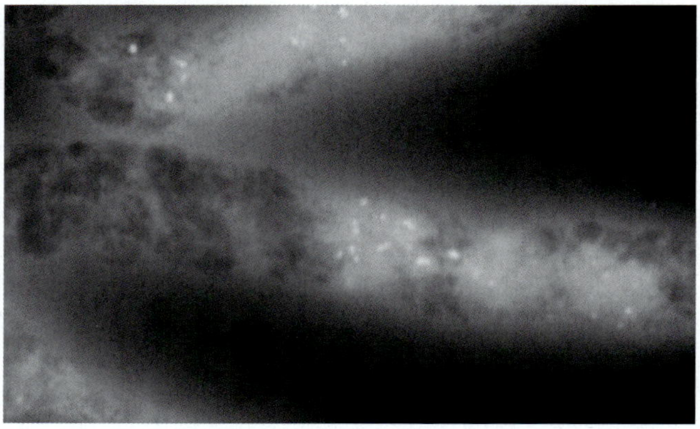

within the suspicious lesion or adjacent to the lesion. The device is activated and tissue is aspirated and collected. After sample retrieval, the biopsy cavity can be aspirated to remove any residual hemorrhage and a radiopaque biopsy marker placed. The biopsy marker can be localized for additional tissue sampling or removal when necessary (Figure 21-4). Direct pressure is applied to the biopsy site until hemostasis is achieved.

An advantage of VAB as compared to CNB with a spring-loaded device is the increased volume of tissue obtained; however, the samples obtained by VAB may be more fragmented than those obtained via CNB without vacuum assistance.[32] The larger volume samples increase retrieval of microcalcifications and may decrease histologic underestimation and false-negative findings.[33] The accuracy of VAB is higher than CNB without vacuum assistance with false-negative rates ranging from 0.05% to 4.6% with the lowest false-negative rate in biopsies performed with a larger gauge needle and image guidance.[34–37] VABs are associated with higher rates of hematoma formation than CNB given increased size of the sample.[7]

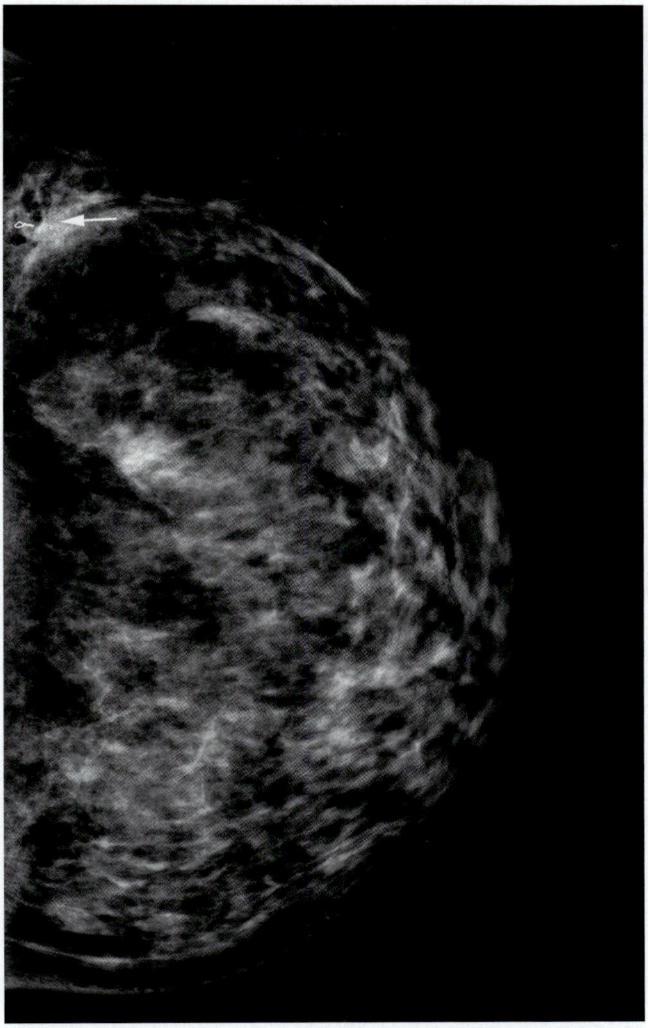

FIGURE 21-4: Left craniocaudal image depicts radiopaque biopsy marker (*arrow*) placed post-stereotactic biopsy that removed the majority of left lateral breast calcifications. Biopsy showed ductal carcinoma *in situ*.

Needle-Localized Excisional Biopsy

Preoperative localization of nonpalpable breast lesions by image-guided needle localization is commonly used in the diagnosis and surgical management of nonpalpable breast lesions. After skin cleansing and administration of local anesthesia, a rigid introducer needle containing a hook wire is advanced into the suspicious lesion using two-view mammographic (Figure 21-5), sonographic (Figure 21-6), or MRI guidance. When the needle is positioned within or near the lesion, the wire is advanced and the needle is withdrawn leaving the hook wire in place. The radiologist describes the lesion location in relation to the wire for the surgeon with images. After excision, the specimen is oriented by the surgeon using suture, clips, or indelible ink, and a specimen radiograph (Figure 21-7) is obtained to verify that the targeted lesion has been removed with direction for reexcision as indicated by specimen radiography.

Although surgical biopsies with needle localization have low false-negative and miss rates,[38] excisional surgical biopsy is not standard of care for initial diagnosis in most cases. A tissue diagnosis of malignancy prior to surgical intervention allows for more informed discussions related to definitive surgery and nodal assessment and is associated with fewer positive surgical margins.[39]

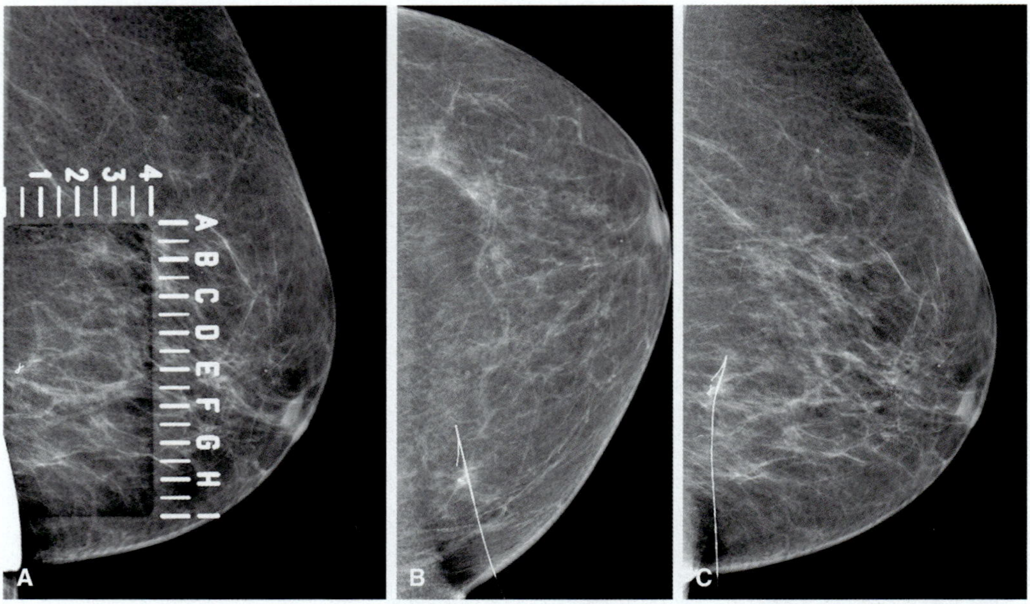

FIGURE 21-5: Mammographic guidance for biopsy marker at site of prior biopsy that revealed invasive carcinoma. Biopsy marker is localized by grid at 0.5 and E through opening of compression paddle in view. After position confirmation of needle in the craniocaudal (CC) view, the wire is deployed and needle removed (**A**). Wire localizing the biopsy clip is documented in CC (**B**) and mediolateral (ML) (**C**) views.

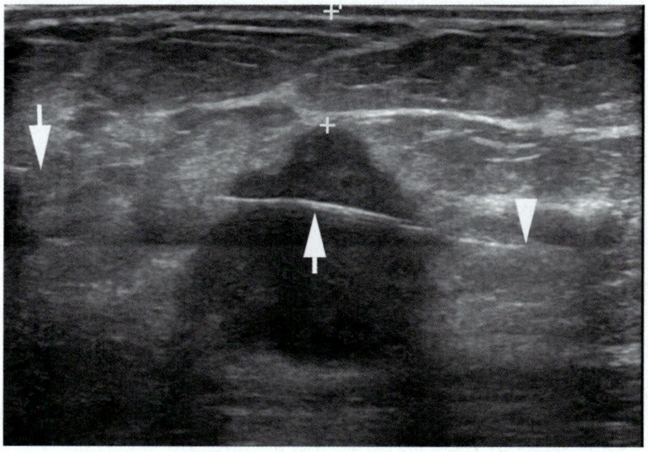

FIGURE 21-6: US-guided wire localization. Note the wire (*arrows*) passes through the hypoechoic round mass with indistinct margins that proved to be invasive ductal carcinoma. Wire tip (*arrowhead*) is just past the mass. Overlying skin surface nearest mass is marked with indelible ink and measured by calipers at 9 mm.

IMAGE GUIDANCE

Ultrasound

The equipment required for US-guided biopsy includes a US machine with a high-frequency transducer, a biopsy device, and a trained physician to obtain the samples, allowing for its use in a variety of clinical settings. The patient is usually placed in a comfortable lateral oblique position with the ipsilateral arm elevated overhead. After review of prior imaging and localization of the suspicious lesion via US, the area is marked, prepped, and anesthetized. A small incision is made if the biopsy will be taken via spring-loaded or VAB device. Utilizing real-time imaging, the needle is advanced to the lesion and several cores are obtained under direct observation. US-guided biopsy is unique since it provides real-time visualization of the procedure and results in accurate samples with reported agreement between biopsy results and surgical excision results and follow-up of 95.8% with a false-negative rate of 1.6%.[40]

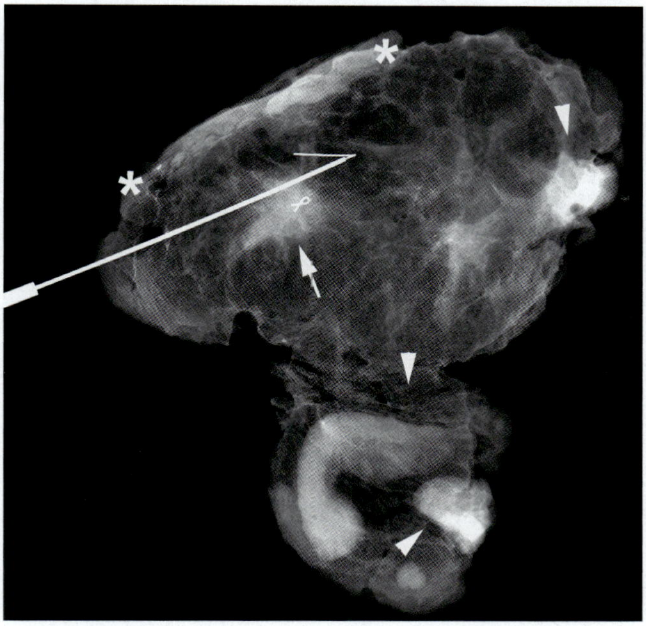

FIGURE 21-7: Specimen radiograph demonstrates excision of the targeted spiculated mass and clip (*arrows*) with localization wire through the mass. Overlying skin (*asterisk*) was excised given the close proximity to the mass. Also, note sentinel lymph nodes (*arrowheads*) biopsied within the same specimen given the mass location in the axillary tail.

US-guided procedures are better tolerated by patients, since the procedure is usually performed while the patient is in a comfortable position, requires no breast compression, has no radiation exposure, and does not require intravenous contrast administration.[27,41]

Stereotactic

Stereotactic-guided biopsy techniques were first developed in the 1970s. Stereotactic breast biopsies can be performed with the patient seated or prone depending on stereotactic equipment. The breast is compressed and a scout image is obtained to verify that the suspicious lesion is visible through the compression paddle opening. Stereo images are then obtained 15 degrees from the midline in both the positive and negative directions with 3D coordinates of the lesion calculated by computerized triangulation formulas. Adequate stroke margin, the distance between the tip of the needle and opposite skin surface of the breast, is required to avoid striking the opposing compression plate possibly resulting in damage to the breast tissue or biopsy equipment. Tissue samples are usually obtained with vacuum assistance as discussed in the sampling techniques section. A radiopaque marker is placed before biopsy device removal to identify the biopsy site within the breast. A specimen radiograph is obtained to assess for adequate sampling (Figure 21-3). The false-negative rates of stereotactic biopsy range from 0.05% to 8.9% and vary based on sampling method and needle gauge.[35,42]

There are specific limitations of stereotactic biopsy including weight restrictions for stereotactic biopsy tables that may limit this option for certain patients; additionally, patients with petite breasts may not have adequate breast tissue thickness when in compression (~3 to 4 cm) to allow for safe biopsy.

Magnetic Resonance Imaging

The increased utilization of breast MRI prompted the development of biopsy techniques for lesions that can only be visualized by this imaging modality. A suspicious lesion identified on MRI usually prompts a targeted US for localization since US-guided biopsy is less expensive and more comfortable for the patient. If no sonographic or mammographic correlate is identified, an MRI-guided biopsy can be performed. For MRI-guided biopsy, the patient is placed in the prone position on the imaging table with the breast dependent in a dedicated interventional breast imaging coil, and the targeted breast is placed in mild compression for stabilization. Localization,

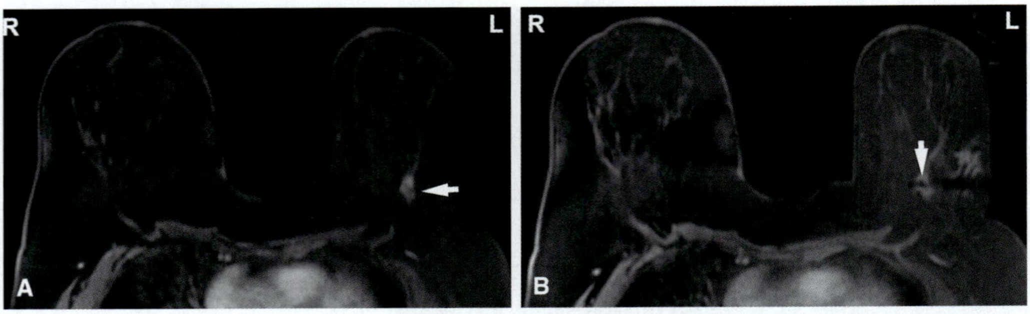

FIGURE 21-8: Axial T1 fat-saturated image demonstrates enhancing mass in the left posterior breast targeted for MR biopsy (**A**). Axial T1 fat-saturated image confirms successful placement of coaxial needle through the lesion for vacuum-assisted biopsy that revealed invasive lobular carcinoma (**B**).

fiducial, and precontrast images are obtained. Intravenous gadolinium is administered for lesion identification, and postcontrast imaging is obtained. Images are reviewed, and the exact location of the lesion in relation to the overlying skin grid is determined. The overlying skin is cleansed and anesthetized, and the biopsy trocar is placed with an overlying sheath through a small skin incision. The trocar is removed and a plastic introducer is placed. Subsequently, imaging is obtained to document proper positioning (Figure 21-8). The patient is again removed from the magnetic bore, and the biopsy device is inserted through the plastic sheath. Tissue samples are obtained as determined by the sampling technique usually with vacuum assistance and a biopsy marker placed. MRI-guided vacuum-assisted biopsies have reported false-negative rates of 2% to 4%.[43–45] There are certain limitations related to MRI-guided biopsies as guidance with MRI is more time consuming, more expensive, and technically more complicated than other imaging modalities utilized to biopsy breast lesions. The biopsy must be performed within a designated time period because adjacent breast parenchyma shows persistent enhancement that could obscure a lesion. Additionally, certain suspicious lesions show rapid contrast wash-out limiting the time of visualization.

Radiologic and Pathologic Concordance

Correlating pathology results with imaging findings is essential to ensure appropriate patient diagnosis and tissue sampling. In cases of discordant results, additional tissue sampling should be obtained. A limitation of percutaneous image-guided core biopsy is related to sampling error or underestimation of disease. This is more common with certain high-risk lesions with underestimation rates ranging from 3.4% to 26%.[42,46] Image-guided core biopsies of ductal carcinoma *in situ* (DCIS) also reveal underestimation of disease with up to 36.5% lesions being upgraded from DCIS on CNB to invasive cancer after surgical resection.[40] Excisional biopsy is recommended following diagnosis on core biopsy of atypical hyperplasia, mucin-producing lesions, cellular fibroepithelial lesions, papillary lesions, and radial scars to exclude higher-grade lesions and rule out sampling error.[47–56] However, there may be instances when close observation may be substituted for excision.[57–63]

References

1. Levin DC, Rao VM, Frangos AJ, et al. Current practice patterns and recent trends in breast biopsy among radiologists and surgeons. *J Am Coll Radiol* 2006;3:707–709.
2. Burbank F. Mammography findings after 14-gauge automated needle and 14-gauge directional, vacuum-assisted stereotactic breast biopsies. *Radiology* 1997;204:153–156.
3. Kaye MD, Vicinanza-Adami CA, Sullivan ML. Mammographic findings after stereotaxic biopsy of the breast performed with large-core needles. *Radiology* 1994;192:149–151.

4. Liberman L. Percutaneous image-guided core breast biopsy. *Radiol Clin North Am* 2002;40:483–500.
5. Friese CR, Neville BA, Edge SB, et al. Breast biopsy patterns and outcomes in surveillance, epidemiology, and end results-Medicare data. *Cancer* 2009;115:716–724.
6. Smith DN, Christian R, Meyer JE. Large-core needle biopsy of non-palpable breast cancers. The impact on subsequent surgical excisions. *Arch Surg* 1997;132:256–259.
7. Bruening W, Fontanarosa J, Tiptonn K, et al. Systematic review: comparative effectiveness of core-needle and open surgical biopsy to diagnose breast lesions. *Ann Intern Med* 2010;152:238–246.
8. Hillner BE, Bear HD, Fajardo LL. Estimating the cost-effectiveness of stereotaxic biopsy for non-palpable breast abnormalities: a decision analysis model. *Acad Radiol* 1996;3:351–360.
9. Lee CH, Egglin TK, Philpots L, et al. Cost-effectiveness of stereotactic core needle biopsy: analysis by means of mammographic findings. *Radiology* 1997;202:849–854.
10. Liberman L, Fahs MC, Dershaw DD, et al. Impact of stereotaxic core breast biopsy on cost of diagnosis. *Radiology* 1995;195:633–637.
11. Liberman L, Feng TL, Dershaw DD, et al. US-guided core breast biopsy: use and cost-effectiveness. *Radiology* 1998;208:717–723.
12. Liberman L, Sama MP. Cost-effectiveness of stereotactic 11-gauge directional vacuum-assisted breast biopsy. *AJR Am J Roentgenol* 2000;175:53–58.
13. Hatmaker AR, Donahue RM, Tarpley JL, et al. Cost effective use of breast biopsy techniques in a veterans health care system. *Am J Surg* 2006;192:37–41.
14. Rubin E, Mennemeyer ST, Desmond RA, et al. Reducing the cost of diagnosis on a clinical breast practice. *Cancer* 2001;91:324–332.
15. Martin HE, Ellis EB. Biopsy by needle puncture and aspiration. *Ann Surg* 1930;92:169–181.
16. Stewart FW. The diagnosis of tumors by aspiration. *Am J Pathol* 1933;9:901–912.
17. Bolmgren J, Jacobson B, Nordenstrom B. Stereotaxic instrument for needle biopsy of the mamma. *AJR Am J Roentgenol* 1977;129:121–125.
18. Fornage BD, Faroux MJ, Simatos A. Breast masses. US-guided fine-needle aspiration biopsy. *Radiology* 1987;162:409–414.
19. Ariga R, Bloom K, Reddy VB, et al. Fine-needle aspiration of clinically suspicious palpable breast masses with histopathologic correlation. *Am J Surg* 2002;184:410–413.
20. Ljung BM, Drejet A, Chiampi N, et al. Diagnostic accuracy of fine-needle aspiration biopsy is determined by physician training in sampling technique. *Cancer* 2001;93:263–268.
21. Mitnick JS, Vazquez MF, Roses DF, et al. Stereotaxic localization for fine-needle aspiration breast biopsy. Initial experience with 300 patients. *Arch Surg* 1991;126:1137–1140.
22. Liao J, Davey DD, Warren G, et al. Ultrasound-guided fine-needle aspiration biopsy remains a valid approach in the evaluation of non-palpable breast lesions. *Diagn Cytopathol* 2004;30:325–331.
23. Boerner S, Fornage BD, Singletary E, et al. Ultrasound-guided fine-needle aspiration (FNA) of nonpalpable breast lesions: a review of 1885 FNA cases using the National Cancer Institute- supported recommendations on the uniform approach to breast FNA. *Cancer* 1999;87:19–24.
24. Mainiero MB, Cinelli CM, Koelliker SL, et al. Axillary ultrasound and fine-needle aspiration in the preoperative evaluation of the breast cancer patient: an algorithm based on tumor size and lymph node appearance. *AJR Am J Roentgenol* 2010;195:1261–1267.
25. Koelliker SL, Chung MA, Mainiero MB, et al. Axillary lymph nodes: US-guided fine-needle aspiration for initial staging of breast cancer—correlation with primary tumor size. *Radiology* 2008;246:81–89.
26. Robert JG, Preece PE, Balton PM, et al. The "tru-cut" biopsy in breast cancer. *Clin Oncol* 1975;1:297–303.
27. Parker SH, Burbank F. A practical approach to minimally invasive breast biopsy. *Radiology* 1996;200:11–20.
28. Parker SH, Jobe WE, Dennis MA, et al. US-guided automated large-core breast biopsy. *Radiology* 1993;187:507–511.
29. Rich PM, Michell MJ, Humphreys S, et al. Stereotactic 14G core biopsy of non-palpable breast cancer: what is the relationship between the number of core samples taken and the sensitivity of detection of malignancy? *Clin Radiol* 1999;54:384–389.
30. Brenner RJ, Fajardo L, Fisher PR, et al. Percutaneous core biopsy of the breast: effect of operator experience and number of samples on diagnostic accuracy. *AJR Am J Roentgenol* 1996;166:341–346.
31. Liberman L, Dershaw DD, Rosen PP, et al. Stereotaxic 14-gauge breast biopsy: how many core biopsy specimens are needed? *Radiology* 1994;192:793–795.
32. Berg WA, Krebs TL, Campassi C, et al. Evaluation of 14-and 11-gauge directional, vacuum-assisted biopsy probes and 14-gauge biopsy guns in a breast parenchymal model. *Radiology* 1997;205:203–208.

33. Liberman L, Smolkin JH, Dershaw DD, et al. Calcification retrieval at stereotactic, 11-gauge directional, vacuum-assisted breast biopsy. *Radiology* 1998;208:251–260.
34. Shah VI, Raju U, Chitale D, et al. False-negative core needle biopsies of the breast: an analysis of clinical, radiologic, and pathologic findings in 27 consecutive cases of missed breast cancer. *Cancer* 2003;97:1824–1831.
35. Kettritz U, Rotter K, Schreer I, et al. Stereotactic vacuum-assisted breast biopsy in 2874 patients: a multicenter study. *Cancer* 2004;100:245–251.
36. Jackman RJ, Marzoni FA, Rosenberg J. False-negative diagnoses at stereotactic vacuum-assisted needle breast biopsy: long-term follow-up of 1,280 lesions and review of the literature. *AJR Am J Roentgenol* 2009;192:341–351.
37. Pfrarl G, Helbich TH, Riedl CC, et al. Stereotactic 11-gauge vacuum-assisted breast biopsy: a validation study. *AJR Am J Roentgenol* 2002;179:1503–1507.
38. Riedl CC, Pfarl G, Memarsadeghi M, et al. Lesion miss rates and false-negative rates for 1115 consecutive cases of stereotactically guided needle-localized open breast with long-term follow-up. *Radiology* 2005;237:847–853.
39. White RR, Halperin TJ, Olsen JA Jr, et al. Impact of core-needle breast biopsy on the surgical management of mammographic abnormalities. *Am Surg* 2001;233:769–777.
40. Schueller G, Jaromi S, Ponhold L, et al. US-guided 14-gauge core-needle breast biopsy: results of a validation study in 1352 cases. *Radiology* 2008;248:406–413.
41. Bassett LW, Mahoney MC, Apple SK. Interventional breast imaging: current procedures and assessing for concordance with pathology. *Radiol Clin North Am* 2007;45:881–894.
42. Dillon MF, Hill AD, Quinn CM, et al. The accuracy of ultrasound, stereotactic and clinical core biopsies in the diagnosis of breast cancer, with an analysis of false-negative cases. *Ann Surg* 2005;242:701–707.
43. Helbich TH. Localization and biopsy of breast lesions by magnetic resonance imaging guidance. *J Magn Reson Imaging* 2001;13:903–911.
44. Carbognin G, Girardi V, Brandalise A, et al. MR-guided vacuum-assisted breast biopsy in the management of incidental enhancing lesions detected by breast MR imaging. *Radiol Med* 2011;116:876–885.
45. Orel SG, Rosen M, Mies C, et al. MR imaging-guided 9-gauge vacuum-assisted core-needle breast biopsy: initial experience. *Radiology* 2006;238:54–61.
46. Lourenco AP, Mainiero MB, Lazarus E, et al. Stereotactic breast biopsy: comparison of histologic underestimation rates with 11- and 9-gauge vacuum-assisted breast biopsy. *AJR Am J Roentgenol* 2007;189:W275–W279.
47. Tea M-KM, Grimm C, Fink-Retter A, et al. The validity of complex breast cysts after surgery. *Am J Surg* 2009;197:199–202.
48. Levine P, Simsir A, Cangiarella J. Management issues in breast lesions diagnosed by fine-needle aspiration and percutaneous core breast biopsy. *Am J Clin Pathol* 2006;125:S124–S134.
49. Verkooijen HM. Diagnostic accuracy of stereotactic large-core needle biopsy for nonpalpable breast disease: results of a multicenter prospective study with 95% surgical confirmation. *Int J Cancer* 2002;99:853–859.
50. Egyed Z, Pentek Z, Jaray B, et al. Radial scar-significant diagnostic challenge. *Pathol Oncol Res* 2008;14:123–129.
51. Cangiarella J, Guth A, Axelrod D, et al. Is surgical excision necessary for the management of atypical lobular hyperplasia and lobular carcinoma in situ diagnosed on core needle biopsy?: a report of 38 cases an review of the literature. *Arch Pathol Lab Med* 2008;132:979–983.
52. Elsheikh TM, Silverman JF. Follow-up surgical excision is indicated when breast core biopsies show atypical lobular hyperplasia or lobular carcinoma in situ: a correlative study of 33 patients with review of the literature. *Am J Surg Pathol* 2005;29:534–543.
53. Frouge C, Tristant H, Guinebretiere JM, et al. Mammographic lesions of radial scars: microscopic findings in 40 cases. *Radiology* 1995;195:623–625.
54. Margenthaler JA, Duke D, Monsees BS, et al. Correlation between core biopsy and excisional biopsy in breast high-risk lesions. *Am J Surg* 2006;192:534–537.
55. Parker SH, Burbank F, Jackman RJ, et al. Percutaneous large-core breast biopsy: a multi-institutional study. *Radiology* 1994;193:359–364.
56. Lineel F, Pinder SE, Ellis IO. Precursor lesions of breast carcinoma. *Breast J* 1993;2:220–223.
57. Middleton LP, Grant S, Stephens T, et al. Lobular carcinoma in situ diagnosed by core needle biopsy: when should it be excised? *Mod Pathol* 2003;16:120–129.
58. Sohn VY, Arthurs ZM, Kim FS, et al. Lobular neoplasia: is surgical excision warranted? *Am Surg* 2008;74:172–177.

59. Bowman K, Munoz A, Mahvi DM, et al. Lobular neoplasia diagnosed at core biopsy does not mandate surgical excision. *J Surg Res* 2007;142:275–280.
60. Kopans DB. LCIS found at core needle biopsy may not need surgical excision. *AJR Am J Roentgenol* 2008;191:W152.
61. O'Neil M, Madam R, Tawfik OW, et al. Lobular carcinoma in situ/atypical lobular hyperplasia on breast needle biopsies: does it warrant surgical excisional biopsy? A study of 27 cases. *Ann Diagn Pathol* 2010;14:251–255.
62. Rendi MH, Dintzis SM, Lehman CD, et al. Lobular in-situ neoplasia on breast core needle biopsy: imaging indication and pathologic extent can identify which patients require excisional biopsy. *Ann Surg Oncol* 2012;19:914–921.
63. Nagi CS, O'Donnell JE, Tismenetsky M, et al. Lobular neoplasia on core needle biopsy does not require excision. *Cancer* 2008;112:2152–2158.

SECTION

IV

Molecular Pathology, Predictive and Prognostic Markers

Molecular Classification of Breast Cancer

22

For many decades, the classification of breast cancer has been based solely on the histomorphologic appearance of breast cancer as described in Section II. While some of these histologic subtypes are proved to be prognostically significant (i.e., tubular carcinoma and mucinous carcinoma), a disadvantage of this classification system is that it often provides limited information on clinical decision making. In fact, the latter is largely based on the combination of clinicopathologic parameters with prognostic significance along with predictive biomarkers, including histologic grade, the presence/absence of lymphovascular invasion or nodal metastasis, and receptor (ER/PR/HER2) status.

Over the last decade, advances in gene microarray technology have enabled researchers to characterize the heterogeneous nature of breast cancer by classifying the disease into a number of molecular subtypes with prognostic significance. In 2000, Perou et al. initially identified a set of 496 genes that demonstrated significantly greater variation between individual tumors than within paired tumor samples from the same individual. When this intrinsic gene set was utilized in hierarchical clustering of their tumor samples, four "intrinsic subtypes" were identified[1,2]:

1. Luminal
2. HER2-enriched
3. Basal-like
4. Normal breast–like

These molecular subtypes were so named based on the similarities in gene expression to luminal and basal epithelial cells in the normal breast (luminal and basal-like, respectively), increased expression of genes in the *HER2* amplicon (HER2-enriched), and the inclusion of three normal, nonmalignant breast samples (normal breast–like). Subsequent studies from the same group further separated the luminal subtypes into luminal A, luminal B, and luminal C, with the latter two demonstrating lower expression of ER-related genes and poorer outcomes compared to luminal A tumors.[2] Further studies failed to reproduce the luminal C subtype; thus, the luminal classification was collapsed to include only luminal A and luminal B subtypes. Extension of the molecular subtype studies by other groups with larger data sets has resulted in discovery of additional rare molecular subtypes, including claudin low, molecular apocrine, and interferon rich.[3–6]

CHARACTERISTICS OF BREAST CANCER MOLECULAR SUBTYPES

Luminal Subtypes

Luminal A is the most common subtype of breast cancer. These tumors highly express ER-related genes and typically demonstrate ER- and/or PR-positive and HER2-negative receptor profile and low Ki-67 proliferation index.[2,7–12]

Luminal B subtype is less common than luminal A. The luminal B tumors express ER (often low levels), while PR levels may be low or negative. These tumors tend to be of higher histologic grade and consistently display high expression levels of proliferation-related genes, thus demonstrating higher Ki-67 proliferation index when compared to those of the luminal A subtype. Some of the luminal B tumors show HER2 amplification/overexpression.[2,7–12]

The luminal tumors, constituting 60% to 70% of invasive breast cancers, typically respond to endocrine therapy although the response to tamoxifen and aromatase inhibitors may be different for luminal A and luminal B tumors. These tumors show variable response to chemotherapy but typically greater in the luminal B subtype. The latter generally confers an increased risk of early relapse with endocrine therapy when compared with the luminal A tumors, likely related to higher histologic grade, larger tumor size, and more frequent lymph node metastasis at presentation.[13,14]

While the ER+ and/or PR+ receptor profile has been used as surrogate for luminal subtypes, there is no universally accepted definition to discriminate luminal A and luminal B tumors. Ki-67 proliferation index has been commonly used as the discriminating factor between the two subtypes in numerous studies, with variable cut-points.[14] The ER+/HER2+ profile has also been used to designate the luminal B subtype. However, the currently available evidence on the analytical validity and clinical utility of Ki-67 was found to be inadequate in subtype classification and that the luminal A and B subtypes may be misclassified based on the ER/HER2 profiles.[13,15] Further, there are several lines of evidence to demonstrate that the levels of expression of proliferation-related genes constitute a continuum rather than a bimodal distribution. Therefore, there are theoretically no natural cutoffs of Ki-67 proliferation index to separate the two subtypes.

HER2 Enriched

This subtype, constituting 15% to 20% of all breast cancers, demonstrates high expression of genes in HER2 amplicon and low expression of ER and related genes. Tumors of this subtype are typically ER/PR negative and HER2 amplified/overexpressed; thus, the ER−/PR−/HER+ profile is commonly used as surrogate for HER2-enriched subtype. It should be emphasized, however, that tumors of HER2-enriched subtype defined by gene expression profiling studies are not always equivalent to the HER2+ tumors identified by the FDA-approved methods following the American Society of Clinical Oncology (ASCO)/College of American Pathologists (CAP) guidelines.[16] The ER status and HER2 status alone are not accurate surrogates for true intrinsic subtype status, as most of ER+/HER2+ tumors lie within the luminal B cluster, and some ER−/HER2+ tumors fall into the basal-like clusters.[11]

HER2-positive tumors can be treated with trastuzumab (Herceptin), a monoclonal antibody, as well as other newer drugs that target the HER2 receptor. The patient outcomes are generally poor.[2,7–14]

Basal-like

Basal-like carcinomas (15% to 20%) highly express genes of basal epithelium and demonstrate low expression of ER-related genes and HER2. Thus, they typically show "triple-negative" phenotype (ER−/PR−/HER2−). These tumors are prevalent in younger women and tend to occur in patients of African American and Hispanic descent and in those harboring *BRCA1* germline mutations. This group shows the greatest diversity with regard to histopathologic features, molecular profiling, response to chemotherapy, and survival outcomes.

Histologically, these tumors are almost always high grade, frequently have a pushing margin with extensive lymphocytic infiltrate and central necrosis. They frequently harbor TP53 gene mutations and characteristically express high molecular weight cytokeratins (i.e., CK5/6 and CK14), p63, and epidermal growth factor receptor (EGFR). Thus, the "triple-negative" phenotype along with expression of one of aforementioned markers is commonly used to identify basal-like carcinomas clinically. However, there has been increased evidence that the definition of basal-like carcinoma based on morphology, expression of basal markers, and gene profiling varies significantly and does not reproducibly identify the same lesion.[17] Therefore, subclassification of triple-negative breast cancers into basal-like and nonbasal based on the immunoexpression of aforesaid markers may be of limited value.

Basal-like carcinomas do not respond to endocrine therapy or trastuzumab but appear to be more sensitive to cytotoxic chemotherapy. As a group, these tumors generally (but not uniformly) have a poor prognosis.[2,7–14]

Normal Breast–Like

This subtype was so named because of higher expression of many genes known to be expressed by adipose tissue and other nonepithelial cell types. The presence of normal breast–like cancers remains controversial. Some authorities have questioned the existence of this subtype and argue that most normal breast–like cancers, if not all, constitute a significant proportion of nontumoral breast stroma and epithelium given the low cellularity of these tumors (<50%), thus most likely representing artifacts of tissue procurement.[18] Therefore, proposing to assess the existence of this subtype must include true normal samples in the analyses, and further larger studies, such as The Cancer Genome Atlas project, are needed to address this issue.[19]

Additional Rare Subtypes

Claudin Low

This subtype is characterized by low to absent expression of luminal differentiation markers, high enrichment for epithelial-to-mesenchymal transition markers (such as *vimentin*, *Snail-1*, and *TWIST1*), immune response genes (i.e., *CD79b*, *CD14*, and *vav1*), down-regulation of genes involved in cell adhesion (i.e., *E-Cadherin* and *claudins 3*, *4*, and *7*), and acquisition of undifferentiated mammary stem cell–like features ($CD44^+/CD24^{-/low}$ antigenic phenotype).[3,19] Most of these tumors are triple-negative carcinomas, with a high frequency of metaplastic and medullary histomorphologic features. Controversies remain with regard to this phenotype as a significant proportion of the claudin-low tumors defined by gene microarray displayed moderate-to-strong expression of E-Cadherin and claudin 3 at protein levels, thus raising the possibility of contamination with stromal cells. Moreover, preliminary data show that these tumors demonstrate an intermediate response rate to standard neoadjuvant chemotherapy between basal-like and luminal tumors.[19]

Molecular Apocrine

This subtype was initially characterized by a gene microarray analysis and hierarchical clustering that divided 49 tumor samples into basal, luminal, and molecular apocrine groups.[6] These tumors are androgen receptor positive and display HER2 overexpression/amplification more commonly than the luminal and basal-like tumors. A subsequent study identified a subgroup of ER/PR-negative tumors with transcriptomic characteristics similar to those of molecular apocrine tumors.[20] These tumors showed paradoxical expression of genes known to be direct targets of ER, responsive to estrogen, or typically expressed in ER+ tumors. The differentially expressed genes included *SPDEF*, *FOXA1*, *XBP1*, *CYB5*, *TFF3*, *NAT1*, *APOD*, *ALCAM*, and *AR*.[20] Another study showed that almost all molecular apocrine tumors had the immunoprofile of HER2+ or GCDFP15+.[21] While this group of tumors display strong apocrine features histologically, including abundant eosinophilic cytoplasm and prominent nucleoli, they do not always fulfill the histologic criteria for apocrine carcinoma and hence termed *molecular apocrine tumors*. A recent study showed that this group of tumors had a good response to neoadjuvant chemotherapy, although they were associated with early recurrence.[22]

Interferon Rich

This subtype is characterized by a subgroup of triple-negative tumors displaying high expression of interferon-regulated genes including *STAT1*. Patients with these tumors had a considerably better prognosis than those associated with other triple-negative breast cancers.[4]

The biologic and clinical significance of these rare subtypes (probably more yet to be characterized) remains to be determined. The impact of identification of these subtypes on clinical decision making and management abides to be defined.

The clinicopathologic characteristics of the breast cancer molecular subtypes are summarized in Table 22-1.

Table 22-1 Molecular Subtypes of Breast Cancer

Molecular Subtype	Gene Expression Pattern	Typical Immunophenotype	Clinicopathologic Features
Luminal A	High expression of ER-related genes	ER+ and/or PR+, HER2−, low Ki-67	Low histologic grade Respond to endocrine therapy Variable response to chemotherapy Good prognosis
Luminal B	High expression of ER-related genes (<luminal A)	ER+ and/or PR+, HER2−/+, high Ki-67	Often high grade Respond to endocrine therapy Variable response to chemotherapy (>luminal A) Poorer prognosis than luminal A
HER2 enriched	High expression of HER2 and related genes Low expression of ER-associated genes	ER−, PR−, HER2+	High grade Respond to trastuzumab Generally poor prognosis
Basal-like	Low expression of the ER and HER2 gene clusters High expression of genes of basal epithelium	ER−, PR−, HER2−, CK5/6+, p63+, and/or EGFR+	High grade May be associated with germline *BRCA1* mutations No response to endocrine therapy or trastuzumab Appears to be more sensitive to cytotoxic chemotherapy Generally poor prognosis
Normal breast–like[a]	Highest expression of genes known to be expressed by adipose tissue and other stromal cells	Typically ER−, PR−, HER2−	Usually small tumors with low tumor cellularity and tend to have a good prognosis
Claudin low	Low expression of cell–cell adhesion proteins Enriched with immune system response genes	ER−, PR−, HER2−	High grade High frequency of metaplastic and medullary differentiation Intermediate response rate to neoadjuvant chemotherapy
Molecular apocrine	AR-related genes	ER−, PR−, HER2+/−, AR+, GCDFP15+	High grade Poor prognosis
Interferon rich	Interferon-regulated genes	ER−, PR−, HER2−	Better prognosis than other triple-negative breast cancers

[a]Controversial as to the existence of this subtype (see text).

LIMITATIONS OF CURRENT BREAST CANCER CLASSIFICATION

The rapidly evolving field of molecular genetic techniques has been progressively taking its place in routine pathology practice. The molecular classification of breast cancer furnishes information regarding the genomic complexity, key genetic alterations, and prognosis, thus is expected to lead to superior patient management. Despite this, however, molecular classification can only supplement the morphology-based approach and has not found a way to replace it. Foremost of all, there is a lack of standardization for the molecular classification methods used in the literature. Hierarchical clustering, multidimensional scaling, and self-organizing maps are among the most commonly used methods to discover and display structure in high-dimensional gene expression data, and all have limitations due to their inherited disadvantage. For example, in the clustering study, the investigators select the genes that show the greatest between-sample variability, and the results are displayed as a dendrogram. Clustering algorithms always detect clusters, even in random data, and may be difficult to define how many true clusters a particular dendrogram tree has.[23] Thus, it is easy to misinterpret the results of clustering analysis, especially when novel molecular subsets are proposed but lack robustness and reproducibility.[23] Another commonly encountered issue in practice is tissue sampling, as discussed previously in normal breast–like and claudin-low subtypes.

On the other hand, while a classification based on surrogate marker studies does not consistently represent the true intrinsic subtype status, such surrogate markers are currently being used to place a patient in one of these intrinsic subtypes for both routine clinical management as well as for enrollment in clinical trials.[24,25]

In summary, molecular testing in breast cancer is still in evolution. The molecular classification of breast cancer remains a working model rather than a true classification at this point of time. Further insights into the underlying molecular events with therapeutic significance may become of preeminent importance.

References

1. Perou CM, Sorlie T, Eisen MB, et al. Molecular portraits of human breast tumours. *Nature* 2000;406:747–752.
2. Sorlie T, Perou CM, Tibshirani R, et al. Gene expression patterns of breast carcinomas distinguish tumor subclasses with clinical implications. *Proc Natl Acad Sci U S A* 2001;98:10869–10874.
3. Prat A, Parker JS, Karginova O, et al. Phenotypic and molecular characterization of the claudin-low intrinsic subtype of breast cancer. *Breast Cancer Res* 2010;12:R68.
4. Hu Z, Fan C, Oh DS, et al. The molecular portraits of breast tumors are conserved across microarray platforms. *BMC Genomics* 2006;7:96.
5. Foulkes WD, Smith IE, Reis-Filho JS. Triple-negative breast cancer. *N Engl J Med* 2010;363:1938–1948.
6. Farmer P, Bonnefoi H, Becette V, et al. Identification of molecular apocrine breast tumours by microarray analysis. *Oncogene* 2005;24:4660–4671.
7. Sorlie T, Tibshirani R, Parker J, et al. Repeated observation of breast tumor subtypes in independent gene expression data sets. *Proc Natl Acad Sci U S A* 2003;100:8418–8423.
8. Koboldt D, Fulton, RS, McLellan, MD, et al. Comprehensive molecular portraits of human breast tumours (for the Cancer Genome Atlas Network). *Nature* 2012;490:61–70.
9. Goldhirsch A, Winer EP, Coates AS, et al. Personalizing the treatment of women with early breast cancer: highlights of the St. Gallen International Expert Consensus on the Primary Therapy of Early Breast Cancer 2013. *Ann Oncol* 2013;24:2206–2223.
10. Brenton JD, Carey LA, Ahmed AA, et al. Molecular classification and molecular forecasting of breast cancer: ready for clinical application? *J Clin Oncol* 2005;23:7350–7360.
11. Parker JS, Mullins M, Cheang MC, et al. Supervised risk predictor of breast cancer based on intrinsic subtypes. *J Clin Oncol* 2009;27:1160–1167.

12. Sotiriou C, Pusztai L. Gene-expression signatures in breast cancer. *N Engl J Med* 2009;360:790–800.
13. Carey LA, Perou CM, Livasy CA, et al. Race, breast cancer subtypes, and survival in the Carolina Breast Cancer Study. *JAMA* 2006;295:2492–2502.
14. Dowsett M, Nielsen TO, A'Hern R, et al. Assessment of Ki67 in breast cancer: recommendations from the International Ki67 in Breast Cancer working group. *J Natl Cancer Inst* 2011;103:1656–1664.
15. Guiu S, Michiels S, Andre F, et al. Molecular subclasses of breast cancer: how do we define them? The IMPAKT 2012 Working Group Statement. *Ann Oncol* 2012;23:2997–3006.
16. Wolff AC, Hammond ME, Hicks DG, et al. Recommendations for human epidermal growth factor receptor 2 testing in breast cancer: American Society of Clinical Oncology/College of American Pathologists clinical practice guideline update. *J Clin Oncol* 2013;31:3997–4013.
17. Gazinska P, Grigoriadis A, Brown JP, et al. Comparison of basal-like triple-negative breast cancer defined by morphology, immunohistochemistry and transcriptional profiles. *Mod Pathol* 2013;26:955–966.
18. Peppercorn J, Perou CM, Carey LA. Molecular subtypes in breast cancer evaluation and management: divide and conquer. *Cancer Invest* 2008;26:1–10.
19. Prat A, Perou CM. Deconstructing the molecular portraits of breast cancer. *Mol Oncol* 2011;5:5–23.
20. Doane AS, Danso M, Lal P, et al. An estrogen receptor-negative breast cancer subset characterized by a hormonally regulated transcriptional program and response to androgen. *Oncogene* 2006;25:3994–4008.
21. Lehmann-Che J, Hamy AS, Porcher R, et al. Molecular apocrine breast cancers are aggressive estrogen receptor negative tumors overexpressing either HER2 or GCDFP15. *Breast Cancer Res* 2013;15:R37.
22. Guedj M, Marisa L, de Reynies A, et al. A refined molecular taxonomy of breast cancer. *Oncogene* 2012;31:1196–1206.
23. Pusztai L, Mazouni C, Anderson K, et al. Molecular classification of breast cancer: limitations and potential. *Oncologist* 2006;11:868–877.
24. Chen X, Sun L, Cong Y, et al. Baseline staging tests based on molecular subtype is necessary for newly diagnosed breast cancer. *J Exp Clin Cancer Res* 2014;33:28.
25. Falck AK, Ferno M, Bendahl PO, et al. St. Gallen molecular subtypes in primary breast cancer and matched lymph node metastases—aspects on distribution and prognosis for patients with luminal A tumours: results from a prospective randomised trial. *BMC Cancer* 2013;13:558.

Predictive Markers and Targeted Therapies

23

A predictive marker is usually a gene or protein that, based on its presence or expression at a certain level, can predict a particular response (or lack thereof) to a specific treatment or management. These markers allow for better identification of patient candidates for a particular treatment, thus assisting the oncologists greatly in clinical decision making to achieve optimal patient management and to minimize the potential adverse side effects.[1] Predictive markers are sometimes confused with prognostic markers, although some molecules are both predictive and prognostic (i.e., estrogen receptor [ER]). The prognostic markers provide information on patients' outcomes independent of systemic therapy (see Chapter 24).

In invasive breast cancer, ER and/or progesterone receptor (PR) expression is a powerful predictive marker for response to tamoxifen and other hormonal therapies, while the presence of HER2 amplification/overexpression predicts response to specific anti-HER2 antibodies such as trastuzumab and also indicates an enhanced sensitivity for anthracycline-based chemotherapy regiments. The American Society of Clinical Oncology (ASCO) and the College of American Pathologists (CAP) convened an international Expert Panel that conducted a systemic review and evaluation of the literature and developed recommendation for optimal ER/PR testing.[2,3] The Panel recommends that ER, PR, and HER2 status be determined on all invasive breast cancers and breast cancer recurrences. The Panel also acknowledges that all newly diagnosed ductal carcinoma *in situ* (DCIS) are also commonly being tested for ER and PR, a practice based on the results of a retrospective subset analysis of the National Surgical Adjuvant Breast and Bowel Project (NSABP) B-24 clinical trial.[2] The Panel did not make a formal recommendation on ER testing in patients with DCIS but rather suggests clinician–patient discussion due to lack of validation studies. While it is not mandatory, the current National Comprehensive Cancer Network (NCCN) task force recommends that both ER and PR status should be determined for DCIS, although hormonal therapy in patients with DCIS is not routine because of much less benefit.[4] In practice, perhaps most medical oncologists recommend hormonal therapy in a substantial proportion of patients with receptor-positive DCIS. Thus, hormonal receptor studies are typically performed in DCIS to predict response to prophylactic hormonal therapy.

HORMONE RECEPTORS

Estrogen Receptor

ER-alpha (ER-α; ER) is a nuclear transcription factor activated by estrogen (17β-estradiol) and is essential in regulating cell proliferation and differentiation of breast tissue and also plays a key role in the mammary tumorigenesis.[5] ER is probably the most powerful predictive marker in breast cancer. Up to 70% of breast cancers are ER positive by immunohistochemistry (IHC) and use its ligand estradiol as the main stimulator for tumor growth. Thus, targeting ER signaling has naturally become the object of endocrine therapies, either directly using weak ER antagonists such as tamoxifen or indirectly by blockade of conversion of androgens to estrogen through aromatase inhibitors.

Endocrine therapies have become the mainstay of systemic therapies in the adjuvant and metastatic setting for ER-positive breast cancers.[6,7] It should be noted that the predictive value of ER is not ideal, and up to 30% to 40% of metastases from ER-positive primary breast cancer do not respond to endocrine therapy, because of either development of resistance to ER-targeted therapy or loss of ER expression due to tumor heterogeneity.[8] Although ER-β binds to estradiol to the same extent, its function has been controversial and far less characterized, and the currently utilized clinical data exclusively pertain to ER-α.

Progesterone Receptor

The value of assessing PR status in breast cancer is a matter of ongoing debate. As an ER-dependent gene product, PR expression is theoretically a surrogate marker for a functioning ER pathway. Therefore, assessment of PR should probably assist in predicting response to ER-targeted hormonal therapy more accurately. In fact, there are several lines of evidence to demonstrate that PR-positive tumors are more likely to respond to endocrine therapy, both in the adjuvant setting and in the metastatic disease,[9–11] although others have shown that ER-expressing tumors respond to endocrine therapy irrespective of PR expression levels.[12]

PR is reportedly expressed by IHC in up to two-thirds of breast cancers with variable intensity, thus slightly less than the frequency of ER-positive tumors.[13,14] A small subset of tumors (~16%) possess an ER+/PR− immunophenotype, and an even smaller proportion of cases (~4%) demonstrate an ER−/PR+ profile.[14] The mechanism of ER−/PR+ expression pattern remains to be defined, and the potential explanations include a false-negative ER assay, very low level of ER, and variants of ER unable to be recognized by the antibody but capable of constitutively activating the downstream signaling pathways.[15] Nonetheless, the predictive value of ER−/PR+ immunoprofile in breast cancer remains controversial.[9,16]

Testing Hormonal Receptors and ASCO/CAP Guidelines

In 2008, ASCO and CAP convened an international Expert Panel that conducted a systematic review and evaluation of the literature, to develop a guideline to improve the accuracy of immunohistochemical testing of ER and PR in breast cancer and the utility of these receptors as predictive markers. The Panel found that up to 20% of IHC determinations of ER and PR testing worldwide might be inaccurate (i.e., false negative or false positive). Most of the issues with testing have occurred because of variation in preanalytic variables, thresholds for positivity, and interpretation criteria. To this end, the Panel recommended that ER and PR status be determined on all invasive breast cancers and breast cancer recurrences. A testing algorithm that relies on accurate, reproducible assay performance was proposed. The essential elements of the guidelines were specified to reliably reduce assay variation, including comprehensive validation of IHC results, quantitative scoring, interpretation, and reporting of the results. Participation in proficiency testing, quality assurance, and use of external controls are integral components of these guidelines.[2] Adherence to these regulations is mandatory for laboratory accreditation and better patient care.[3] Some of these guideline recommendations were revised per the 2011 ASCO/CAP Clinical Notice on ER/PR and HER2 testing.[17] The summary of the key elements of the ER and PR guideline recommendations is shown in Table 23-1.

With regard to reporting, the Panel recommends that ER and PR results be reported with three required result elements (Figures 23-1 and 23-2):

1. The percentage/proportion of tumor cells staining
2. The intensity of staining (reported as weak, moderate, or strong)
3. An interpretation of the assay

Two optional report elements are recommended by the panel but not required:

1. A cautionary statement to negative ER and PR interpretations when the histopathology of the tumor is almost always associated with ER+ and PR+ results, including tubular, lobular, and mucinous histologic types or other tumors of low histologic grade (Figure 23-3)
2. A composite score (such as the H-score, Allred score, or Quick score) using the percentage and intensity measurements provided

Table 23-1 Summary of Key ASCO/CAP ER and PR Test Guideline Recommendations

Topic	Recommendation
Optimal algorithm for ER/PR testing	• Positive for ER/PR: ≥1% of tumor cell nuclei are immunoreactive • Negative for ER/PP: <1% of tumor cell nuclei are immunoreactive • Uninterpretable: no tumor nuclei are immunoreactive and that internal epithelial elements present in the sample or separately submitted from the same sample lack any nuclear staining
Optimal testing conditions[a]	Large, preferably multiple core biopsies of tumor are preferred for testing if they are representative of the tumor (grade and type) at resection
Optimal tissue handling	• Time from tissue acquisition to fixation (cold ischemic time): ≤1 hour • Fixation time: 6–72 hours (10% neutral buffered formalin)
Optimal internal validation procedure	• Validation must be done before test is offered, using a clinically validated ER or PR test method[38] • Revalidation should be done whenever there is a significant change to the test system
Optimal internal QA procedures	For initial test validation, ongoing quality control, laboratory personnel training, and competency assessment
Optimal external proficiency assessment	• Mandatory participation, at least two testing events per year • Satisfactory performance requires at least 90% correct responses
Optimal laboratory accreditation	• Optimal laboratory accreditation every other year • Annual requirement for self-inspection

[a]The guidelines recommend to reject the specimen in cases that the external controls are not as expected or artifacts involve most of sample or in conditions such as lack of staining of internal or external controls, decalcified specimen using strong acids, ER–/PR+ phenotype (to rule out a false-negative ER or false-positive PR), or negative ER/PR in samples with prolonged cold ischemia time or fixation duration (<6 or >72 hours) in the absence of internal control elements.

Data from Hammond ME, Hayes DF, Wolff AC. Clinical notice for American Society of Clinical Oncology-College of American Pathologists guideline recommendations on ER/PgR and HER2 testing in breast cancer. *J Clin Oncol* 2011;29:e458. and Wolff AC, Hammond ME, Hicks DG, et al. Recommendations for human epidermal growth factor receptor 2 testing in breast cancer: American Society of Clinical Oncology/College of American Pathologists clinical practice guideline update. *J Clin Oncol* 2013;31:3997–4013.

H-score is a method of assessing the extent of immunoreactivity and takes into consideration the staining intensity in conjunction with the percentage of cells staining positively in tumor cells.[18] The score gives a range of 0 to 300 and is obtained from the following formula:

$$3 \times \%\,\text{strongly staining cells} + 2 \times \%\,\text{moderately staining cells} + 1 \times \%\,\text{weakly staining cells}$$

Allred scoring system also utilizes the percentage and the intensity of tumor cell staining as follows:

Proportion Score	Intensity Score
0, No positive cells	0, Negative
1, ≤ 1%	1, Weak
2, 1% to 1/10	2, Intermediate
3, 1/10 to 1/3	3, Strong
4, 1/3 to 2/3	
5, 2/3 to 1	

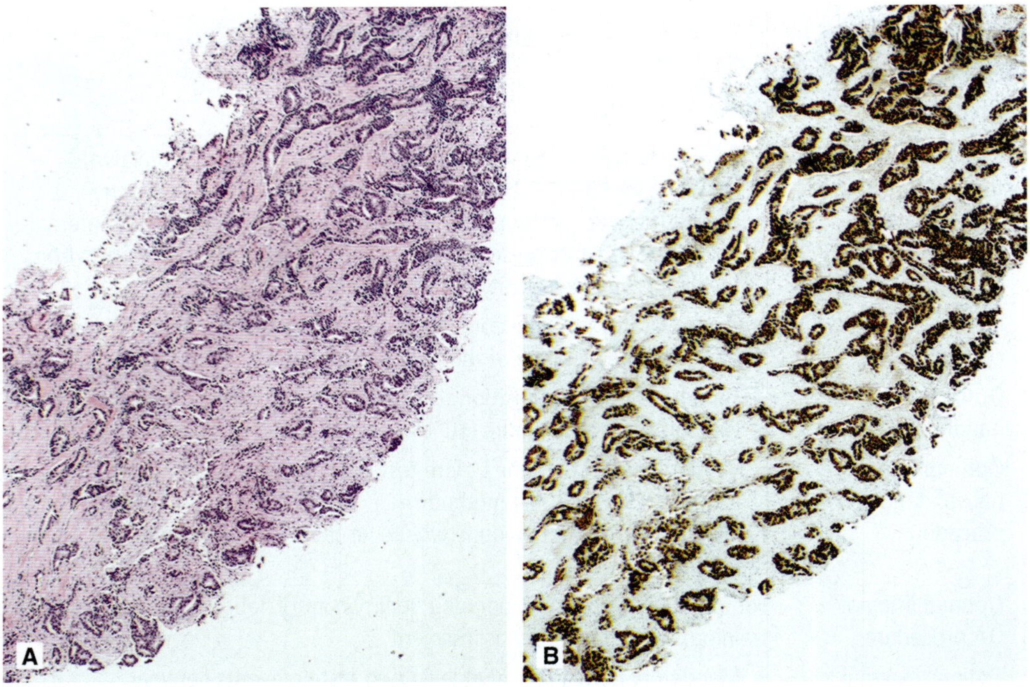

FIGURE 23-1: An invasive tubular carcinoma (**A**) demonstrates strong (3+) estrogen receptor expression by immunohistochemistry in virtually 100% of tumor cells (**B**).

FIGURE 23-2: An example of DCIS showing a heterogeneous ER expression by immunohistochemistry (approximately 20% weak, 20% intermediate, and 30% strong) in 70% of tumor cells.

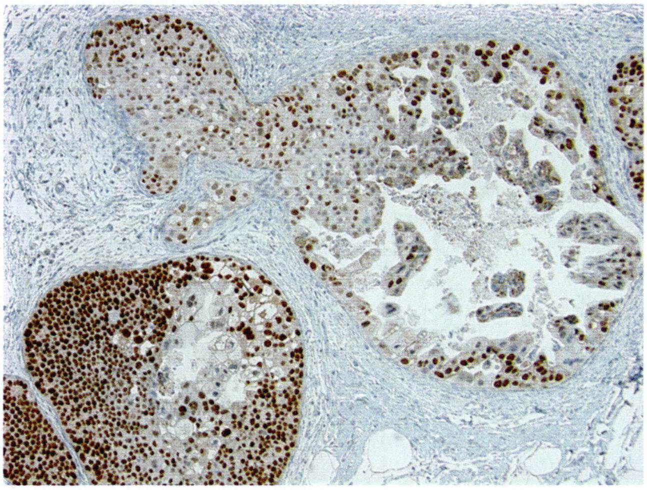

The total Allred score = proportion score + intensity score, giving a range of 0, 2 to 8.[19] The Allred scoring stratifies breast cancers into those that are likely to respond to endocrine therapy.[20]

Quick score is also based on both the intensity (A; 0 to 3) and the proportion (B; 1 to 6) of tumor cell staining.[21] The total score is obtained by either addition (A + B; range 1 to 9) or multiplication (A × B; range 0 to 18) of the two scores. No difference was found between the additive and multiplicative approaches when compared to the H-score, while the latter was favored by the original study given that it provides a wider range of score while permitting a completely negative result.[21]

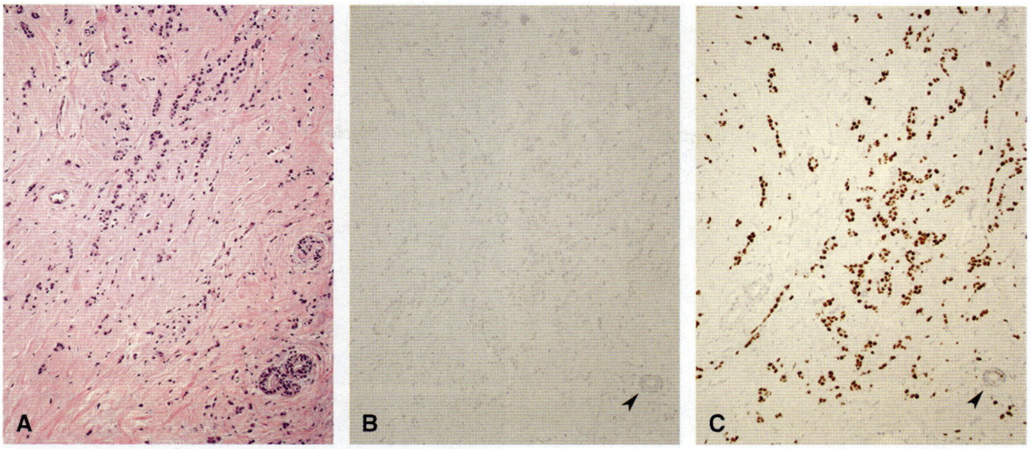

FIGURE 23-3: False-negative ER expression by immunohistochemistry in a low-grade carcinoma. The H&E-stained section shows a low-grade carcinoma (**A**). The tumor was negative for ER expression while there was a complete lack of staining in a benign gland (*arrowhead*) in lower right of image (**B**). The repeated ER stain demonstrated a strong and diffuse ER expression in the tumor while the aforesaid benign gland (*arrowhead*) showed weak ER expression (**C**).

HUMAN EPIDERMAL GROWTH FACTOR RECEPTOR 2 (HER2, ERBB2)

HER2 is a protein that in humans is coded by *ERBB2*, a known protooncogene located at the long arm of human chromosome 17 (17q12). The ErbB family proteins are a group of receptor tyrosine kinases. HER2 can form a heterodimer with any of the other family members. The resulting dimerization leads to autophosphorylation of tyrosine residues and initiates a variety of downstream signaling pathways. Other members of the family include epidermal growth factor receptor, erbB-3 (neuregulin binding; lacks kinase domain), and erbB-4.[22]

The HER2 gene is amplified and/or the HER2 protein is overexpressed in approximately 15% to 20% of primary breast cancers.[23] While HER2-positive tumors are typically high-grade carcinomas of no special type and were generally associated with a worse prognosis before the era of HER2-targeted therapy, the development of trastuzumab (Herceptin) has had a major impact in the treatment of HER2+ breast cancer, either in the early stage or in the metastatic setting.[24,25] Moreover, the combination of trastuzumab with chemotherapy has been shown to increase both survival and response rate, in comparison to trastuzumab alone.[26] Newer drugs that target HER2 include pertuzumab, another anti-HER2 humanized monoclonal antibody; lapatinib, a small-molecule HER2 inhibitor; and T-DM1, an antibody–drug conjugate consisting of trastuzumab linked to the cytotoxic agent mertansine.[23] Because of this, HER2 testing has also become mandatory for all newly diagnosed invasive breast cancers (primary and/or metastatic sites).

Testing HER2 and ASCO/CAP Guidelines

Among other methods, HER2 gene amplification and protein overexpression are usually tested by *in situ* hybridization (ISH) or IHC, respectively (Figure 23-4). As with hormonal receptor testing, the ASCO/CAP developed guidelines to test for HER2 in 2007.[27] The guideline recommendations were updated in 2013 to further improve the accuracy of HER2 testing and its utility as a predictive marker in invasive breast cancer.[23,28] The key elements of the current guidelines are summarized in Table 23-2, and the interpretation criteria for HER2 testing results are summarized in Table 23-3.

More than 10 IHC/ISH assays for HER2 testing have been developed thus far, among which a few are FDA approved.[29] In general, the concordance between unequivocal IHC and ISH results

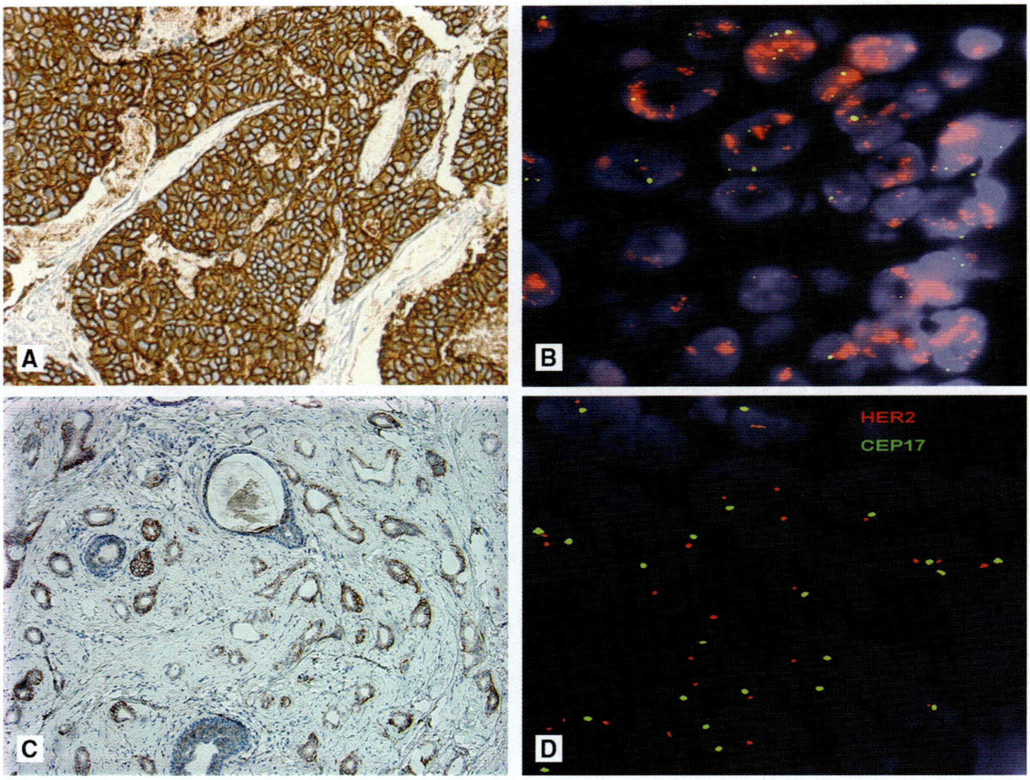

FIGURE 23-4: HER2 testing by immunohistochemistry and fluorescent *in situ* hybridization (FISH). Positive (3+) HER2 overexpression (**A**); HER2 gene amplification by FISH showing multiple copies of the HER2 gene (red signal) compared to CEP 17 centromere (*green signal*) (**B**); IHC showing an equivocal HER2 (2+) result in a tubular carcinoma (**C**) with nonamplification by subsequent FISH test (**D**).

Table 23-2 Summary of Key ASCO/CAP HER2 Test Guideline Recommendations

Topic	Recommendation
Specimens to test	• All newly diagnosed breast cancer • Metastatic breast cancer (if tissue sample is available)
Optimal algorithm	See Table 23-3
ISH rejection criteria	Report as indeterminate if: • Controls not as expected • Cannot find and count at least two areas of invasive tumor • >25% unscorable signals • >10% signals over cytoplasm • Poor nuclear resolution • Strong autofluorescence
ISH interpretation	• Scan the entire ISH slide prior to counting at least 20 cells. • Report a second population (>10% tumor cells) with increased HER2 signals/cell, if any. • Compare patterns in normal breast and tumor cells for bright-field ISH to avoid artifactual results
Acceptable tests	Use an FDA-approved IHC, bright-field ISH, or FISH assay

(*Continued*)

Table 23-2 Summary of Key ASCO/CAP HER2 Test Guideline Recommendations (*Continued*)

Topic	Recommendation
IHC interpretation criteria	See Table 23-3
IHC rejection criteria	Rejected and repeated or tested by FISH if: • Controls not as expected • Artifacts in most of sample • Strong membrane staining of normal breast ducts
Optimal tissue handling requirements	Duration of fixation: 6–72 hours
Optimal tissue sectioning requirements	Not to use sections cut >6 weeks earlier
Optimal internal validation procedure	Validation of test must be done before test is offered
Optimal initial test validation	• 20 negative and 20 positive for FDA-approved assays and 40 negative and 40 positive for laboratory developed tests • Compliance with accreditation and proficiency testing requirements for HER2 testing assays
Optimal internal QA procedures	• Review and document external and internal controls with each test and each batch of tests • Ongoing quality control and equipment maintenance • Initial and ongoing laboratory personnel training and competency assessment • Use of standardized operating procedures including routine use of control materials • Revalidation of procedure if changed • Perform ongoing competency assessment and document the actions taken
Optimal external proficiency assessment	• Participation in and successful completion of external proficiency testing program at least twice a year • Satisfactory performance requires at least 90% correct responses
Optimal laboratory accreditation	Onsite inspection every other year with annual requirement for self-inspection

Data from Wolff AC, Hammond ME, Hicks DG, et al. Recommendations for human epidermal growth factor receptor 2 testing in breast cancer: American Society of Clinical Oncology/College of American Pathologists clinical practice guideline update. *J Clin Oncol* 2013;31:3997–4013; and Wolff AC, Hammond ME, Hicks DG, et al. Recommendations for human epidermal growth factor receptor 2 testing in breast cancer: American Society of Clinical Oncology/College of American Pathologists clinical practice guideline update. *Arch Pathol Lab Med* 2014;138:241–56.

is near satisfactory in large central laboratories.[30] One study found that IHC interpretation was the major cause of the IHC-positive, ISH-negative discordance, with overinterpretation of weak membranous staining intensity, crush and sample edge artifacts, and inclusion of granular cytoplasmic staining as the causes of likely original false-positive IHC results, whereas IHC-negative/ISH-positive discordance was likely driven by loss of chromosome 17 signals.[30] It is generally accepted that equivocal HER2 results by IHC (2+) should be retested by ISH methods, which typically improve consistency among observers/institutions.[31]

Table 23-3 Interpretation of HER2 Testing Results by IHC and ISH

	IHC	ISH
Positive	**IHC 3+:** • Circumferential membrane staining that is complete, intense, observed in a homogeneous and contiguous population and within ≥10% of the invasive tumor cells	• Single-probe average HER2 copy number ≥6.0 signals/cell • Dual-probe HER2/CEP17 ratio ≥2.0; with an average HER2 copy number ≥4.0 signals/cell • Dual-probe HER2/CEP17 ratio ≥2.0; with an average HER2 copy number <4.0 signals/cell • Dual-probe HER2/CEP17 ratio < 2.0; with an average HER2 copy number ≥6.0 signals/cell
Equivocal	**IHC 2+:** • Circumferential membrane staining that is incomplete and/or weak/moderate and within >10% of the invasive tumor cells • Complete and circumferential membrane staining that is intense and within ≤10% of the invasive tumor cells	• Single-probe ISH average HER2 copy number ≥4.0 and <6.0 signals/cell • Dual-probe HER2/CEP17 ratio <2.0 with an average HER2 copy number ≥4.0 and <6.0 signals/cell
Negative	**IHC 1+:** • Incomplete membrane staining that is faint/barely perceptible and within >10% of the invasive tumor cells **IHC 0:** • No staining observed • Membrane staining that is incomplete and is faint/barely perceptible and within ≤10% of the invasive tumor cells	• Single-probe average HER2 copy number <4.0 signals/cell • Dual-probe HER2/CEP17 ratio <2.0 with an average HER2 copy number <4.0 signals/cell
Indeterminate	Technical issues prevent IHC and/or ISH from being reported as positive, negative, or equivocal	

Data from Wolff AC, Hammond ME, Hicks DG, et al. Recommendations for human epidermal growth factor receptor 2 testing in breast cancer: American Society of Clinical Oncology/College of American Pathologists clinical practice guideline update. *J Clin Oncol* 2013;31:3997–4013; and Wolff AC, Hammond ME, Hicks DG, et al. Recommendations for human epidermal growth factor receptor 2 testing in breast cancer: American Society of Clinical Oncology/College of American Pathologists clinical practice guideline update. *Arch Pathol Lab Med* 2014;138:241–56.

The HER2 gene is located on chromosome 17q12-21. Thus, the ratio of HER2 to CEP17 by ISH with the centromeric probe CEP17 is used to determine HER2 gene amplification status. Some recent findings have suggested that true polysomy 17 is uncommon, [32] while tumors with extra copies of HER2 as a result of polysomy 17 may be fundamentally different from those with

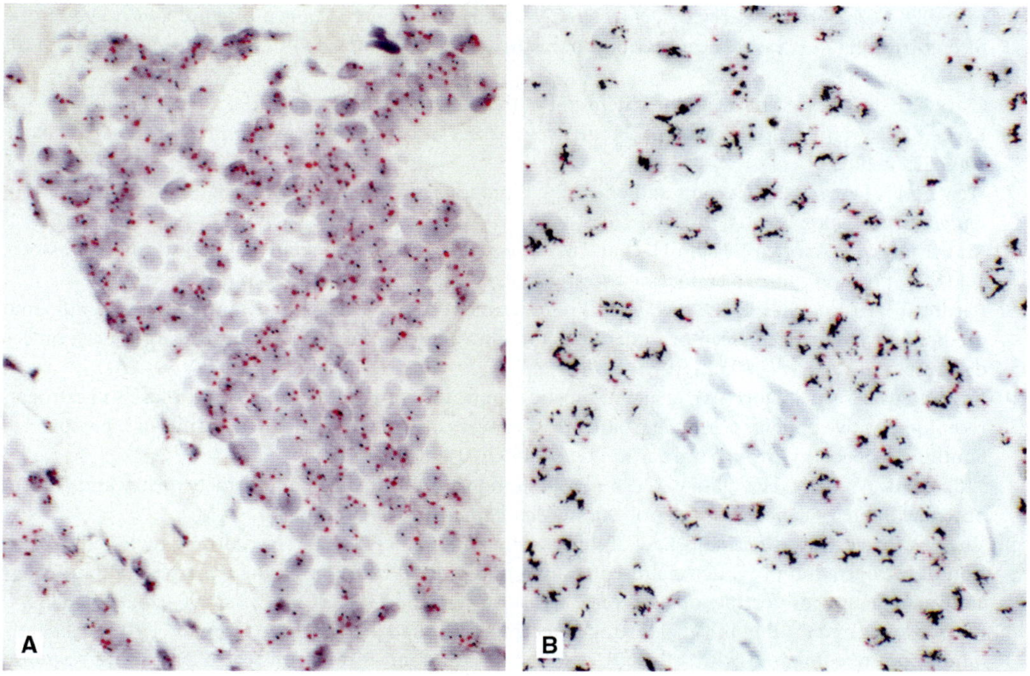

FIGURE 23-5: Illustration of a negative (**A**) and a positive (**B**) HER2 gene amplification by dual-color *in situ* hybridization.

extra copies resulting from gene amplification.[33] HER2-targeted therapy benefit seemed independent of HER2/centromere 17 ratio and chromosome 17 copy number.[34]

ISH determines the HER2 gene copy numbers using a DNA probe coupled to a fluorescent, chromogenic, or silver detection system (fluorescent *in situ* hybridization [FISH], CISH, or SISH), or a combination of CISH and SISH (i.e., dual-color ISH; Figure 23-5). CISH/SISH is a relatively new method for detection of gene amplification using a peroxidase reaction, with the advantage of using a standard light microscope. Recent studies have shown high level of concordance between these methods; thus, the later has become a viable alternative methodology in HER2 testing algorithm.[35,36]

Despite strict regulatory guidelines, however, discrepancies remain, including intraobserver and interobserver variability, inconsistency between different methods, and discrepancy between testing laboratories.[37] While it is arguable that false-positive HER2 results may not have as serious an impact on patient outcome as do false-negative results, there is no doubt that improving the accuracy of HER2 testing and reducing the incidence of false-negative results are vital in patient care. Some authorities proposed that sequencing might give us the final answer once inexpensive-enough techniques become available.[29]

References

1. Duffy MJ. Predictive markers in breast and other cancers: a review. *Clin Chem* 2005;51:494–503.
2. Hammond ME, Hayes DF, Dowsett M, et al. American Society of Clinical Oncology/College of American Pathologists guideline recommendations for immunohistochemical testing of estrogen and progesterone receptors in breast cancer. *J Clin Oncol* 2010;28:2784–2795.
3. Hammond ME, Hayes DF, Dowsett M, et al. American Society of Clinical Oncology/College of American Pathologists guideline recommendations for immunohistochemical testing of estrogen and progesterone receptors in breast cancer. *Arch Pathol Lab Med* 2010;134:907–922.

4. Allred DC, Carlson RW, Berry DA, et al. NCCN Task Force Report: estrogen receptor and progesterone receptor testing in breast cancer by Immunohistochemistry. *J Natl Compr Canc Netw* 2009;7(suppl 6): S1–S21; quiz S2–S3.
5. Clarke RB. Steroid receptors and proliferation in the human breast. *Steroids* 2003;68:789–794.
6. Payne SJ, Bowen RL, Jones JL, et al. Predictive markers in breast cancer—the present. *Histopathology* 2008;52:82–90.
7. Weigel MT, Dowsett M. Current and emerging biomarkers in breast cancer: prognosis and prediction. *Endocr Relat Cancer* 2010;17:R245–R262.
8. Kuukasjarvi T, Kononen J, Helin H, et al. Loss of estrogen receptor in recurrent breast cancer is associated with poor response to endocrine therapy. *J Clin Oncol* 1996;14:2584–2589.
9. Bardou VJ, Arpino G, Elledge RM, et al. Progesterone receptor status significantly improves outcome prediction over estrogen receptor status alone for adjuvant endocrine therapy in two large breast cancer databases. *J Clin Oncol* 2003;21:1973–1979.
10. Ravdin PM, Green S, Dorr TM, et al. Prognostic significance of progesterone receptor levels in estrogen receptor-positive patients with metastatic breast cancer treated with tamoxifen: results of a prospective Southwest Oncology Group study. *J Clin Oncol* 1992;10:1284–1291.
11. Mohsin SK, Weiss H, Havighurst T, et al. Progesterone receptor by immunohistochemistry and clinical outcome in breast cancer: a validation study. *Mod Pathol* 2004;17:1545–1554.
12. Viale G, Regan MM, Maiorano E, et al. Prognostic and predictive value of centrally reviewed expression of estrogen and progesterone receptors in a randomized trial comparing letrozole and tamoxifen adjuvant therapy for postmenopausal early breast cancer: BIG 1–98. *J Clin Oncol* 2007;25:3846–3852.
13. Elledge RM, Green S, Pugh R, et al. Estrogen receptor (ER) and progesterone receptor (PgR), by ligand-binding assay compared with ER, PgR and pS2, by immuno-histochemistry in predicting response to tamoxifen in metastatic breast cancer: a Southwest Oncology Group Study. *Int J Cancer* 2000;89: 111–117.
14. Hefti MM, Hu R, Knoblauch NW, et al. Estrogen receptor negative/progesterone receptor positive breast cancer is not a reproducible subtype. *Breast Cancer Res* 2013;15:R68.
15. Fuqua SA, Wolf DM. Molecular aspects of estrogen receptor variants in breast cancer. *Breast Cancer Res Treat* 1995;35:233–241.
16. Early Breast Cancer Trialists' Collaborative Group. Tamoxifen for early breast cancer: an overview of the randomised trials. *Lancet* 1998;351:1451–1467.
17. Hammond ME, Hayes DF, Wolff AC. Clinical notice for American Society of Clinical Oncology-College of American Pathologists guideline recommendations on ER/PgR and HER2 testing in breast cancer. *J Clin Oncol* 2011;29:e458.
18. McClelland RA, Finlay P, Walker KJ, et al. Automated quantitation of immunocytochemically localized estrogen receptors in human breast cancer. *Cancer Res* 1990;50:3545–3550.
19. Allred DC, Harvey JM, Berardo M, et al. Prognostic and predictive factors in breast cancer by immunohistochemical analysis. *Mod Pathol* 1998;11:155–168.
20. Allred DC, Anderson SJ, Paik S, et al. Adjuvant tamoxifen reduces subsequent breast cancer in women with estrogen receptor-positive ductal carcinoma in situ: a study based on NSABP protocol B-24. *J Clin Oncol* 2012;30:1268–1273.
21. Detre S, Saclani Jotti G, Dowsett M. A "quickscore" method for immunohistochemical semiquantitation: validation for oestrogen receptor in breast carcinomas. *J Clin Pathol* 1995;48:876–878.
22. Olayioye MA. Update on HER-2 as a target for cancer therapy: intracellular signaling pathways of ErbB2/HER-2 and family members. *Breast Cancer Res* 2001;3:385–389.
23. Wolff AC, Hammond ME, Hicks DG, et al. Recommendations for human epidermal growth factor receptor 2 testing in breast cancer: American Society of Clinical Oncology/College of American Pathologists clinical practice guideline update. *J Clin Oncol* 2013;31:3997–4013.
24. Moja L, Tagliabue L, Balduzzi S, et al. Trastuzumab containing regimens for early breast cancer. *Cochrane Database Syst Rev* 2012;4:CD006243.
25. Hudis CA. Trastuzumab—mechanism of action and use in clinical practice. *N Engl J Med* 2007;357:39–51.
26. Nahta R, Esteva FJ. HER-2-targeted therapy: lessons learned and future directions. *Clin Cancer Res* 2003;9:5078–5084.
27. Wolff AC, Hammond ME, Schwartz JN, et al. American Society of Clinical Oncology/College of American Pathologists guideline recommendations for human epidermal growth factor receptor 2 testing in breast cancer. *J Clin Oncol* 2007;25:118–145.

28. Wolff AC, Hammond ME, Hicks DG, et al. Recommendations for human epidermal growth factor receptor 2 testing in breast cancer: American Society of Clinical Oncology/College of American Pathologists clinical practice guideline update. *Arch Pathol Lab Med* 2014;138:241–256.
29. Allison M. The HER2 testing conundrum. *Nat Biotechnol* 2010;28:117–119.
30. Grimm EE, Schmidt RA, Swanson PE, et al. Achieving 95% cross-methodological concordance in HER2 testing: causes and implications of discordant cases. *Am J Clin Pathol* 2010;134:284–292.
31. Umemura S, Osamura RY, Akiyama F, et al. What causes discrepancies in HER2 testing for breast cancer? A Japanese ring study in conjunction with the global standard. *Am J Clin Pathol* 2008;130:883–891.
32. Tse CH, Hwang HC, Goldstein LC, et al. Determining true HER2 gene status in breast cancers with polysomy by using alternative chromosome 17 reference genes: implications for anti-HER2 targeted therapy. *J Clin Oncol* 2011;29:4168–4174.
33. Rosenberg CL. Polysomy 17 and HER-2 amplification: true, true, and unrelated. *J Clin Oncol* 2008;26:4856–4858.
34. Perez EA, Reinholz MM, Hillman DW, et al. HER2 and chromosome 17 effect on patient outcome in the N9831 adjuvant trastuzumab trial. *J Clin Oncol* 2010;28:4307–4315.
35. van de Vijver M, Bilous M, Hanna W, et al. Chromogenic in situ hybridisation for the assessment of HER2 status in breast cancer: an international validation ring study. *Breast Cancer Res* 2007;9:R68.
36. Hanna WM, Kwok K. Chromogenic in-situ hybridization: a viable alternative to fluorescence in-situ hybridization in the HER2 testing algorithm. *Mod Pathol* 2006;19:481–487.
37. Roche PC, Suman VJ, Jenkins RB, et al. Concordance between local and central laboratory HER2 testing in the breast intergroup trial N9831. *J Natl Cancer Inst* 2002;94:855–857.
38. Fitzgibbons PL, Murphy DA, Hammond ME, et al. Recommendations for validating estrogen and progesterone receptor immunohistochemistry assays. *Arch Pathol Lab Med* 2010;134:930–935.

24 Prognostic Markers

A prognostic marker is a variable that can be used to predict outcome of a disease, independent of therapy. Prognostic factors should be distinguished from predictive factors, although some pathologic parameters demonstrate both predictive and prognostic utilities, such as ER/PR/HER2 status in breast cancer (see Chapter 23). The introduction of mammographic screening programs has resulted in early detection and diagnosis of breast cancer, thus substantially improving the survival outcomes over the last few decades.

The field of biomarker discovery has been evolving rapidly owing to our accelerated understanding of tumor biology. The prognostic markers in breast cancer (and other cancers) can be largely divided into patient-related and tumor-related markers. As discussed in other chapters, younger age is particularly a poor prognostic indicator for women with newly diagnosed nonmetastatic breast cancer.[1,2] Race is another independent prognosticator. Being African American is associated with an excess mortality when compared to Caucasians.[1,3] Other patient characteristics significantly associated with survival outcomes largely include comorbidity and socioeconomic status.[1] This chapter is focused on the tumor-related characteristics that demonstrate prognostic significance, including histomorphologic factors and tissue biomarkers. Most of the former are incorporated into staging (Chapter 25). Some prognostic markers utilize the combination of clinical and pathologic information, such as Adjuvant! Online.

PATHOLOGIC PROGNOSTIC FACTORS

Axillary Lymph Node Status

The presence or absence of axillary lymph node (ALN) involvement is arguably the most significant prognostic factor in breast carcinoma.[4] The presence of macrometastasis, defined as tumor deposit greater than 2 mm in size, has been clearly shown to be associated with a worse outcome in multiple studies.[1,4] While the prognostic significance of micrometastasis (tumor deposit >0.2 mm and ≤2 mm in size) and isolated tumor cells (≤0.2 mm or <200 cells in a single nodal cross-section) was originally controversial,[5] the consensus from the most recent data is that neither micrometastasis nor isolated tumor cells convey any significant survival difference compared to node-negative disease and, if detected in sentinel lymph nodes (SLNs) (see below), does not require completion ALN dissection (ALND).[6–8] The majority of patients with nodal metastatic disease are candidates for systemic adjuvant therapy.

The SLNs are the first few lymph nodes into which a tumor drains and are identified by injecting a radioactive tracer and/or blue dye into the tissue near the tumor. The solution is taken up by the surrounding lymphatics and travels to the SLNs. SLN biopsy (SLNB) has been widely accepted as an appropriate initial alternative to routine staging of ALND for patients with early-stage breast cancer with clinically negative axillary nodes, given that the former is associated with a significantly lower rate of lymphedema, although there are no sufficient data on the effect of SLNB on long-term survival of patients with breast cancer.[9,10] The American Society of Clinical Oncology (ASCO) guidelines recommend that the SLNs are inspected for blue color, measured, and cut into sections no thicker than 2.0 mm through and parallel to the longest meridian. Each SLN is submitted in a separate cassette or identified by colored ink to permit accurate assessment of the total number of lymph nodes and number of involved lymph nodes.[10] All SLN sections should be submitted for microscopic examination, as failure to examine all nodal tissue can result in missing metastases in up to 40% of positive nodes.[11] Importantly, SLNB can be falsely positive due to iatrogenic displacement and transport of benign epithelial cells.[12] Conversely, SLNB results may be false negative, more often associated with a lobular or poorly differentiated ductal histologic type, or partial-to-complete replacement of non-SLNs with tumor, or the combination of both.[13]

Nodal metastases can be reliably detected by H&E-stained thin sections prepared following the ASCO guidelines. The utility of molecular techniques (i.e., RT-PCR) in routine practice remains unclear given the substantial false-positive and false-negative results.[10]

Lymphatic/Vascular Invasion

The presence of peritumoral lymphatic/vascular invasion (LVI) has long been considered a poor prognostic indicator, although controversies remain as to whether it is a factor independent of other variables (tumor size, grade, nodal status, hormonal receptor status, and adjuvant endocrine therapy).[14–16] LVI in the dermis, however, is associated with a particularly poor prognosis and, when extensive, often causes the skin changes characteristics of inflammatory carcinoma, although the definition of the latter does not require the finding of dermal LVI.[17]

The presence of LVI can be reliably identified on routine H&E-stained sections. Immunohistochemistry (IHC) stains for endothelial markers may be occasionally needed for ambiguous cases. When lymphatic or vascular spaces are completely filled and extended by tumor cells, distinction between LVI and ductal carcinoma *in situ* (DCIS) can be challenging and may require myoepithelial and/or endothelial markers. It is of particular importance that D2-40 (Podoplanin), an antibody thought to be specific for lymphatic endothelial cells, also react with myoepithelial cells and myofibroblasts in the breast.[18] Thus, caution should be exercised when interpreting the D2-40–labeled cells surrounding DCIS and carcinoma with retraction artifact. It is unnecessary to distinguish the vessel type in practice as both are prognostically significant. Moreover, the currently available markers are not entirely specific to any of the vessel types.

Tumor Size

Tumor size is defined by the greatest diameter of the primary tumor and has long been recognized as an independent prognostic factor.[4,19] Early studies have shown that tumor size is correlated with nodal status, but its prognostic value is independent of the latter,[19] although the correlation of tumor size and nodal status was found to be weaker in triple-negative breast cancers.[20]

Histologic Grade

The most popularized grading system for breast cancer is the modified Scarff-Bloom-Richardson system (also known as Nottingham grading system).[21] This modification provides somewhat objective criteria for its three components (tubule formation, nuclear pleomorphism, and mitotic count), and its prognostic significance has been confirmed by multiple studies.[21,22]

Histologic Subtypes

Certain histologic subtypes of breast cancer are generally associated with a favorable outcome, including tubular, cribriform, and mucinous carcinomas and adenoid cystic carcinoma. Conversely, a few subtypes are commonly associated with an unfavorable prognosis, such as micropapillary carcinoma and metaplastic carcinoma (see Section II for details).

Nottingham Prognostic Index

The Nottingham prognostic index (NPI), initially proposed in 1982, utilizes three pathologic variables and is calculated using the following formula:

$$NPI = [0.2 \times S] + N + G$$

where S is the size of tumor in cm, N is the number of lymph nodes involved, and G is the histologic grade of the tumor (1, 2, or 3).[23] The NPI scores stratify patients into four prognostic groups: excellent (≤2.4; 5-year survival 93%), good (2.4 to 3.4; 5-year survival 85%), moderate (3.4 to 5.4; 5-year survival 70%), and poor (>5.4; 5-year survival 50%). The prognostic value of NPI was subsequently validated after long-term follow-up of 1,629 patients by the authors' group[24] and independently in large multicenter studies.[25] Recently, it has been felt that the NPI cannot fully reveal the heterogeneity in clinical outcomes currently observed in breast cancer; thus, NPI plus (NPI+) has been proposed for greater sophistication and more personalized management of breast cancer patients.[26] The NPI+ utilizes a selective IHC panel of 10 biomarkers (ER, PR, CK5/6, CK7/8, EGFR/HER1, HER2, HER3, HER4, p53, and Mucin 1) and stratifies patients into seven core molecular classes: luminal A, luminal N, luminal B, basal p53 altered, basal p53 normal, HER2+/ER+, and HER2+/ER−.[26]

Adjuvant! Online

Adjuvant! Online can be accessed at http://www.adjuvantonline.com and is an tool for assessing the 10-year risk of breast cancer–related mortality or relapse without therapy and risk reduction with therapy on the basis of a number of clinicopathologic factors including age, comorbidity, tumor size, histologic grade, hormonal receptor status, and nodal involvement.[27] Adjuvant! Online provides a decision aid and does not direct toward a specific treatment regimen. It is also sensitive to patients' comorbidity levels, and the model outputs have been shown to be significant enough to affect physician recommendations and patients' treatment choices.[28] Yet, the National Cancer Center Network (NCCN) Task Force Report has indicated its imperfect estimates generated based on the available data sets, along with lack of long-term data about widely used adjuvant therapies as another uncertainty.[29]

TISSUE BIOMARKERS

The tumor-related prognostic markers in breast cancer with clinical utility largely include a number of single biomarkers, such as hormonal receptor and HER2 status, and a growing number of emerging combinatorial indices derived from gene expression profiles. The prognostic significance of the intrinsic subtypes of breast cancer is discussed in details in Chapter 22.

Hormone Receptors and HER2 Status

While the prognostic importance of the hormonal receptor status has been a matter of debate for the last few decades, it is now generally accepted, by most authorities, that both ER and PR are prognostically significant.[30] Moreover, hormonal receptor status is also associated with specific sites of metastatic spread. For example, ER/PR-positive tumors are more likely to develop bone relapse and much more significantly associated isolated bone metastasis, whereas ER/PR-negative tumors more frequently metastasize to visceral organs, including the brain.[31,32]

HER2 amplification/overexpression confers a poor prognosis, particularly if patients are not treated with HER2-targeted therapy.[33,34] However, the accuracy of this information remains indeterminate as the patients' outcomes may have been largely influenced by the administration of the therapeutic agents.

Ki-67

Ki-67 is a nuclear nonhistone protein universally expressed among proliferating cells (G1, S, and G2 phases of the cell cycle) and absent in quiescent cells (G0 phase), thus is among the best validated marker of proliferation.[35] The possible prognostic role for Ki-67 in breast cancer has been explored in many studies. The ability of Ki-67 as a single variable to distinguish between a good and unfavorable outcome in early breast cancer has been demonstrated by a number of large-scale studies, but its independent significance has not been established.[36–39] This is likely due to the association of Ki-67 and common histopathologic parameters and, more importantly, lack of standardization of Ki-67 measurement and interpretation methods. Currently, Ki-67 is still not recommended as a prognostic marker for routine clinical use.

IHC4 Score

The IHC4 score is a prognostic tool based on quantitative assessment of ER, PR, HER2, and Ki-67% and is derived from an analytically validated test using strict methodologies for staining and reading.[40] It has been shown that the prognostic information contained in this IHC-based assay is similar to that in the Oncotype DX.[40]

Mammostrat

The Mammostrat is an IHC-based assay of five gene products, including solute carrier family 7 member 5 (SLC7A5), p53, HTF9C (cell cycle molecule), *N*-myc downstream regulated 1 (NDRG1), and carcinoembryonic antigen–related cell adhesion molecule 5 (CEACAM5).[41] A prognostic index based on the expression of these proteins is calculated, and patients are stratified into low, moderate, and high risk of recurrence (ROR). The clinical utility of this test in risk stratification of postmenopausal patients with ER-positive breast cancer has been shown in a multicenter trial.[42]

Urokinase Plasminogen Activator/Plasminogen Activator Inhibitor-1

The serine protease urokinase plasminogen activator (uPA) and its inhibitor, plasminogen activator inhibitor-1 (PAI-1), play an important role in angiogenesis, invasion, and metastasis.[43] Early studies indicated that overexpression of uPA and PAI-1 emerged as independent poor prognostic indicators.[44] However, the needs of fresh/frozen tissue and enzyme-linked immunosorbent assay have limited its widespread uptake in the clinical practice and thus is not of much use currently.

Other Tissue Biomarkers

Among many others, single biomarkers proposed in the literature include p53 mutations, DNA ploidy, cyclin D1, cyclin E, topoisomerase IIα, circulating tumor cells, and circulating DNA.[45] The prognostic utility of these markers remains controversial, and none of them are routinely analyzed in clinical practice.

GENE EXPRESSION–BASED MARKERS

Oncotype DX Recurrence Score

Oncotype DX is a quantitative RT-PCR (qRT-PCR)–based assay utilizing formalin-fixed paraffin-embedded (FFPE) tissues, initially developed to estimate the risk of distant recurrence for patients with ER-positive, lymph node–negative breast cancers. The assay quantifies the expression of 21 genes, including 16 cancer-related genes largely grouped into the estrogen, proliferation, HER2, and invasion groups, and five reference genes. [46] Derived from the reference-normalized expression measurements, the result is reported as a recurrence score (RS), on a scale from 0 to 100, that predicts likelihood of recurrence at 10 years. Patients are classified into three categories based on RS: low risk (RS < 18), intermediate risk (RS 18 to 30), and high risk (RS ≥ 31). Oncotype DX testing has been endorsed by NCCN and ASCO guidelines for breast cancer care.[47]

MammaPrint (Amsterdam 70-Gene Profile)

MammaPrint is a supervised DNA microarray analysis.[48] The 70 genes in the MammaPrint signature were selected from genome-wide expression data using a data-driven approach. Different from Oncotype DX, it can be used to determine the prognosis in patients with breast

Table 24-1 Commercially Available Multigene Prognostic Tests for Breast Cancer

Test	Manufacturer	Technique	Tissue Requirements	Indication	Output	Guidelines
Oncotype DX	Genomic Health Inc. (Redwood City, CA)	qRT-PCR (21 genes)	FFPE	Patients with ER+, node-negative disease	**RS** Continuous score that predict 10-year distant recurrence	NCCN and ASCO
MammaPrint	Agendia Inc. (Irvine, CA)	DNA microarray (70 genes)	Fresh or frozen	T1-T2, node-negative disease	**Low risk/high risk** Predict 10-year distant metastasis	FDA approved
PAM50/ Prosigna	NanoString Technologies, Inc. (Seattle, WA)	qRT-PCR and nCounter technology (55 genes)	Fresh frozen or FFPE	Postmenopausal women with node-negative (stage I or II) or node-positive (stage II) disease	**ROR** Continuous risk of recurrence at 10 years	FDA approved
MapQuant Dx	Ipsogen (Marseille, France)	DNA microarray (97 genes)	Fresh frozen or FFPE	Invasive, primary, ER positive, grade 2 tumors To restratify grade 2 tumors into grade 1 or grade 3	**GGI** Low grade/high grade	
Breast Cancer Index[SM]	bioTheranostics (San Diego, CA)	Multigene qRT-PCR (combination of the HOXB13:IL17BR index and MGI)	Fresh frozen or FFPE	ER+, node-negative disease	**BCI score** Continuous score that predicts risk of recurrence and potential benefit of extended endocrine therapy	

HR, hormonal receptor; qRT-PCR, quantitative reverse transcriptase–polymerase chain reaction; FFPE, formalin-fixed, paraffin-embedded; MGI, molecular grade index; RS, recurrence score; ROR, risk of recurrence; GGI, genomic grade index; BCI, breast cancer index; NCCN, National Cancer Center Network; FDA, Food and Drug Administration.

cancer regardless of hormone receptor status and in patients with HER2-positive disease. This FDA-approved assay is based on fresh frozen tissue that limits its application. Validation using FFPE tissue has been performed recently.[49]

PAM50 Risk of Recurrence Score

The Predictor Analysis of Microarray 50 (PAM50) employees the expression of 50 prespecified classifier genes and 5 control genes that incorporate the intrinsic subtypes of breast cancer.[50] This FDA-approved assay utilizes qRT-PCR technique and can be performed on fresh frozen or FFPE tissue and has recently been implanted on the nanotechnology-based nCounter digital gene expression platform, thus can be performed in any pathology laboratory.[47] The results of the assay are used to generate the ROR score, which predicts distant relapse-free survival and likelihood of recurrence at 10 years in the setting of ER-positive disease.

Other Gene Expression–Based Assays

There are a number of additional gene expression profile–based assays proposed to predict breast cancer prognosis. *Rotterdam 76-gene signature* consists of separate gene sets developed for ER-negative (16 genes) and ER-positive (60 genes) diseases.[51] *Genomic grade index* (GGI) is a 97-gene signature found to improve the prognostic value of histologic grade.[52] Subsequent studies showed that GGI was prognostic independently from classical markers and performed equally well as the RS for ER-positive tumors.[53] *Breast cancer index* (BCI) is a combination of two profiles, the *HOXB13-to-IL17BR* expression index (the ratio of two ER-regulated genes) and the five-gene *Molecular Grade Index* (MGI), of which the latter is derived from GGI.[54] *Endopredict* is an RNA-based assay utilizing RT-PCR of 11 genes (including three reference genes) to calculate a prognostic score.[55] These assays have not been validated by large-scale independent studies; thus, their clinical utilities remain to be determined.

In summary, numerous new gene expression–based prognostic markers have been proposed in the last two decades, of which the Oncotype DX, MammaPrint, and PAM50 are among the best validated and commercially available assays in the clinic setting at this point of time.[47,56] The major multigene prognostic tests commercially available and their clinical utility are summarized in Table 24-1.

NEXT-GENERATION SEQUENCING

The revolution in next-generation sequencing has enabled genome sequencing studies on hundreds of individual human malignancies, including breast cancer.[57,58] By utilizing these techniques, the somatic DNA changes in the cancer can be identified through comparing the DNA sequences of the primary tumor and the patient's normal tissue. Moreover, the evolutional changes during metastatic spread can be identified through comparing the DNA of the primary tumor and the metastasis. Thus, it is highly anticipated that genome sequencing will play a growing role in the near future in the pursuit of personalized medicine.

References

1. Soerjomataram I, Louwman MW, Ribot JG, et al. An overview of prognostic factors for long-term survivors of breast cancer. *Breast Cancer Res Treat* 2008;107:309–330.
2. Arriagada R, Le MG, Dunant A, et al. Twenty-five years of follow-up in patients with operable breast carcinoma: correlation between clinicopathologic factors and the risk of death in each 5-year period. *Cancer* 2006;106:743–750.
3. Ren Z, Li Y, Hameed O, et al. Prognostic factors in patients with metastatic breast cancer at the time of diagnosis. *Pathol Res Pract* 2014;210:301–306.

4. Carter CL, Allen C, Henson DE. Relation of tumor size, lymph node status, and survival in 24,740 breast cancer cases. *Cancer* 1989;63:181–187.
5. de Boer M, van Deurzen CH, van Dijck JA, et al. Micrometastases or isolated tumor cells and the outcome of breast cancer. *N Engl J Med* 2009;361:653–663.
6. Gobardhan PD, Elias SG, Madsen EV, et al. Prognostic value of lymph node micrometastases in breast cancer: a multicenter cohort study. *Ann Surg Oncol* 2011;18:1657–1664.
7. Maaskant-Braat AJ, van de Poll-Franse LV, Voogd AC, et al. Sentinel node micrometastases in breast cancer do not affect prognosis: a population-based study. *Breast Cancer Res Treat* 2011;127:195–203.
8. Houvenaeghel G, Classe JM, Garbay JR, et al. Prognostic value of isolated tumor cells and micrometastases of lymph nodes in early-stage breast cancer: a French sentinel node multicenter cohort study. *Breast* 2014;23(5):561–566.
9. McLaughlin SA, Wright MJ, Morris KT, et al. Prevalence of lymphedema in women with breast cancer 5 years after sentinel lymph node biopsy or axillary dissection: objective measurements. *J Clin Oncol* 2008;26:5213–5219.
10. Lyman GH, Giuliano AE, Somerfield MR, et al. American Society of Clinical Oncology guideline recommendations for sentinel lymph node biopsy in early-stage breast cancer. *J Clin Oncol* 2005;23: 7703–7720.
11. Smith PA, Harlow SP, Krag DN, et al. Submission of lymph node tissue for ancillary studies decreases the accuracy of conventional breast cancer axillary node staging. *Mod Pathol* 1999;12:781–785.
12. Bleiweiss IJ, Nagi CS, Jaffer S. Axillary sentinel lymph nodes can be falsely positive due to iatrogenic displacement and transport of benign epithelial cells in patients with breast carcinoma. *J Clin Oncol* 2006;24:2013–2018.
13. Wei S, Bleiweiss IJ, Nagi C, et al. Characteristics of breast carcinoma cases with false-negative sentinel lymph nodes. *Clin Breast Cancer* 2014;14:280–284.
14. Pinder SE, Ellis IO, Galea M, et al. Pathological prognostic factors in breast cancer. III. Vascular invasion: relationship with recurrence and survival in a large study with long-term follow-up. *Histopathology* 1994;24:41–47.
15. Ejlertsen B, Jensen MB, Rank F, et al. Population-based study of peritumoral lymphovascular invasion and outcome among patients with operable breast cancer. *J Natl Cancer Inst* 2009;101:729–735.
16. Viale G, Giobbie-Hurder A, Gusterson BA, et al. Adverse prognostic value of peritumoral vascular invasion: is it abrogated by adequate endocrine adjuvant therapy? Results from two International Breast Cancer Study Group randomized trials of chemoendocrine adjuvant therapy for early breast cancer. *Ann Oncol* 2010;21:245–254.
17. Edge SB; American Joint Committee on Cancer. *AJCC Cancer Staging Manual*. 7th ed. New York: Springer; 2010.
18. Ren S, Abuel-Haija M, Khurana JS, et al. D2-40: an additional marker for myoepithelial cells of breast and the precaution in interpreting tumor lymphovascular invasion. *Int J Clin Exp Pathol* 2011;4:175–182.
19. Koscielny S, Tubiana M, Le MG, et al. Breast cancer: relationship between the size of the primary tumour and the probability of metastatic dissemination. *Br J Cancer* 1984;49:709–715.
20. Foulkes WD, Grainge MJ, Rakha EA, et al. Tumor size is an unreliable predictor of prognosis in basal-like breast cancers and does not correlate closely with lymph node status. *Breast Cancer Res Treat* 2009;117:199–204.
21. Elston CW, Ellis IO. Pathological prognostic factors in breast cancer. I. The value of histological grade in breast cancer: experience from a large study with long-term follow-up. *Histopathology* 1991;19:403–410.
22. Rakha EA, El-Sayed ME, Lee AH, et al. Prognostic significance of Nottingham histologic grade in invasive breast carcinoma. *J Clin Oncol* 2008;26:3153–3158.
23. Haybittle JL, Blamey RW, Elston CW, et al. A prognostic index in primary breast cancer. *Br J Cancer* 1982;45:361–366.
24. Galea MH, Blamey RW, Elston CE, et al. The Nottingham Prognostic Index in primary breast cancer. *Breast Cancer Res Treat* 1992;22:207–219.
25. Balslev I, Axelsson CK, Zedeler K, et al. The Nottingham Prognostic Index applied to 9,149 patients from the studies of the Danish Breast Cancer Cooperative Group (DBCG). *Breast Cancer Res Treat* 1994;32:281–290.
26. Rakha EA, Soria D, Green AR, et al. Nottingham Prognostic Index Plus (NPI+): a modern clinical decision making tool in breast cancer. *Br J Cancer* 2014;110:1688–1697.
27. Ravdin PM, Siminoff LA, Davis GJ, et al. Computer program to assist in making decisions about adjuvant therapy for women with early breast cancer. *J Clin Oncol* 2001;19:980–991.

28. Ozanne EM, Braithwaite D, Sepucha K, et al. Sensitivity to input variability of the Adjuvant! Online breast cancer prognostic model. *J Clin Oncol* 2009;27:214–219.
29. Carlson RW, Brown E, Burstein HJ, et al. NCCN task force report: adjuvant therapy for breast cancer. *J Natl Compr Canc Netw* 2006;4(suppl 1):S1–S26.
30. Bartlett JM, Brookes CL, Robson T, et al. Estrogen receptor and progesterone receptor as predictive biomarkers of response to endocrine therapy: a prospectively powered pathology study in the Tamoxifen and Exemestane adjuvant multinational trial. *J Clin Oncol* 2011;29:1531–1538.
31. Insa A, Lluch A, Prosper F, et al. Prognostic factors predicting survival from first recurrence in patients with metastatic breast cancer: analysis of 439 patients. *Breast Cancer Res Treat* 1999;56:67–78.
32. Wei S, Li Y, Siegal GP, et al. Breast carcinomas with isolated bone metastases have different hormone receptor expression profiles than those with metastases to other sites or multiple organs. *Ann Diagn Pathol* 2011;15:79–83.
33. Gusterson BA, Gelber RD, Goldhirsch A, et al. Prognostic importance of c-erbB-2 expression in breast cancer. International (Ludwig) Breast Cancer Study Group. *J Clin Oncol* 1992;10:1049–1056.
34. Chia S, Norris B, Speers C, et al. Human epidermal growth factor receptor 2 overexpression as a prognostic factor in a large tissue microarray series of node-negative breast cancers. *J Clin Oncol* 2008;26:5697–5704.
35. Lopez F, Belloc F, Lacombe F, et al. Modalities of synthesis of Ki67 antigen during the stimulation of lymphocytes. *Cytometry* 1991;12:42–49.
36. Urruticoechea A, Smith IE, Dowsett M. Proliferation marker Ki-67 in early breast cancer. *J Clin Oncol* 2005;23:7212–7220.
37. de Azambuja E, Cardoso F, de Castro G Jr., et al. Ki-67 as prognostic marker in early breast cancer: a meta-analysis of published studies involving 12,155 patients. *Br J Cancer* 2007;96:1504–1513.
38. Stuart-Harris R, Caldas C, Pinder SE, et al. Proliferation markers and survival in early breast cancer: a systematic review and meta-analysis of 85 studies in 32,825 patients. *Breast* 2008;17:323–334.
39. Inwald EC, Klinkhammer-Schalke M, Hofstadter F, et al. Ki-67 is a prognostic parameter in breast cancer patients: results of a large population-based cohort of a cancer registry. *Breast Cancer Res Treat* 2013;139:539–552.
40. Cuzick J, Dowsett M, Pineda S, et al. Prognostic value of a combined estrogen receptor, progesterone receptor, Ki-67, and human epidermal growth factor receptor 2 immunohistochemical score and comparison with the Genomic Health recurrence score in early breast cancer. *J Clin Oncol* 2011;29:4273–4278.
41. Ring BZ, Seitz RS, Beck R, et al. Novel prognostic immunohistochemical biomarker panel for estrogen receptor-positive breast cancer. *J Clin Oncol* 2006;24:3039–3047.
42. Bartlett JM, Bloom KJ, Piper T, et al. Mammostrat as an immunohistochemical multigene assay for prediction of early relapse risk in the tamoxifen versus exemestane adjuvant multicenter trial pathology study. *J Clin Oncol* 2012;30:4477–4484.
43. Andreasen PA, Kjoller L, Christensen L, et al. The urokinase-type plasminogen activator system in cancer metastasis: a review. *Int J Cancer* 1997;72:1–22.
44. Duffy MJ. Urokinase plasminogen activator and its inhibitor, PAI-1, as prognostic markers in breast cancer: from pilot to level 1 evidence studies. *Clin Chem* 2002;48:1194–1197.
45. Patani N, Martin LA, Dowsett M. Biomarkers for the clinical management of breast cancer: international perspective. *Int J Cancer* 2013;133:1–13.
46. Paik S, Shak S, Tang G, et al. A multigene assay to predict recurrence of tamoxifen-treated, node-negative breast cancer. *N Engl J Med* 2004;351:2817–2826.
47. Goncalves R, Bose R. Using multigene tests to select treatment for early-stage breast cancer. *J Natl Compr Canc Netw* 2013;11:174–182; quiz 82.
48. van't Veer LJ, Dai H, van de Vijver MJ, et al. Gene expression profiling predicts clinical outcome of breast cancer. *Nature* 2002;415:530–536.
49. Sapino A, Roepman P, Linn SC, et al. MammaPrint molecular diagnostics on formalin-fixed, paraffin-embedded tissue. *J Mol Diagn* 2014;16:190–197.
50. Nielsen TO, Parker JS, Leung S, et al. A comparison of PAM50 intrinsic subtyping with immunohistochemistry and clinical prognostic factors in tamoxifen-treated estrogen receptor-positive breast cancer. *Clin Cancer Res* 2010;16:5222–5232.
51. Wang Y, Klijn JG, Zhang Y, et al. Gene-expression profiles to predict distant metastasis of lymph-node-negative primary breast cancer. *Lancet* 2005;365:671–679.

52. Sotiriou C, Wirapati P, Loi S, et al. Gene expression profiling in breast cancer: understanding the molecular basis of histologic grade to improve prognosis. *J Natl Cancer Inst* 2006;98:262–272.
53. Loi S, Haibe-Kains B, Desmedt C, et al. Definition of clinically distinct molecular subtypes in estrogen receptor-positive breast carcinomas through genomic grade. *J Clin Oncol* 2007;25:1239–1246.
54. Ma XJ, Wang Z, Ryan PD, et al. A two-gene expression ratio predicts clinical outcome in breast cancer patients treated with tamoxifen. *Cancer Cell* 2004;5:607–616.
55. Filipits M, Rudas M, Jakesz R, et al. A new molecular predictor of distant recurrence in ER-positive, HER2-negative breast cancer adds independent information to conventional clinical risk factors. *Clin Cancer Res* 2011;17:6012–6020.
56. Arpino G, Generali D, Sapino A, et al. Gene expression profiling in breast cancer: a clinical perspective. *Breast* 2013;22:109–120.
57. Shah SP, Morin RD, Khattra J, et al. Mutational evolution in a lobular breast tumour profiled at single nucleotide resolution. *Nature* 2009;461:809–813.
58. Ding L, Ellis MJ, Li S, et al. Genome remodelling in a basal-like breast cancer metastasis and xenograft. *Nature* 2010;464:999–1005.

SECTION

V

Staging

25 General Staging Guidelines

As is the case for tumors of other organs, TNM staging of breast carcinoma is based on the characteristics of the primary tumor (T), status of regional lymph nodes (N), and distant metastases (M). Such staging is based on the American Joint Committee on Cancer (AJCC) criteria, which is currently in its seventh edition.[1] In contrast to clinical staging (cTNM) that is based on physical examination and imaging findings, pathologic staging (pTNM) is dependent on findings obtained from *microscopic* evaluation of breast and axillary lymph node biopsy and excisional material, as well as material from possible metastatic sites. In other words, although pathologic staging is usually performed after surgical resection, findings from all available specimens should be utilized for staging. The primary focus of discussion is on pathologic staging, where these general guidelines most apply.

In the case of bilateral breast carcinoma, each tumor should have its own separate stage.[1] Metachronous primary carcinomas should also be separately staged as a new tumor. Multiple tumors within the same breast are handled differently (see below). The "y" prefix is used to designate staging following neoadjuvant therapy,[2,3] whereas the "r" prefix is used to designate staging of recurrent tumors. The presence of residual tumor after surgical or neoadjuvant therapy may be described by the symbol "R" to indicate the tumor status after treatment. This, as well as T and N, could be categorized as "X" when the status is not known.

PATHOLOGIC TUMOR SIZE (pT)

In the pTNM staging system, a "T" is followed by a number that, for invasive tumors, is primarily based on the size of the primary tumor and/or chest wall/skin involvement.[1] The size is based on the greatest dimension of contiguous tumor and, in the presence of more than one simultaneous tumor in the same breast, the tumor with the highest pT category should be used for staging. The "m" modifier or the actual number of tumors can be used to denote multiple (>1) foci of invasive carcinoma, for example, pT1(m) or T1(4) for four tumors.

REGIONAL LYMPH NODES (pN)

In the pTNM staging system, an "N" status is based on the number and location of involved regional lymph nodes (if any) in patients with breast cancer. If applicable, the (pN) may be preceded with an "sn" modifier to specifically designate staging of (<6) sentinel nodes.[1]

DISTANT METASTASIS (pM)

In the pTNM staging system, a designation of "pM1" is used in the presence of histologically proven distant metastasis larger than 0.2 mm. Although there is a clinical "cM0(i+)" for cases with smaller metastasis or isolated tumor cells (ITCs) including circulating tumor cells or bone marrow micrometastases detected by IHC or molecular techniques, there are no "pM0" or "pMX" categories.[1,4]

BREAST CANCER STAGE GROUPING

The information obtained from the T, N, and M categories is combined to obtain stage grouping, which is expressed in Roman numerals from 0 to IV.[1,4]

Common Dilemmas in Staging, Including Assessment of Tumor Size and Lymph Node Status

Pathologic assessment is critical for the accurate assessment of breast carcinoma. This includes determination of the correct staging elements especially the size of invasive tumor and nodal status. Such assessment is not always straightforward, and this chapter addresses the most common pitfalls.

TUMOR SIZE ASSESSMENT AND PITFALLS

- Size by gross evaluation of excision specimen must always be correlated with that determined by microscopic evaluation, obviously excluding any *in situ* component. In case of discrepancy, tumor size should be based on microscopic determination.[2]
- Categorization of tumor size is generally applicable after resection of the primary tumor from a single specimen; however, as noted earlier, it takes into consideration other specimens including needle biopsy material and potentially other excision/reexcision specimens, where clinicopathologic correlation is even more important for accurate size determination and stage categorization.[4] In any case, adding the sizes from more than one specimen should be avoided.
- Unless there has been neoadjuvant therapy, tumor size should be based on needle biopsy extent when larger than that found on excision. This is because size could be underestimated in a significant proportion of cases otherwise.[5]
- Determination of tumor size following neoadjuvant therapy should be based on the largest focus of residual contiguous tumor excluding areas of fibrosis secondary to treatment. Tumors with complete pathologic response are categorized as ypT0 or ypTis depending on whether there is residual DCIS.
- Tumor extension into pectoralis muscles should not be considered chest wall involvement (pT4a), as only rib and intercostal muscle invasion is classified as such. Similarly, invasion of the dermis alone does not qualify for pT4b, as skin ulceration, satellite nodules, and/or erythema/edema (not diagnostic of inflammatory carcinoma) are required for such a designation.
- In contrast to other pT categories, a determination of inflammatory carcinoma (pT4d) is based on the clinical finding of erythema and edema (peau d'orange) of at least one-third of the breast skin, independent from whether tumor emboli are identified in dermal lymphatics pathologically.[4,6]

REGIONAL LYMPH NODE ASSESSMENT AND PITFALLS

- Regional lymph nodes include ipsilateral axillary, transpectoral, internal mammary, and supraclavicular nodes. Ipsilateral intramammary lymph nodes are also considered axillary nodes for staging purposes. On the other hand, metastasis to any other nodes including contralateral axillary and contralateral internal mammary lymph nodes is considered distant metastasis (pM1).[1]
- At least one positive or negative node by pathologic examination is required for nodal (pN) staging.
- Involvement of lymph node parenchyma by tumor and the presence of nodule with smooth contour in regional lymph node area without lymph node remnants are both considered positive.

- The size of a tumor deposit is generally determined by the largest *contiguous* focus of tumor without including tissue between the clusters. Micrometastases measure between 0.2 and 2 mm and/or greater than 200 cells, while macrometastasis are greater than 2 mm in extent.
- Lymph nodes with individual cells or small clusters of cells that are less than 0.2 mm in greatest extent with fewer than 200 cells are considered to have ITCs. These need to be documented, but for staging purposes, they are counted as negative nodes (e.g., pN0 in the absence of micro- or macrometastasis elsewhere).
- For a designation of pN1a or higher, at least one regional lymph node should contain a macrometastasis (see below). Multiple nodes with only micrometastatic disease would still be staged as pN1mi.
- Although not a component of staging, the presence/absence of extranodal extension of tumor and, when present, counted toward the size of the metastatic deposit.
- Similar to primary tumors, fibrotic foci within lymph nodes secondary to neoadjuvant therapy should be excluded from size measurements of metastatic deposits.

References

1. Edge B, Byrd RD, Compton CC, et al. *AJCC Cancer Staging Manual (Edge, AJCC Cancer Staging Manual)*. 7th ed. New York: Springer; 2011.
2. Sahoo S, Lester SC. Pathology of breast carcinomas after neoadjuvant chemotherapy: an overview with recommendations on specimen processing and reporting. *Arch Pathol Lab Med* 2009;133(4):633–642.
3. Kuroi K, Toi M, Tsuda H, et al. Issues in the assessment of the pathologic effect of primary systemic therapy for breast cancer. *Breast Cancer* 2006;13(1):38–48.
4. NHS Cancer Screening Programmes. *Pathology Reporting of Breast Disease. A Joint Document Incorporating the Third Edition of the NHS Breast Screening Programme's Guidelines for Pathology Reporting in Breast Cancer Screening and the Second Edition of the Royal College Of Pathologists' Minimum Dataset for Breast Cancer Histopathology*. NHS Cancer Screening Programmes jointly with The Royal College of Pathologists. http://www.cancerscreening.nhs.uk/breastscreen/publications/nhsbsp58.html. January 2005 edition, Vol. NHSBSP. Publication No 582009.
5. Edwards HD, Oakley F, Koyama T, et al. The impact of tumor size in breast needle biopsy material on final pathologic size and tumor stage: a detailed analysis of 222 consecutive cases. *Am J Surg Pathol* 2013;37(5):739–744.
6. Dawood S, Merajver SD, Viens P, et al. International expert panel on inflammatory breast cancer: consensus statement for standardized diagnosis and treatment. *Ann Oncol* 2011;22(3):515–523.

SECTION

VI

Precursor/Associated Lesions

26 Atypical Ductal Hyperplasia

The term atypical ductal hyperplasia (ADH) is used to define a monomorphic neoplastic population that architecturally and cytologically resembles, but does not fulfill the criteria of, low-grade ductal carcinoma *in situ* (DCIS).[1] While the diagnostic criteria are imperfect, ADH reportedly accounts for at least 10% of benign biopsies in mammographic series.[2] There is a moderately increased risk for subsequent development of invasive carcinoma (relative risk 3.0 to 5.0) in patients diagnosed with ADH.[3] The recognition of ADH is crucial since its diagnosis in a biopsy warrants a subsequent surgical excision because of the high potential for the presence of associated DCIS.

ATYPICAL DUCTAL HYPERPLASIA, IMAGING AND GROSS FEATURES

There are no specific radiographic findings for ADH apart from commonly associated calcifications. Thus, in the absence of other lesions, ADH is most frequently identified in breast biopsies for calcifications detected by screening mammography (Figure 26-1).[4] ADH lesions are not grossly identifiable.

ATYPICAL DUCTAL HYPERPLASIA, HISTOLOGY

The cytologic features of ADH are indistinguishable from those in low-grade DCIS. The lesional cells are uniform with distinct cell borders and hyperchromatic, usually round and monomorphic nuclei. Mitoses and focal necrosis may be seen but are rare; atypical mitoses are typically absent. Architecturally, most areas of ADH show evenly spaced cells and may form bridges and arcades of uniform thickness, micropapillae, cribriform, and solid patterns, similar to what can be seen in low-grade DCIS (Figures 26-2 and 26-3).

The distinction between ADH and low-grade DCIS is solely based on histologic assessment of the extent of the process. ADH may partially involve a limited number of ducts or terminal duct lobular units (TDLUs) with the remainder of the cell population showing cytologic and architectural features of usual ductal hyperplasia (UDH). Alternatively, ADH may uniformly display all the features of low-grade DCIS but is limited in extent. Different quantitative criteria have been proposed in distinguishing ADH from low-grade DCIS. Page et al.[5] initially proposed that a diagnosis of low-grade DCIS be rendered when the uniform neoplastic epithelial proliferation completely involves two or more TDLUs. Tavassoli et al.[6] subsequently proposed that lesions that fulfill all features of low-grade DCIS and comprise a size of less than 2 mm be given a diagnosis of ADH. It should be noted that neither of these quantitative criteria has been universally accepted and, in fact, many pathologists use combinations of both in their practice. The WHO Working Group did not consider that it was possible to recommend one approach rather than another, given the unacceptable levels of concordance and consistency for ADH classification.[1] Moreover, these

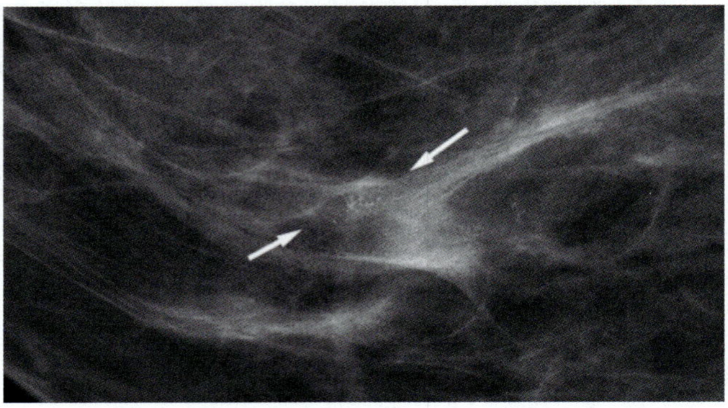

FIGURE 26-1: Mammography shows grouped fine calcifications (*arrows*). A core needle biopsy demonstrated ADH.

criteria should apply solely to distinguish ADH from low-grade DCIS; lesions with cytologic features of intermediate- or high-grade DCIS should be categorized as DCIS regardless of size and extent.

An issue frequently encountered in daily practice is the presence of borderline lesions in a needle biopsy specimen that fall short of overt DCIS, but a low-grade DCIS of limited extent cannot be ruled out. A descriptive diagnosis, such as "ADH bordering on low-grade DCIS," is appropriate to avoid overdiagnosis. A definitive diagnosis should be rendered in the subsequent surgical excision.

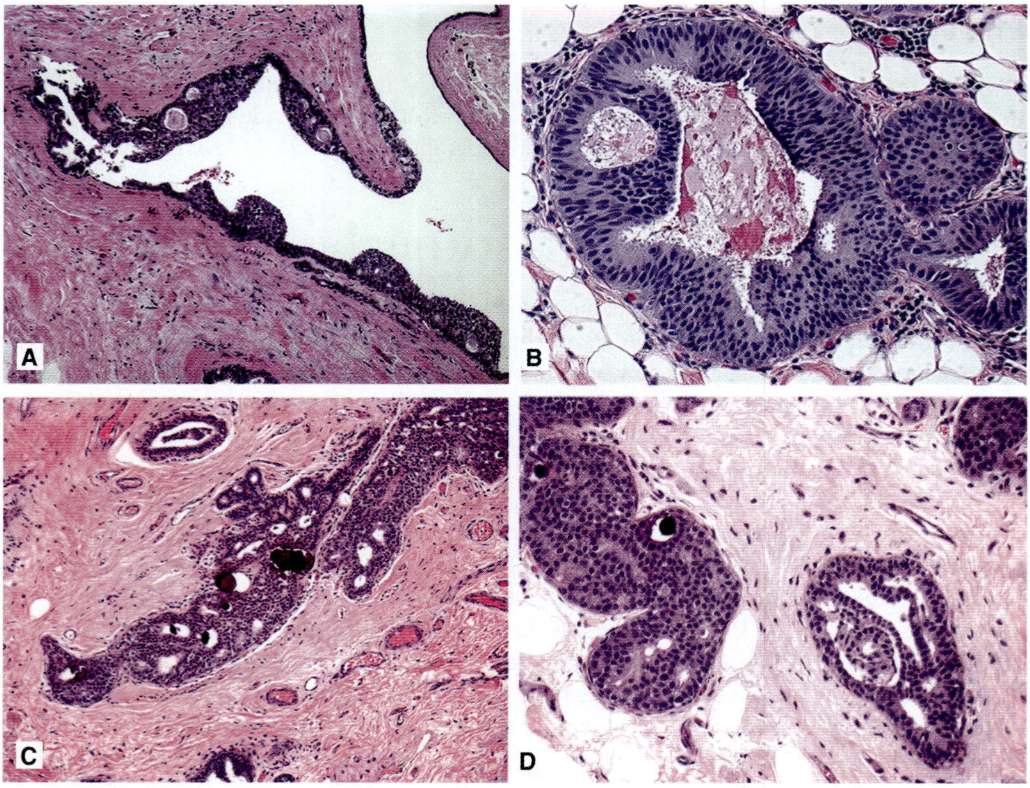

FIGURE 26-2: The cells constituting ADH may form variable architectural patterns, including cribriform with round, punched-out spaces surrounded by polarized epithelial cells (**A**), bridges and arcades of uniform thickness (**B**), and solid with or without microacini (**C, D**). Note that ADH may partially or completely involve a duct space, with or without associated microcalcifications. The lesional cells are small, round, and monotonous with hyperchromatic nuclei that are evenly spaced.

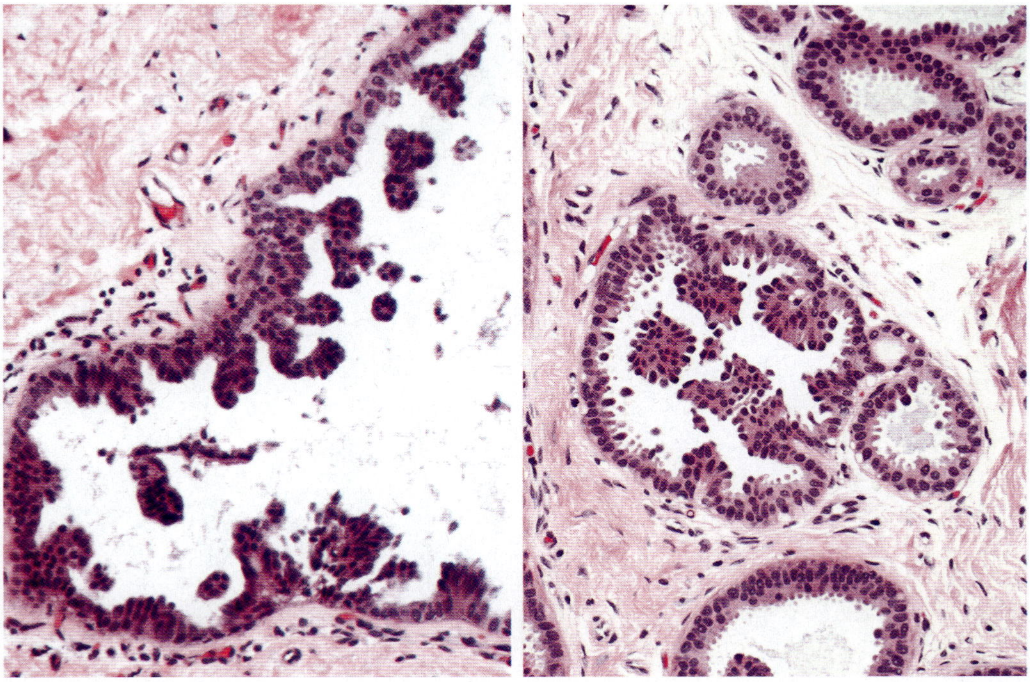

FIGURE 26-3: Additional examples of ADH showing micropapillations that are typically club shaped, with epithelial projections narrower at the base than at the apex. Note the micropapillae may become detached from the wall of duct or acinar spaces.

ATYPICAL DUCTAL HYPERPLASIA, IMMUNOHISTOCHEMISTRY

Similar to low-grade DCIS, the cells constituting ADH typically show strong and diffuse expression of estrogen receptor and lack high molecular weight cytokeratin expression. Although there are no markers that readily distinguish ADH from low-grade DCIS, the pattern of expression of the above markers has occasional utility in the differential diagnosis, especially when UDH is being considered.

ATYPICAL DUCTAL HYPERPLASIA, DIFFERENTIAL DIAGNOSIS

The differential diagnosis of ADH essentially includes UDH, low-grade DCIS and, less frequently, flat epithelial atypia.

UDH is composed of a heterogeneous population of epithelial cells, which are unevenly distributed and demonstrate overlapping of cells and nuclei. The cellular proliferation frequently shows one or more types of architecture including swirling and streaming, epithelial bridges that are stretched and uneven in thickness, and irregular, often slit-like fenestrations more prominent at the periphery. In contrast to ADH, the cells of UDH characteristically show a mosaic staining pattern of CK5/6 and patchy, variable intensity of ER (Figure 26-4).

Flat epithelial atypia is composed of cells with cytologic features that resemble those seen in ADH/low-grade DCIS without the architectural complexity (see Chapter 27).

ATYPICAL DUCTAL HYPERPLASIA, MOLECULAR GENETICS

Common cytogenetic alterations have been identified in ADH, low-grade DCIS, and invasive carcinoma in the same breast, supporting the model of linear progression of breast cancer with

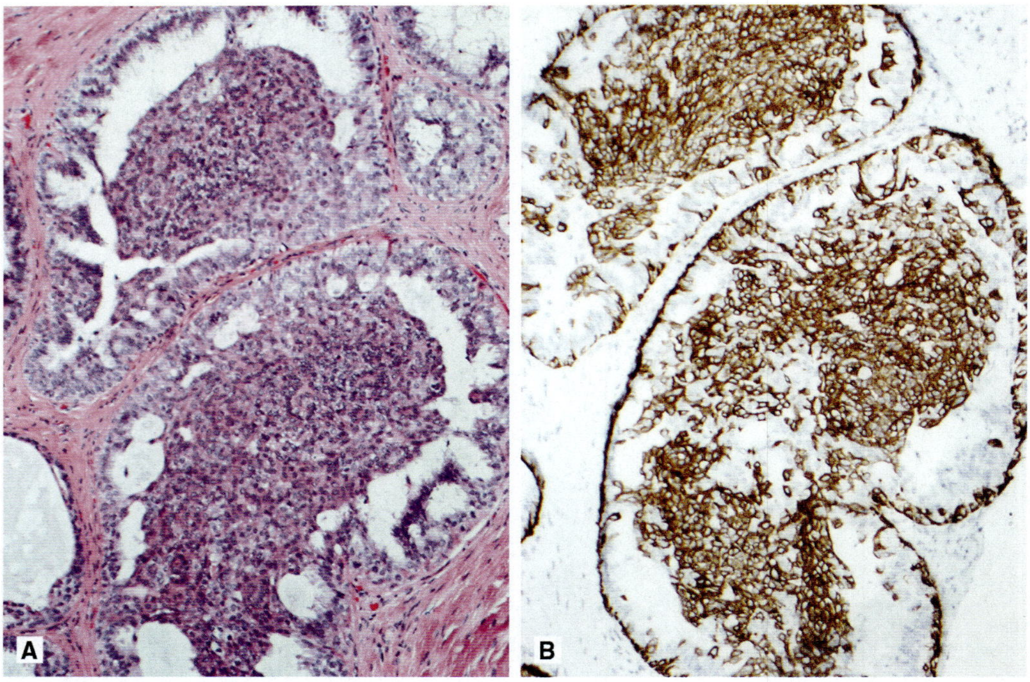

FIGURE 26-4: Usual ductal hyperplasia. Note the unevenly distributed, heterogeneous population of epithelial cells with overlapping nuclei. The proliferating epithelial cells often form bridges that are stretched and variable in thickness, and irregular, slit-like fenestrations more prominent at the periphery (**A**). A mosaic staining pattern of CK5/6 is characteristic (**B**).

ADH lesions as direct precursors.[7–9] In particular, ADH and low-grade DCIS both frequently exhibit losses of 16q and 17p.[10,11] Conversely, high-grade DCIS frequently demonstrated more complex genomic alterations, such as losses of 8p, 11q, 13q, and 14q; gains of 1q, 5p, 8q, and 17q; and high-level amplifications of 17q12 and 11q13, suggesting that the progression to high-grade DCIS may be through other pathways.[12] It is of great interest that losses involving chromosome 16q were also seen in the majority of LCIS lesions.[13,14] Few studies have examined the molecular genetic abnormalities in ADH as the most advanced lesion. Notably, phosphatidylinositol-3-kinase catalytic subunit (*PIK3CA*) mutations are more frequently seen in ADH but are also found in a significant proportion of UDH lesions.[15]

References

1. Simpson JF, Schnitt SJ, Visscher DW, et al. Atypical ductal hyperplasia. In: Lakhani SR, Ellis IO, Schnitt SJ, et al., eds. *WHO Classification of Tumours of the Breast*. Lyon, France: IARC; 2012:88–89.
2. Rubin E, Visscher DW, Alexander RW, et al. Proliferative disease and atypia in biopsies performed for nonpalpable lesions detected mammographically. *Cancer* 1988;61:2077–2082.
3. Fitzgibbons PL, Henson DE, Hutter RV. Benign breast changes and the risk for subsequent breast cancer: an update of the 1985 consensus statement. Cancer committee of the College of American Pathologists. *Arch Pathol Lab Med* 1998;122:1053–1055.
4. Pinder SE, Ellis IO. The diagnosis and management of pre-invasive breast disease: ductal carcinoma in situ (DCIS) and atypical ductal hyperplasia (ADH)—current definitions and classification. *Breast Cancer Res* 2003;5:254–257.
5. Page DL, Dupont WD, Rogers LW, et al. Atypical hyperplastic lesions of the female breast. A long-term follow-up study. *Cancer* 1985;55:2698–2708.

6. Tavassoli FA, Norris HJ. A comparison of the results of long-term follow-up for atypical intraductal hyperplasia and intraductal hyperplasia of the breast. *Cancer* 1990;65:518–529.
7. Lakhani SR. The transition from hyperplasia to invasive carcinoma of the breast. *J Pathol* 1999;187:272–278.
8. Larson PS, de las Morenas A, Cerda SR, et al. Quantitative analysis of allele imbalance supports atypical ductal hyperplasia lesions as direct breast cancer precursors. *J Pathol* 2006;209:307–316.
9. Moulis S, Sgroi DC. Re-evaluating early breast neoplasia. *Breast Cancer Res* 2008;10:302.
10. Lakhani SR, Collins N, Stratton MR, et al. Atypical ductal hyperplasia of the breast: clonal proliferation with loss of heterozygosity on chromosomes 16q and 17p. *J Clin Pathol* 1995;48:611–615.
11. Amari M, Suzuki A, Moriya T, et al. LOH analyses of premalignant and malignant lesions of human breast: frequent LOH in 8p, 16q, and 17q in atypical ductal hyperplasia. *Oncol Rep* 1999;6:1277–1280.
12. Buerger H, Otterbach F, Simon R, et al. Comparative genomic hybridization of ductal carcinoma in situ of the breast-evidence of multiple genetic pathways. *J Pathol* 1999;187:396–402.
13. Etzell JE, Devries S, Chew K, et al. Loss of chromosome 16q in lobular carcinoma in situ. *Hum Pathol* 2001;32:292–296.
14. Green AR, Krivinskas S, Young P, et al. Loss of expression of chromosome 16q genes DPEP1 and CTCF in lobular carcinoma in situ of the breast. *Breast Cancer Res Treat* 2009;113:59–66.
15. CAng D, Warrick AL, Shilling A, et al. Frequent phosphatidylinositol-3-kinase mutations in proliferative breast lesions. *Mod Pathol* 2014;27:740–750.

27 Flat Epithelial Atypia

Flat epithelial atypia (FEA) is a constituent of the spectrum of columnar cell lesions (CCLs), which also include columnar cell change (CCC) and columnar cell hyperplasia (CCH). FEA is characterized by low-grade (monomorphic) cytologic atypia involving the terminal duct lobular units (TDLUs) and the absence of architectural features of ADH or low-grade DCIS.[1]

There has been a diverse published descriptions and a wide assortment of names applied to "flat" breast lesions that would currently be categorized as FEA, including atypical cystic lobules, atypical lobules type A, atypical cystic duct, columnar alteration with prominent apical snouts and secretion, small ectatic ducts lined by atypical cells with apocrine snouts, ductal intraepithelial neoplasia-flat type, enlarged lobular units with columnar alteration, CCC with atypia, and CCH with atypia.[2–4] Of important note, the two types of "clinging carcinoma" introduced by Azzopardi more than three decades ago are now considered two separate entities: the pleomorphic variant (with high-grade nuclear atypia) to represent high-grade DCIS and the monomorphic variant (with low-grade atypia) to substitute FEA.[1,5,6]

As an emerging entity of uncertain clinical significance, FEA has long been of great scientific interest. The sparse available data from small, respective studies suggest that FEA may progress to invasive cancer at a risk substantially lower than other well-established breast cancer precursors (ADH and ALH).[7,8] Moreover, the outcome data are hampered by the limitation of study design and the diverging reported upgrade rates. Thus, the need for surgical excision following a diagnosis of FEA as the most advanced lesion on needle biopsy remains controversial. The general consensus at this point of time is that FEA should not be regarded as an obligate breast cancer precursor for patient management purposes.

FLAT EPITHELIAL ATYPIA, IMAGING AND GROSS FEATURES

FEA lesions are frequently incidental histologic findings but are more commonly identified due to the associated microcalcifications detected on screening mammography.[9] FEA is not discernible macroscopically.

FLAT EPITHELIAL ATYPIA, HISTOLOGY

Histologically, FEA is characterized by variably enlarged and dilated acini lined by one or several layers of monomorphic cells that replace the native luminal epithelium. The lesional cells are small and uniform with round, hyperchromatic nuclei and inconspicuous nucleoli, thus are similar to that seen in ADH and low-grade DCIS. The affected enlarged and distended terminal ducts or acini often have a more rounded configuration. The high nuclear-to-cytoplasmic ratio results in a more basophilic appearance at lower magnification. The cells lack polarity but often exhibit apical cytoplasmic snouts. Granular and densely stained luminal secretions are common and may become prominent and calcified (Figures 27-1 and 27-2). It should be

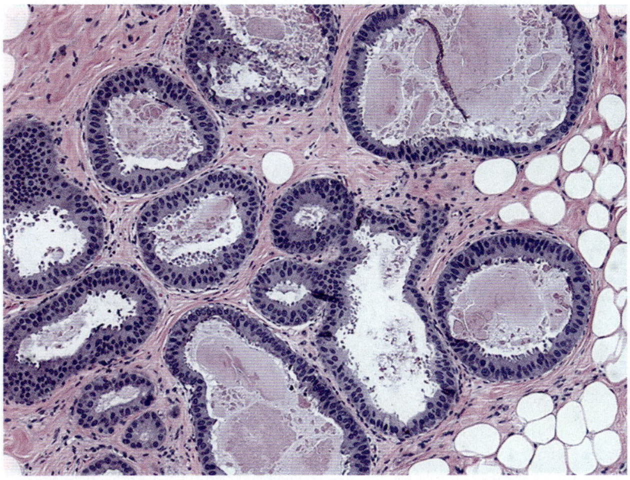

FIGURE 27-1: A low-power view of flat epithelial atypia involving the entire TDLU. Note the variably dilated and distended acini lined by one or several layers of a monotonous population of cells devoid of architectural complexity. Many cells exhibit apical cytoplasmic snouts. Abundant luminal secretions are present.

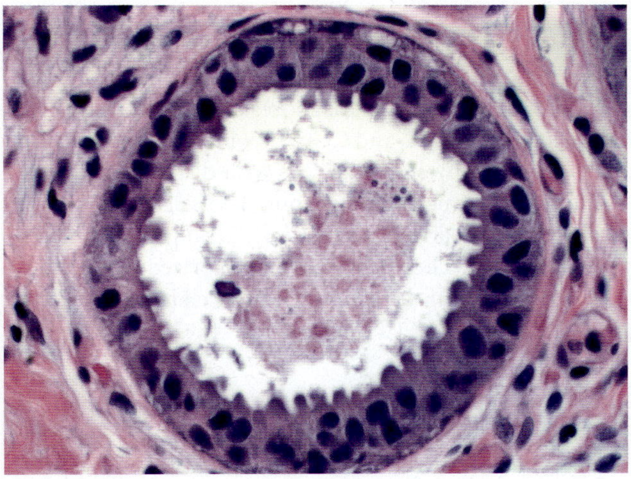

FIGURE 27-2: At higher magnification, the lesional cells demonstrate small and hyperchromatic nuclei and inconspicuous nucleoli. Secretory materials containing microcalcifications are evident.

emphasized that flat lesions comprising cells with severe nuclear atypia should be classified as high-grade DCIS.[1]

One should be aware that FEA is essentially a "flat" lesion, as its name implies. Thus, the presence of any architectural complexity, such as arcades, cellular bridges, or well-formed micropapillae, should prompt a diagnosis of ADH or low-grade DCIS based on the extent of disease. Moreover, ADH or low-grade DCIS may arise in a background of FEA (Figure 27-3). On the other hand, although FEA has not been established as an obligate breast cancer precursor, a convincing association between FEA and other associated and neoplastic lesions, including lobular neoplasia (ALH/LCIS), ADH, low-grade DCIS, and low-grade invasive carcinoma (frequently tubular carcinoma), has been demonstrated by multiple studies.[10–13] In fact, the frequent coexistence of CCLs (including FEA), tubular carcinoma, and LCIS has been proposed as the "Rosen Triad," which has prompted close attention to biopsy specimens containing any one of these lesions to exclude the presence of the other two.[14]

FLAT EPITHELIAL ATYPIA, IMMUNOHISTOCHEMISTRY

The immunophenotype of FEA cells is similar to that of low-grade DCIS.[3] The cells are strongly and diffusely positive for ER and PR, are negative for high molecular weight cytokeratins (such as CK5/6 and CK14), and do not overexpress HER2.[3]

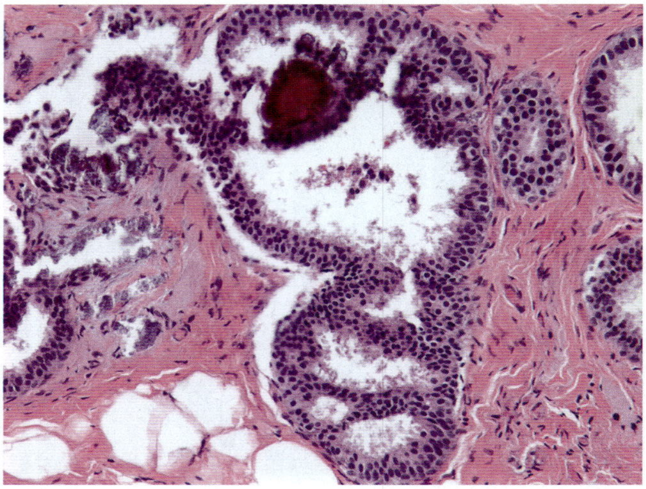

FIGURE 27-3: ADH arising in a background of FEA. The presence of architectural complexity (bridges and arcades in this acinar space) renders a diagnosis of ADH. Note the luminal secretions and prominent calcifications.

FLAT EPITHELIAL ATYPIA, DIFFERENTIAL DIAGNOSIS

In addition to ADH and low-grade DCIS, the chief differential diagnoses of FEA are other components constituting the spectrum of CCLs, including CCC and CCH, of which the characteristic features are variably enlarged and dilated acini lined by epithelial cells with distinct apical cytoplasmic snouts and frequent luminal secretions and microcalcifications. The cells of CCC/CCH have bland oval to elongated nuclei, usually basally polarized and typically arranged perpendicularly to the basement membrane in a regular fashion. These lesions are categorized by the thickness of the lining cells (one- to two-cell layers for CCC and greater than two-cell layers for CCH). In contrast to FEA, cytologic atypia is not a feature of CCC/CCH (Figure 27-4). CCH may exhibit

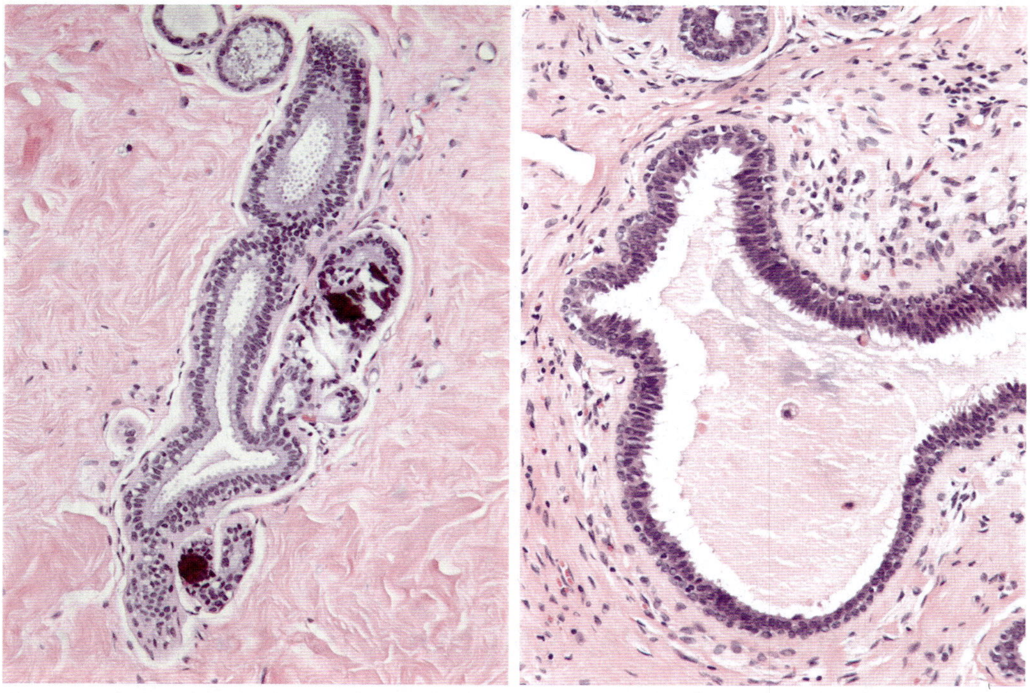

FIGURE 27-4: Illustrations of columnar cell change/hyperplasia. The spaces are lined by epithelial cells with distinct apical cytoplasmic snouts with frequent luminal secretions and microcalcifications. The lining cells display bland oval to elongated nuclei without nuclear atypia, typically basally polarized and arranged perpendicularly to the basement membrane in a regular fashion.

nuclear crowding/overlapping or form small mounds, tufts, and rare short micropapillations but is devoid of architectural complexity, such as rigid bridges or arcades, and cribriform spaces. The cells of CCC and CCH show similar immunoprofile to that of FEA.

Once again, flat lesions exhibiting severe nuclear atypia should be regarded as DCIS (see Figure 2-9). These lesions frequently display comedonecrosis in contrast to the basophilic luminal secretions typically seen in CCLs, including FEA. Thus, the distinction of the flat lesions is based solely on the degree of nuclear atypia.

Distinguishing FEA from usual ductal hyperplasia (UDH) is usually not problematic. The latter is characterized by significant cellular heterogeneity as opposed to the monomorphic cell population characteristic of FEA. With regard to the architecture, the cells of FEA do not pile up to fill the TDLU spaces (as they do in UDH) but rather manifest a single or minimally pseudostratified layer of luminal epithelial cells.

FLAT EPITHELIAL ATYPIA, MOLECULAR GENETICS

The data on molecular genetics in FEA lesions are limited. A particularly high rate of loss of heterozygosity at chromosome 16q in FEA was found in an early study.[15] Comprehensive comparative genomic hybridization–based studies in a limited number of cases further demonstrated low numbers of genetic alterations and recurrent 16q loss in FEA, features significantly overlapping with ADH, low-grade DCIS, and low-grade invasive carcinoma.[3,16] These observations, along with the similar immunoprofile among these lesions, indicate that some of these lesions represent both a morphologic and molecular continuum and suggest that FEA may represent the earliest morphologically identifiable precursor lesion of low nuclear grade breast cancer.[3,13,16,17] Notably, various chromosomal alterations have also been identified in some examples of CCC and CCH, the significance of which remains undefined.[3,18]

References

1. Schnitt SJ, Collins LC, Lakhani SR, et al. Flat epithelial atypia. In: Lakhani SR, Ellis IO, Schnitt SJ, et al., eds. *WHO Classification of Tumours of the Breast.* Lyon, France: International Agency for Research on Cancer; 2013:87.
2. Schnitt SJ. The diagnosis and management of pre-invasive breast disease: flat epithelial atypia—classification, pathologic features and clinical significance. *Breast Cancer Res* 2003;5:263–268.
3. Simpson PT, Gale T, Reis-Filho JS, et al. Columnar cell lesions of the breast: the missing link in breast cancer progression? A morphological and molecular analysis. *Am J Surg Pathol* 2005;29:734–746.
4. Moinfar F. Flat ductal intraepithelial neoplasia of the breast: a review of diagnostic criteria, differential diagnoses, molecular-genetic findings, and clinical relevance—it is time to appreciate the Azzopardi concept! *Arch Pathol Lab Med* 2009;133:879–892.
5. Holland R, Peterse JL, Millis RR, et al. Ductal carcinoma in situ: a proposal for a new classification. *Semin Diagn Pathol* 1994;11:167–180.
6. Schnitt SJ. Clinging carcinoma: an American perspective. *Semin Diagn Pathol* 2010;27:31–36.
7. Bijker N, Peterse JL, Duchateau L, et al. Risk factors for recurrence and metastasis after breast-conserving therapy for ductal carcinoma-in-situ: analysis of European Organization for Research and Treatment of Cancer Trial 10853. *J Clin Oncol* 2001;19:2263–2271.
8. Eusebi V, Feudale E, Foschini MP, et al. Long-term follow-up of in situ carcinoma of the breast. *Semin Diagn Pathol* 1994;11:223–235.
9. Senetta R, Campanino PP, Mariscotti G, et al. Columnar cell lesions associated with breast calcifications on vacuum-assisted core biopsies: clinical, radiographic, and histological correlations. *Mod Pathol* 2009;22:762–769.
10. Brogi E, Oyama T, Koerner FC. Atypical cystic lobules in patients with lobular neoplasia. *Int J Surg Pathol* 2001;9:201–206.

11. Carley AM, Chivukula M, Carter GJ, et al. Frequency and clinical significance of simultaneous association of lobular neoplasia and columnar cell alterations in breast tissue specimens. *Am J Clin Pathol* 2008;130:254–258.
12. Leibl S, Regitnig P, Moinfar F. Flat epithelial atypia (DIN 1a, atypical columnar change): an underdiagnosed entity very frequently coexisting with lobular neoplasia. *Histopathology* 2007;50:859–865.
13. Abdel-Fatah TM, Powe DG, Hodi Z, et al. High frequency of coexistence of columnar cell lesions, lobular neoplasia, and low grade ductal carcinoma in situ with invasive tubular carcinoma and invasive lobular carcinoma. *Am J Surg Pathol* 2007;31:417–426.
14. Brandt SM, Young GQ, Hoda SA. The "Rosen Triad": tubular carcinoma, lobular carcinoma in situ, and columnar cell lesions. *Adv Anat Pathol* 2008;15:140–146.
15. Moinfar F, Man YG, Bratthauer GL, et al. Genetic abnormalities in mammary ductal intraepithelial neoplasia-flat type ("clinging ductal carcinoma in situ"): a simulator of normal mammary epithelium. *Cancer* 2000;88:2072–2081.
16. Stacher E, Boldt V, Leibl S, et al. Chromosomal aberrations as detected by array comparative genomic hybridization in early low-grade intraepithelial neoplasias of the breast. *Histopathology* 2011;59:549–555.
17. Abdel-Fatah TM, Powe DG, Hodi Z, et al. Morphologic and molecular evolutionary pathways of low nuclear grade invasive breast cancers and their putative precursor lesions: further evidence to support the concept of low nuclear grade breast neoplasia family. *Am J Surg Pathol* 2008;32:513–523.
18. Dabbs DJ, Carter G, Fudge M, et al. Molecular alterations in columnar cell lesions of the breast. *Mod Pathol* 2006;19:344–349.

Index

Note: Page numbers followed by *f* indicate figures; those followed by *t* indicate tables.

D